AF552826

NUTRITION

APPLIED SCIENCE SERIES

A TEXT BOOK OF NUTRITION

CHINTAPALLI VIDYA

M.Sc.

DEPARTMENT OF NUTRITION
T.J.P.S. COLLEGE
GUNTUR—522 006

Editor

DIGUMARTI BHASKARA RAO

M.Sc., M.A., M.A., M.Ed., Ph.D.

R.V.R. COLLEGE OF EDUCATION
GUNTUR-522 006
ANDHRA PRADESH
INDIA

DISCOVERY PUBLISHING HOUSE
NEW DELHI—110 002

Published by:

DISCOVERY PUBLISHING HOUSE PVT. LTD.
4383/4B, Ansari Road, Darya Ganj
New Delhi-110 002 (India)
Phone : +91-11-23279245; 23253475; 43596065
E-mail : discoverybooksindia@gmail.com
discoverypublishinghouse@gmail.com
namitwasan9@gmail.com
web : www.discoverypublishinggroup.com

First Published: **1999**

Reprinted: **2022**

ISBN: 978-81-7141-309-6

A Text Book of Nutrition

Printed at:
Infinity Imaging Systems
Delhi

DEDICATED

to

MY PARENTS

MR. C. S. SUNDARA RAO

MRS. C. JAMUNA

—Vidya

Editor's...

Nutrition is now a major task of people and governments. The policy makers, the sociologists, the economists, the educationists, the medical people and the rulers talk about and work for nutritional aspects. As nutrition is one of the basic requirements of human life, the knowledge of it helps the people live better. A good health helps people do better and enjoy life. The concept 'a sound mind in a sound body' becomes a reality by having good dietary habits.

For many more reasons, we need the knowledge of nutrition. So many courses are offered by many universities and professional organisations on nutrition. But the students, as well as general readers and users of nutritional avenues, are lacking a comprehensive book with all nutritional aspects at one point, though a very good standard books are available on one or the other area of nutrition. To fill this gap, we have tried to put before the users such a fine book with all necessary details. We feel our efforts being honoured if this book meets a wide variety of needs of a host of users.

This book—NUTRITION—is a part of my series—APPLIED SCIENCE—of books for ready use in daily life.

Dr. D. Bhaskara Rao

Preface

The present day advances in the field of nutrition clearly expose the ignorance of this subject in the past. People, today, as never before, are increasingly aware of this science. Even the educated people cannot give a right answer about the composition of the food they eat. Medical people also ignored it till the recent past. They did focus on cure of diseases but not on prevention. Human diseases are mostly the result of heredity, environment and food. We cannot change heredity and partly environment, but it is very easy to change food habits. So, knowledge of what we eat is very important not only in health aspect but also in economy.

No doubt that there are a wide variety of good standard books on the subject, nutrition. But the problem for most of the readers is that they have been to go through large volumes in comparatively short period at their disposal. This reason prompted me to undertake this task. Non-medical people, students, and house wives who are interested in nutrition will find this book useful. References are given in the interest of the persons who seek detailed information. This book is an attempt to present the subject in a simplified manner for easy grasp.

The nutritive values given in this book are from a NIN, Hyderabad, publication, i.e., "Nutritive Values of Common Indian Foods" by C. Gopalan, et al. I express my deep gratitude to the publishers of the above book for their generosity in granting permission to use their material.

I would like to express gratitude to all my teachers who made me this able. I am deeply indebted to my parents who induced me to complete this work. My thanks are also due to everyone who tried to discourage me, but it helped a lot in building up my will power. Ms. Himabindu and Mr. Phanibhushan rendered considerable secretarial help, for which I am thankful to them.

If anything I have written sparks enthusiasm atleast in one (I hope for more) I would consider myself successful. All constructive criticism and comments are most welcome and shall form the basis to improve further.

C. Vidya

Contents

Editor's... VII

Preface IX

1. The Science of Food, Nutrition and Health 1
2. Carbohydrates 4
3. Lipids 16
4. Proteins 31
5. Fat Soluble Vitamins 59
6. Water Soluble Vitamins 82
7. Macro-elements 117
8. Micro-elements 137
9. Water and Electrolyte Balance 150
10. Inter-relationship among Nutrients 156
11. Recommended Dietary Allowances 160
12. Cereals 166
13. Pulses 175
14. Nuts and Oil Seeds 178
15. Vegetables 181
16. Fruits 184
17. Milk and Milk Products 192
18. Meat and Fish 196

(Contd.)

Contents (*Contd.*)

19. Eggs 201
20. Beverages 208
21. Spices and Condiments 217
22. Nutritive Values of Indian Food Preparations 221
23. Food Exchange Lists for India 233
24. Food Adulteration 240
25. Food Poisoning and Food Borne Infection 245
26. Toxicants in Foods 260
27. Food Allergy 265
28. Nutrition of Normal Infants 274
29. Nutrition of Pre-school Children 279
30. Nutrition of Children and Adolescents 282
31. Nutrition in Old Age 285
32. Nutrition of Pregnant and Lactating Woman 288

Appendices : 293

1. Nutritive Values of Common Foods 293
2. Vitamin Content : Common Foods 320
3. Mineral and Trace Elements : Common Foods 338
4. Oxalic Acid, Phytin Phosphorus and Dietary Fibre in Foods 349
5. Conversions to and from Metric Measures 354
6. Synopsis of Fat Soluble and Water Soluble Vitamins 355
7. Synopsis of Micro and Macro Elements 370

Glossary 375
Bibliography 405
Index 415

The Science of Food, Nutrition and Health

The science of food, the nutrients in it, their action, interaction and relation to health and disease; the processes by which organism takes in, digests, absorbs and utilizes the nutrients and disposes the ends products is called nutrition. Nutrition is also concerned with social, economic, cultural and psychological implications of food. The nutrients are required for proper growth and functioning of the body. Some are required in large quantities and some in very small amounts. Nutrition is a quantitative science which deals with the amounts of nutrients contributed by different foods and action of each in the functioning of the body.

Eating food is merely a way of staying alive, keeping good health, celebrating an occasion, token of love, a display of prestige, etc. The colour combinations, texture variations, table decorations, varieties of flavours, etc., also play a great role in creating appetite. Chemical analysis of foods showed that food consists of different substances life carbohydrates, proteins, fats, minerals and vitamins. Carbohydrates comprise sugars, starches, fibre and related materials. Proteins are nitrogenous compounds and form the major component of tissues in human body. Fats are present in animals and plants. A variety of vitamins and minerals also accompany the carbohydrates, fats and proteins.

The health of the individual influenced by the utilization of nutrients is called nutritional status of a individual. Through medical checkup, dietary and medical history and laboratory investigations gives an account on nutritional status. The application of knowledge of nutrition in selecting the food, its combination, preparation, storage, serving, modifying according to the need, extending the knowledge of nutrition in selecting the food its combination, preparation, storage, serving, modifying according to the need, extending the knowledge, etc., comprise nutritional care. All this contributes to the health of a person. Health is a state of complete physical, mental and social well being and not merely the absence of any disease or infirmity. This definition of health is given by World Health Organisation. The purpose of nutrition is to support health by means of the food one eats. Obviously, nutrients of foods cannot have any nutritional function if they are not eaten. These nutrients when taken in excess or in deficiency results in malnutrition, under nutrition and over nutrition. Impairment of health resulting from deficiency, excess or imbalance of nutrients is called malnutrition. Under nutrition is deficiency of one or more nutrients. Over nutrition is excess of one or more nutrients.

The science of nutrition began in the late eighteenth century. It was Antoine Lavavoisier a French man who did work on energy metabolism. He is often called Father of the science of nutrition. Though observation on relationship of food and health are made throughout the history some withstood scientific scrutiny and some of the remaining still persists even to this day. Work was done and is going on from the last two centuries and the observations were proved. Medical teachers even today refrain from imparting nutrition knowledge to the medical students. That is the reason why doctors very rarely give full dietary prescription. For example they prescribe fat restricted diet but how does a patient know the extent of restriction needed. He may act on his own way. So, doctors should be able to prescribe a complete diet sheet or should have a skilled dietician. While prescribing a diet the economic status, occupation, time of meals, any allergies or intolerance to food, amount of nutrition required, etc., of the patient should be considered. A good diet should provide appropriate measures of all nutrients to satisfy the body needs and should avoid excess of nutrients which increase the risk of diet related diseases.

Normal nutrition means a balance that avoids deficiency on one hand and excess on other hand. Deficiency is of two kinds Primary and

Secondary. Primary deficiency arises due to lack of food, ignorance, diosyncrasy, poverty, food faddism, addiction to drugs and alcohol etc. Secondary deficiency occurs due to malabsorption, increased excretion, lefective metabolism, etc. Deficiency whether primary or secondary eads to tissue depletion which in turn shows biochemical lesions like educed nutrient levels and finally clinical signs appear.

Wife and mother are principal decision makers concerning family's ood. So woman folk should be educated first. Women plan the menu, urchases the food and prepares the diet. Next comes nutrition education for children. This step helps in formulating good food habits, wise election of foods, preparation of balanced diets, etc. these children when rown up unlike the yesterday teenagers select good balanced diet for heir development and growth. These people when they establish a amily can teach and practice good food habits.

2
Carbohydrates

Carbohydrates contain carbon with oxygen and hydrogen. Carbohydrates occur abundantly in nature. Starches are present in Cereals, roots, tubers, sugar cane, milk, etc. Plants manufacture carbohydrate from a process called photosynthesis. Sunlight is absorbed by the pigments of plants especially chlorophyll and is utilised in transferring two atoms of hydrogen from water to carbon and the oxygen is liberated. The carbon is converted to carbohydrate in this process.

$$6CO_2 + 6H_2O + \text{(Sun) light} \xrightarrow[\text{Plant enzymes}]{\text{Chlorophyll}} C_6 H_{12} O_6 + 6O_2$$

Plants use some of the carbohydrate for its own needs and rest is stored in its various parts. Carbohydrates form the principle constituent of most of the normal diets. It is the most important energy source. Human beings have recognised the importance of Carbohydrate long back. So, we pray Oh God ! Give us daily bread. But carbohydrate alone is not sufficient for body. Protein, fat, vitamins and minerals are also important. Presently in this chapter the composition, classification, digestion, metabolism, etc., are discussed

COMPOSITION

Carbohydrates are simple sugars or polymers of sugars like starch. These sugars may be glucose. fructose, galactose, etc. These units of sugars may be bonded in pairs or small groups. There may be complex structures like starch built from thousands of sugar units. The Greek word 'Sakcharon' means 'Sugar' so, they are called saccharides.

CLASSIFICATION AND DISTRIBUTION

Carbohydrates are classified into three groups

1. Monosaccharides
2. Disaccharides
3. Polysaccharides

Monosaccharides

These are the simplest forms of carbohydrates which cannot be hydrolysed to simpler compounds. All the Carbohydrates should be reduced to this form for absorption and utilisation. These are compounds with two to ten carbons per molecule. They are called bioses, trioses, tetroses, pentoses, hexoses and so on. Sugars which contain aldehyde group (CHO) are called aldoses, e.g. : glucose, galactose, mannose and sugars which contain ketone group (CO) are called ketoses, e.g. : fructose and sorbose. Hexoses have a formula $C_6 H_{12} O_6$ and are important for human nutrition. Though all hexoses have same empirical formula they differ in the arrangement of carbon atoms and so they have distinctive physical properties. Hexoses important for human nutrition are discussed below. For structures see Figures 2.1, 2.2 and 2.3.

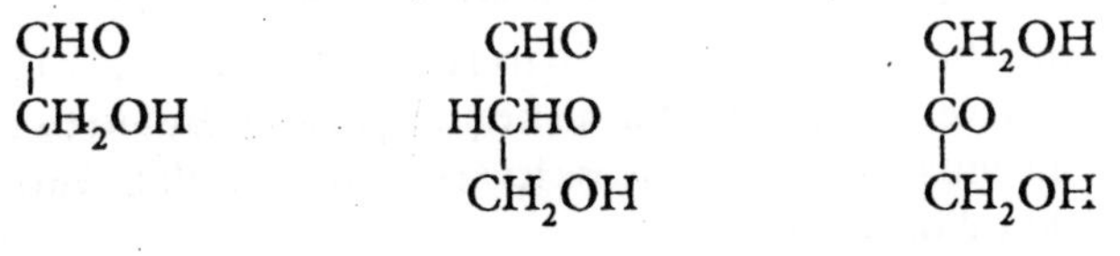

GLYCOLIC ALDENYDE (BIOSE)	GLYCERALDEHYDE (TRIOSE)	DINYDROXY ACETONE (TRIOSE)
CHO	CHO	CH_2OH
CH_2OH	HCHO	CO
	CH_2OH	CH_2OH

Fig. 2.1 : Structures of Biose and Triose

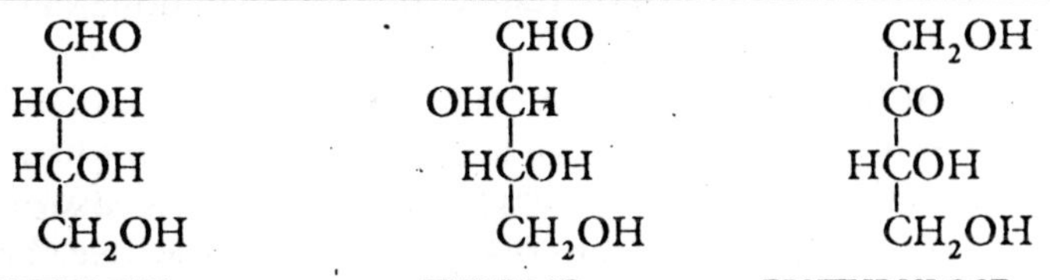

ERYTHROSE	THREOSE	ERYTHRULOSE
CHO	CHO	CH_2OH
HCOH	OHCH	CO
HCOH	HCOH	HCOH
CH_2OH	CH_2OH	CH_2OH

(TETROSES)

Fig. 2.2 : Structures of Tetroses

RIBOSE (PENTOSE)	GLUCOSE	GALACTOSE	MANNOSE	FRUCTOSE
CHO	CHO	CHO	CHO	CH_2OH
HCOH	HCOH	HCOH	OHCH	CO
HCOH	OHCH	OHCH	OHCH	OHCH
HCOH	HCOH	OHCH	HCOH	HCOH
CH_2OH	HCOH	HCOH	HCOH	HCOH
	CH_2OH	CH_2OH	CH_2OH	CH_2OH

(HEXOSES)

Fig. 2.3 : Structures of Pentose and Hexoses

Glucose

It is also called dextrose, or grape sugar. It is soluble in water but is less sweeter than the household sugar, sucrose. The break down product of starch digestion is glucose as many glucose molecules combine to form starch. Glucose is called the carbohydrate currency of the body. It is a white crystalline substance, with sweet taste and is freely soluble in water. Glucose can easily be digested and absorbed. Sweet fruits contain glucose with levulose and sucrose. Vegetables like sweet corn, carrots, onions, etc., and honey also contain glucose. Starch on treating with digestive enzymes or dilute acids give glucose.

Normal human beings have 80 to 100mg of glucose per 100ml of blood. This level is maintained in all healthy persons. But in patients of Diabetes mellitus the blood glucose level may be as high as 180 to 300 mg per 100 ml of blood.

Fructose

Fructose is also called levulose or fruit sugar. Fructose is highly soluble but does not crystallize readily. It is found in honey and ripe fruits. It is twice sweeter than glucose. On hydrolysis sucrose yields glucose and fructose. Fructose is readily absorbed in the body. It is harmless to diabetic patients when taken in limited amount because it enter the body cells and gives energy without the aid of insulin. But excess of fructose is converted to lactate which causes lactic acidosis in Diabetics. It may also rise the level of uric acid in blood which is undesirable in patients with gout.

Galactose

Galactose does not occur in free state in nature. It is combined with glucose to form lactose. Lactose is a milk sugar. Galactose is not found in fruits and vegetables.

Disaccharides

Disaccharides form when two hexoses condense with loss of one molecule of water. Disaccharides are linked with glycosidic linkage. The linkage between first carbon of one hexose with second or fourth carbon of another is called glycosidic linkage. Disaccharides are colorless crystalline substances that are readily soluble in water and sweet to taste. Their sweetness vary widely. They split to simple sugars by acid hydrolysis or digestive enzymes. The disaccharides of nutritional importance are 1. Sucrose 2. Maltose a: 3. Lactose. For structures see figure 2.4.

Sucrose

This is the commonest sugar used in diet. In tropical countries it is made from sugarcane and in western countries it is made from sugar beet. Many fruits and vegetables contain small amounts of sucrose. Sucrose is formed from glucose and fructose. On hydrolysis sucrose gives a mixture of glucose and fructose which is called invert sugar. Bacteria streptococcus mutans ferments sucrose to produce acids that dissolves the minerals in the teeth thus causing dental caries. In order to prevent dental caries one should gargle after every snack.

Maltose

Maltose is a sugar formed in Cereal grains during germination by the hydrolysis of starch by amy-lase. It is also formed when the starch in food is digested by salivary or pancreatic amylase. A molecule of maltose is composed of two linked Glucose units which during digestion can be separated by the action of maltose.

Lactose

It is called milk sugar as it is found in mammal milk. It is not readily soluble in cold water but is more soluble in hot water. Lactose is formed by the condensation of one glucose and one galactose molecules with elimination of one molecule of water. Lactose hydrolyses with the enzyme present in intestinal juice. This sugar can be added to the diet to increase the calories content but not the sweetness, as lactose is one sixth time as sweet as sucrose.

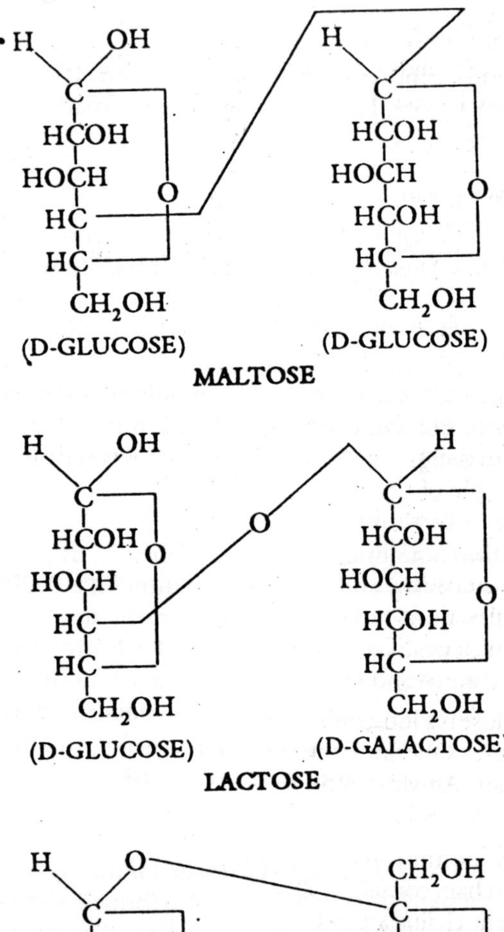

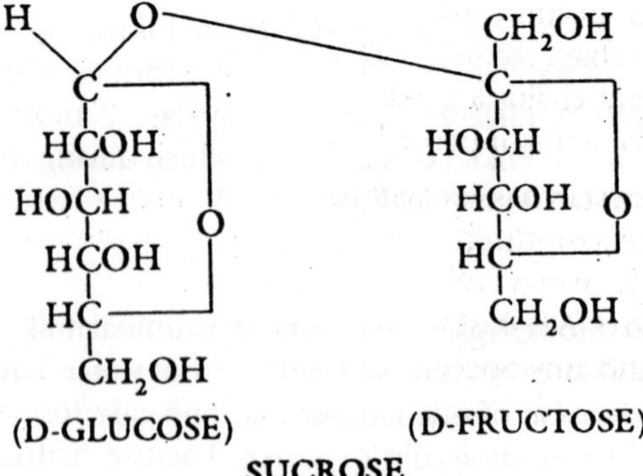

Fig. 2.4 : Structures of Disaccharides

Polysaccharides

Polysaccharides are complex carbohydrates with a formula $(C_6 H_{10} O_5)_n$ and have a high molecular weight. Many monosaccharide molecules are linked together to form a polysaccharide.

Starch

We have already seen sugars with limited number of Monosaccharide molecules like glucose, fructose, etc., on the other hand starch is composed of several hundreds of glucose units linked together into a complex structure. Starch occurs widely in vegetable kingdom. It is the counterpart to glycogen in Animal kingdom. The important sources of starch are: (1) Cereals and millets (2) Roots and tubers.

The starch granules are encased in cellulose type walls and have a distinctive size and shape. Starches derived from different sources have differences in the appearance of the granules. They also behave differently. For example of the rice starch, wheat starch and maize starch, only maize starch is best suited for making a custard. The starch paste from cereal starch sets as a jelly where as starch from tubers remain as thick fluid. These characteristics of starch molecule is dependent on the way in which the molecules are linked i.e, the varying proportions of branched and unbranched chains. Two types of glucose chains are present they are: (1) Amylose (2) Amylopectin.

Amylose is a long unbranched chain of glucose linked together by 1 : 4 linkage. One molecule of Amylose may contain 500 — 5000 glucose units. Amylose accounts for 10 to 20 percent of the molecule. Amylose dissolves in water.

Amylopectin consists of short branched chains of glucose molecules. Each chain consists of 20 – 30 glucose units linked by 1 : 4 linkage. The different chains are linked together by 1 : 6 linkage. Amylopectin accounts for a major part of the molecule.

When starch is cooked the granules swell absorbing water and the cell walls gets ruptured which facilitates better digestion. One molecule of amylopectin may contain 50,000 to 500,000 glucose molecules. The proportion of Amylose to Amylopectin varies from starch to starch. The Amylose and amylopectin contents of some starches are given in Table: 2.1

Table 2.1 : Amylose and Amylopectic Contents of Different Starches

Source of Starch	*Amylose %*	*Amylopectin %*
Rice	25	75
Wheat	24	76
Corn	28	72
Sorghum	22	78
Tapioca	17	83
Potato	22	78
Banana	21	79
Arrow root	20	80
Sweet Potato	18	82

Dextrins

Dextrins are the polysaccharides produces by the partial hydrolysis of starch by amylases or acids i.e. dextrins are the intermediate products of starch hydrolysis and consist shorter chains of glucose units. Dextrins are formed when starch is heated for example when potatoes are fried or bread is toasted.

Glycogen

It is also known as animal starch. Glycogen is the reserve carbohydrate found in animal tissues particularly Liver and muscle. The liver has enzymes which can convert glucose to glycogen and vice versa. In a adult human being liver has about 200g and muscle about 350g of glycogen. Glycogen is a branched chain polysaccharide resembling Amylopectin. It has 5000 to 10,000 glucose units and each chain contain 8 to 12 glucose units.

Cellulose

Cellulose is a polysaccharide made up of glucose. The Cell Walls in vegetables, fruits and cereals is made up of cellulose in which starch is stored. Amyloses cannot digest cellulose. The digestive juices cannot act unless the cellulose barrier is broken. Cooking and mastication aid in the process of digestion.

Cellulose provides an unabsorbable bulk which distends the intestine and stimulates peristalsis. Patients suffering from constipation are benefited by consuming cellulose. Pure forms of cellulose are cotton and paper pulp. Cellulose is insoluble in water.

Hemicellulose

Hemicelluloses are polysaccharide with pentoses, hexoses and uronic acids. Hemicelluloses are soluble in hot water. These can be hydrolysed with hot dilute acids but not by digestive enzymes of human digestive system. Hemicelluloses are found in a variety of plant foods.

Pectins

Pectins are polysaccharides of galacturonic acid, galactose and arabinose. It is soluble in hot water. In the presence of sugar, and citric acid pectin form a gel. Pectin is used as an ingredient in the preparation of jams and Jelles. Apples and citrus fruits are the important sources of pectin.

DIGESTION

The main purpose of carbohydrate digestion is the hydrolysis of disaccharides and polysaccharides to their constituent sugars. This is done by the enzymes present in a digestive juices. The process is as follows:

$$\text{Starch} \xrightarrow{\text{Amylase}} \text{Glucose}$$

$$\text{Sucrose} \xrightarrow{\text{Sucrase}} \text{Glucose + fructose}$$

$$\text{Maltose} \xrightarrow{\text{Maltase}} \text{Glucose + Glucose}$$

$$\text{Lactose} \xrightarrow{\text{Lactase}} \text{Glucose + Galactose.}$$

Mouth

Digestion of carbohydrates begin in the mouth. Because of chewing the cellulose cell wall breaks down and starch is available for digestion. Saliva contains a starch splitting enzyme ptyalin also called salivary amylose which converts starch to dextrins and a little maltose. Ptyalin acts best at a PH of 4 to 9. Salivary amylose does not act on raw starch. In cooked starch the cell walls are ruptured during cooling and so enzymes can act easily.

Stomach

The action of salivary amylose continues in the stomach until the food is acidified.

Small Intestine

The principal site of carbohydrate digestion is small intestine. Amylase acts on both raw and cooked starch. It acts best in alkaline medium. Amylase rapidly converts starch to maltose. Enzymes sucrase, maltase and Lactose are present in the brush border of the intestinal mucosal cells. They act on sucrose, maltose and lactose respectively as shown in the Table 2.2

Table 2.2 : Disaccharide Digestion by Different Enzymes in Small Intestine

Disacharide	*Enzyme*	*Sugars*
Sucrose	Sucrase	Glucose and Fructose
Maltose	Maltase	Glucose and Glucose
Lactose	Lactase	Glucose and Galactose

The end products of carbohydrate digestion is mainly glucose along with fructose and galactose. Cellulose is not digested by human beings because the human digestive system does not have enzvmes to act upon. So, cellulose passes unchanged as fecalbulk.

Absorption

The single sugars first enter the epithelial cell then across the cell they enter the interstitial fluid and reach the blood capillaries From there they enter the portal circulation and liver and are used according to the needs of the body. Fructose diffuses rapidly into the blood from the intestine. Glucose and galactose need sodium for their absorption. After absorption sodium dissociates and reach the brush border of small intestine again. Fructose and galactose from the diet are rapidly synthesized to glucose in the liver. So, any discussion of carbohydrate metabolism in our body is that of glucose only.

Glucose metabolism is inter-linked with protein and fat metabolism. Proteins and fats are potential sources of glucose and glucose can be converted to fatty acids and some amino acids. In some respects of the metabolisms of protein, fat and carbohydrate, one nutrient can substitute for another. When there is an increase in carbohydrate metabolism we can observe a decrease in fatty acid oxidation. Even traces of mineral elements and vitamins are essential for enzyme activity. In this way the metabolism of nutrients is interdependent and the deficiency of one may affect the total metabolism.

Liver and Carbohydrate Metabolism

The monosaccharides from small intestine reach the liver through portal vein. Here fructose and galactose are converted to glucose. Liver synthesizes glycogen from glucose and stores it. This process is called '*Glycogenesis*'. This glycogen can be converted to glucose by the liver which is called '*Glycogenolysis*'. The amino acids can be broken down and the carbon from them is utilized for glucose formation when the stores of glycogen are depleted. This process is called '*Gluconeogenesis*'. Liver also can convert the excess glucose to fatty acids which is called '*Lipogenesis*'. The carbons received from the carbohydrates are utilized by the liver for manufacturing non essential amino acids. The different pathways of carbohydrate metabolism are shown in the Figure 2.5 below:

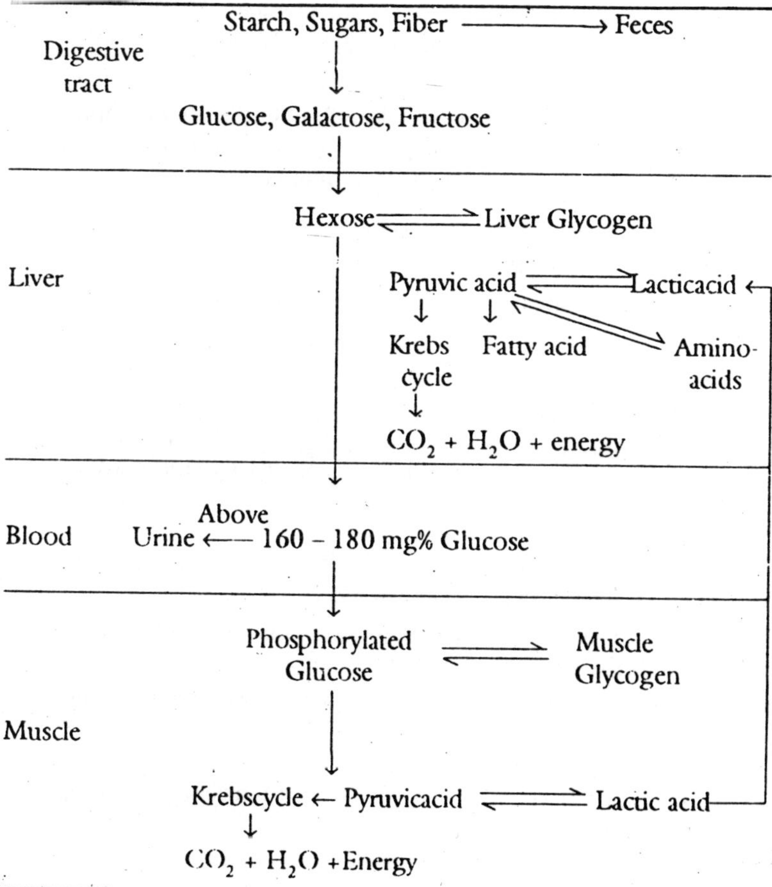

Blood Glucose

Glucose is available to all the cells of the body through blood. Liver replaces the glucose in the blood and maintains a constant controlled glucose level. In the fasting state a normal person has 60 to 100 mg per 100ml of blood. Excess sugar is stored and released when needed. If the blood glucose level exceeds 180/100ml kidneys excrete the sugar. This level varies from person to person and this level is called the renal threshold for glucose. Blood sugar level higher than the normal is called hyperglycemia which is a characteristic symptom in Diabetes mellitus.

Control of Blood sugar Level

Liver is the only organ which supplies glucose to the circulation and removes when it is not needed. Glucose is obtained from 1) Sugars from the diet 2) Glycogenolysis 3) Gluconeogenesis. The blood sugar level is maintained by several hormones like insulin, glucagon, anterior pituitary and epinephrine.

Insulin is produced by the beta cells of is lets of Langerhans of the pancreas. Insulin is the only hormone which reduces the blood sugar level. Insulin reduces the blood sugar level in three ways.

1) It increases the permeability of cell membrane of facilitate active transport,
2) It increases the synthesis of Glycogen in liver, and
3) It help in converting Glucose to fatty acids.

Glucagon is produced by the alpha cells of pancreas. Glucagon initiates glycogenolysis and thereby rises the blood sugar level. Anterior pituitary hormone increases the blood sugar level and prevents the entry of glucose into the tissues. Adrenaline increase the blood sugar level by glycogenolysis.

Glucose level in the blood is constantly maintained by

1. Continuous uptake by the cells
2. Conversion of glucose to glycogen in the liver which is called glycogenesis.
3. Synthesis of fats from glucose which is called Lipogenesis.
4. Synthesis of other Carbohydrate derivatives
5. Glycolysis in red blood cells
6. Removal of glucose from the blood when it crosses the renal threshold level.

Formation of glycogen is limited but formation of fat has no limit so, extra glucose in the body when maximum glycogen reserve is fulfilled is converted to fat.

FUNCTIONS OF CARBOHYDRATE

Energy

Carbohydrates supply approximately 4 k cals of energy. The source of energy after a meal is from carbohydrate. Total body store of carbohydrate is about 300 gms which gives 1200 k cals of energy. When compared to fat stores which last for a month carbohydrates store is sufficient for few hours only. Brain and blood depend on glucose for their metabolism. The blood sugar is maintained continuously even when the carbohydrate store is low. This is because of gluconeogenesis from protein and fats.

Liver

Glycogen is liver protects the liver again toxins. The carbohydrate derivatives produced by liver convert the harmful substances to harmless substance and are carried to excretory organs for excretion.

Brain

Brain is very sensitive for lack of glucose. Lack of glucose for short while creates permanent damage to the brain.

Heart

Glycogen is stored in the heart muscle as a reserve for emergency use. In a normal person with healthy heart low blood sugar level does not alter hearts function. But in a injured heart where glycogen store is low anginal pain may be observed.

Muscle

Carbohydrate is the fuel for muscle movement. With adequate of oxygen the locate is oxidized for energy but with inadequate oxygen lactate cannot be utilized and lactic acid levels rise. Which is called lactic acidosis.

Protein Sparing Action

When the energy needs of a person are met by adequate supply of carbohydrate and fat, protein is utilised for growth and repair of the tissues. This is called the protein sparing action of carbohydrates. When there is inadequate supply of fats and carbohydrates, proteins are utilised for energy needs and nitrogen is excreted by kidneys in the form of urea which is formed in the liver.

3

Lipids

Lipids are organic substances insoluble in water but soluble in solvents such as alcohol, ether, chloroform and benzene. The term Lipids include fatty acids, neutral fats, soaps, phospholipids, steroids and waxes. Lipids form important dietary constituents on account of their high calorific value. Essential fatty acids and fat soluble vitamins are also present. Fats impart flavour to foods. These are retained in stomach for longer time to a sense of satiety is felt. Lipids are present all over the body in each cell. Fat is stored in the body as fat depots which are energy sources. They also provide insulation, padding, synthesis of hormones maintain cell integrity and also carry fat soluble vitamins.

COMPOSITION

Lipids include fats, oils and other fat like substances. They are composed of fatty acids and glycerol. Fats are organic compounds of carbon hydrogen and oxygen. Compared to carbohydrates fats have a very lower proportion of oxygen. Lipids also contain phosphates, carbohydrates or other nitrogenous compounds. All lipids have fatty acids. Most of the naturally occurring fatty acids are straight chain derivatives and have even number of carbon atoms. They have a methyl group (CH_3) at one end and a carboxyl group (COOH) at the other end. The chains may contain as few as two or as many as twenty four carbon atoms. Short chain fatty acids have carbon atoms below 6 in number. Medium chain fatty acids posses eight to twelve carbon atoms and long chain fatty acid have more than twelve carbon atoms.

Fatty acids may be saturated or unsaturated depending on the number of hydrogen atoms attached to each carbon atom. In case of saturated fatty each of the carbon atom has two hydrogen atoms attached to it. In an unsaturated fatty acid one hydrogen atom is missing from each of the two adjoining carbon atoms due to which a double bond is formed between the two carbon atoms.

Saturated fatty acids can be represented by a general formula $CH_3(CH_2)_n$ COOH. The following are some of the saturated fatty acids shown in Table 3.1.

Table 3.1 : Some Saturated Fatty Acids, their Formula and Number of Carbons

Name of the acid	Formula	No. of Carbons
Acetic acid	CH_3 COOH	2
Butyric acid	CH_3 $(CH_2)_2$ COOH	4
Caproic acid	CH_3 $(CH_2)_4$ COOH	6
Caprylic acid	$CH_3(CH_2)_6$ COOH	8
Capric acid	CH_3 $(CH_2)_8$ COOH	10
Lauric acid	CH_3 $(CH_2)_{10}$ COOH	12
Myristic acid	CH_3 $(CH_2)_{12}$ COOH	14
Palmitic acid	CH_3 $(CH_2)_{14}$ COOH	16
Stearic acid	CH_3 $(CH_2)_{16}$ COOH	18
Arachidic acid	CH_3 $(CH_2)_{18}$ COOH	20
Lignoceric acid	CH_3 $(CH_2)_{22}$ COOH	24

Unsaturated fatty acids contain one or more double bonds. Some of them are as follows:

Oleic Acid

This is a derivative of steric acid with double bond between C_9 and C_{10}. It can be represented in the following way:

$$CH_3(CH_2)_7 \boxed{CH = CH} (CH_2)_7 \text{ COOH}$$

Linoleic Acid

This is also a derivative of stearic acid and has two double bonds, one between C_9 and C_{10} and second between C_{12} and C_{13}.

$$CH_3 (CH_2)_4 \boxed{CH = CH} CH_2 \boxed{CH = CH} (CH_2)_7 \text{ COOH}$$

Linolenic Acid

This is also a derivative of stearic acid with three double bonds. They are between C_9 and C_{10} C_{12} and C_{13} and C_{15} and C_{16}.

$$CH_3\,CH_2\boxed{CH=CH}\,CH_2\,\boxed{CH=CH}\,CH_2\,\boxed{CH=CH}(CH_2)_7\,COOH$$

Unsaturated fatty acid occur as geometric isomers. In cis form then can fold back upon itself and in Transform the molecule extends to its maximum length. Food fats and body fats are cis forms. There forms influences the properties of the fat. Structure of some fatty acids is shown in Figure 3.1

```
   H
   |
H—C—OH
   |
H—C—OH
   |
H—C—OH
   |
   H
```

GLYCEROL

```
    O  H  H  H  H  H  H  H  H  H  H  H  H  H
    ‖  |  |  |  |  |  |  |  |  |  |  |  |  |
HO—C—C—C—C—C—C—C—C—C—C—C—C—C—C—H
       |  |  |  |  |  |  |  |  |  |  |  |  |
       H  H  H  H  H  H  H  H  H  H  H  H  H
```

MYRISTIC ACID

```
    O  H  H  H  H  H  H  H  H  H  H  H  H  H  H  H
    ‖  |  |  |  |  |  |  |  |  |  |  |  |  |  |  |
HO—C—C—C—C—C—C—C—C—C—C—C—C—C—C—C—C—H
       |  |  |  |  |  |  |  |  |  |  |  |  |  |  |
       H  H  H  H  H  H  H  H  H  H  H  H  H  H  H
```

PALMITIC ACID

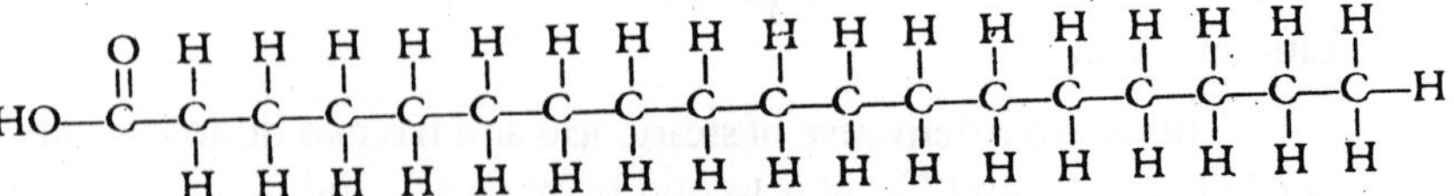

STEARIC ACID

```
     O  H  H  H  H  H  H  H  H
     ‖  |  |  |  |  |  |  |  |
HO — C— C— C— C— C— C— C— C— C— H
        |  |  |  |  |  |  |  ‖
        H  H  H  H  H  H  H  ‖
                             ‖
     H  H  H  H  H  H  H  H  ‖
     |  |  |  |  |  |  |  |  ‖
  H— C— C— C— C— C— C— C— C— C— H
     |  |  |  |  |  |  |  |
     H  H  H  H  H  H  H  H
```

OLEIC ACID

```
     O  H  H  H  H  H  H  H
     ‖  |  |  |  |  |  |  |
HO — C— C— C— C— C— C— C— C— C— H
        |  |  |  |  |  |  |  ‖
        H  H  H  H  H  H  H  ‖
                             ‖
                          H  ‖
                          |  ‖
                    H— C— C— C— H
                       ‖  |
                       ‖  H
                       ‖
                       ‖  H  H  H  H  H
                       ‖  |  |  |  |  |
                    H— C— C— C— C— C— C— H
                          |  |  |  |  |
                          H  H  H  H  H
```

LINOLEIC ACID.

```
     O  H  H  H  H  H  H  H
     ‖  |  |  |  |  |  |  |
HO — C— C— C— C— C— C— C— C— C— H
        |  |  |  |  |  |  |  ‖
        H  H  H  H  H  H  H  ‖
                             ‖
                          H  ‖
                          |  ‖
                    H— C— C— C— H
                       ‖  |
                       ‖  H
                       ‖
                       ‖     H
                       ‖     |
                    H— C     C   C— H
                             |   ‖
                             H   ‖
                       H     H   ‖
                       |     |   ‖
                    H— C     C   C— H
                       |     |
                       H     H
```

LINOLENIC ACID

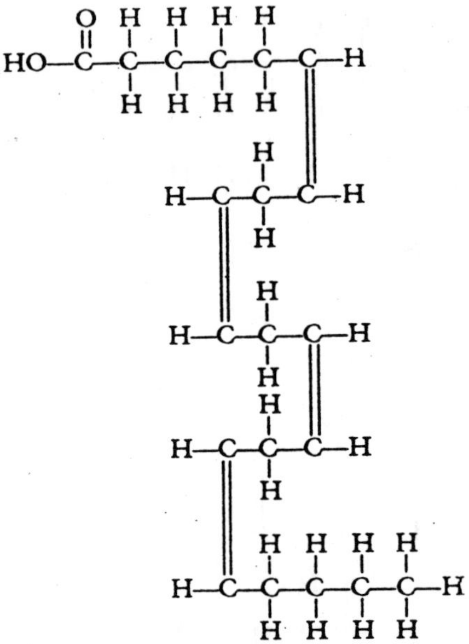

```
    O  H  H  H  H
    ‖  |  |  |  |
HO—C—C—C—C—C—C—H
       |  |  |  |  ‖
       H  H  H  H  ‖
                H  ‖
                |  ‖
          H—C—C—C—H
            ‖   |
            ‖   H
            ‖   H
            ‖   |
          H—C—C—C—H
                |  ‖
                H  ‖
                H  ‖
                |  ‖
          H—C—C—C—H
            ‖   |
            ‖   H
            ‖
            ‖   H  H  H  H
            ‖   |  |  |  |
          H—C—C—C—C—C—H
                |  |  |  |
                H  H  H  H
```

ARACHIDONIC ACID

Fig. 3.1 : Structure of Some Fatty Acids

ESSENTIAL FATTY ACIDS

There are the fatty acid which are nutritionally very important and are to be supplied through diet. These cannot be synthesised in the body. These are linoleic, linoleni and arachidonic acids. Structures are given in figure. Linoleic and Linolenic are present in cotton seeds, ground nut and linseed oils Arachidonic aid is synthesised from linolenic acid in Animals. Safflowel oil, sun flower oil, cotton seed, linseed and soy oils are rich sources of EFA. Fatty acid composition of some fats in given in Table 3.2

CLASSIFICATION

Lipids are usually classified into :

1) Simple lipids
2) Compound lipids
3) Derived lipids.

Table 3.2 : Fatty Acid Composition of Some Edible Oils and Fats

(Values are percentage of total methylester of fatty acid)

S. No.	Oil Fats	Palmitic	Stearic	Arachidic	Bethenic	Lignoseric	Total	Palmitoleic	Oleic	Linoleic	Linolenic	Total
		16:0	18:0	20:0	22:0	24:0	Saturates	16:1	13:1	18:2	18:3	Unsaturates
(1)	(2)	(3)	(4)	(5)	(6)	(7)	(8)	(9)	(10)	(11)	(12)	(13)
1.	Coconut Oil	7.8	2.3	--	--	--	87.9*	--	7.8	0.8	--	8.6
2.	Corn Oil	10.7	1.7	--	--	--	12.7	--	24.6	57.4	--	83.0
3.	Cotton Seed Oil	23.4	1.1	1.3	--	0.1	25.9	--	22.9	47.8	--	70.7
4.	Groundnut Oil	12.6	1.7	4.2	2.1	0.3	20.9	1.4	47.9	29.9	--	79.1
5.	Mustard or Rapeseed Oil	2.9	0.9	6.9	--	--	10.7	0.6	8.9	18.1	14.5	88.6**
6.	Olive Oil	11.5	2.3	--	--	--	14.2	--	71.5	8.2	--	81.4
7.	Palm Oil	42.0	4.3	--	--	--	47.9	--	37.9	9.0	--	47.7
8.	Palmolein	42.3	3.5	--	--	--	47.7	0.4	41.0	10.3	0.3	52.0
9.	Rice Bran Oil	16.5	1.6	--	--	--	19.5	--	39.2	33.3	--	74.6
10.	Saflower Oil	7.8	2.1	0.8	--	--	10.7	--	17.7	78.5	--	92.2
11.	Sesame Oil	9.7	3.4	--	--	--	13.4	0.1	41.2	44.5	--	86.5
12.	Soyabean Oil	9.8	2.4	0.9	--	--	13.1	--	28.9	50.7	6.5	86.1
13.	Sunflower Oil	5.6	2.2	0.9	--	0.4	9.1	--	25.1	66.2	--	8.13
14.	Butter	21.1	9.7	--	--	--	49.8*	--	20.1	1.8	--	--

* Includes lower chain fatty acid

** Includes 46.5% of Erucic acid (22:1)

Simple Lipids

These are esters of glycerol and fatty acids. Glycerol is a 3 carbon alcohol with three hydroxyl groups. A monoglyceride is a combination of a fatty acid with one of the hydroxyl groups of the glycerol molecule. Similarly Diglycerides and triglycerides have two and three fatty acids, bound to the hydroxyl groups of the glycerol molecules respectively. Triglycerides are also called neutral fats. Simple triglyceride is the one with identical fatty acids where as a mixed triglyceride has atleast two different fatty acids. Food Fats usually contain 98 per cent of Mixed triglycerides and body fats have 90 percent. Neutral fats are colour less, odorless and taste less substances. The color and taste of some of the naturally occurring fats in due to extraneous substances.

Compound Lipids

These are the esters of glycerol and fatty acids with substitution of other compound such as carbohydrates, phosphate and/ or nitrogenous grouping. Lecithin and cephalin has a phosphate and Nitrogen group replacing one of the fatty acids in the molecule and called phospholipids. Glycolipids such as cerebrosides contain a molecule of galactore or glucase. Lipoproteins have a variety of lipid molecules bound to protein molecules which facilitates transport in the blood which is a aqueous medium.

Derived Lipids

These are Fatty acids and Sterols.

CHARACTERISTICS OF FATS

Hardness

The hardness of the fat is dependent on the fatty acid composition. Fatty acids with twelve or less carbon atoms and unsaturated fats are liquids at room temperature. Saturated fats and fatty acids that have more than fourteen carbon atoms or more are solids at room temperature. No natural fat is made up of either completely saturated or unsaturated fatty acids. Animal fats have 30 to 60 percent saturated fatty acids in which stearic and palmitic are predominant, 30 to 50 percent sleic acid and a small amount of poly unsaturated fatty acids. Oleic and Linoleic acids are predominant in vegetable fats.

Hydrogenation

Liquid fats can be changed to solid fats by hydrogenation. This is nothing but addition of hydrogen at double bonds of the carbon chain. Nickel acts as catalyst in this reaction.

Emulsification

Fats and oils are lighter than water. They are insoluble in water but can be dispersed into minute globules. This decreases the surface tension and increases surface area. This is called emulsion. In an emulsion fat globules have a lesser tendency to coalesce. In small intestine bile salts emulsify trigly cerides to fatty acids. Lecithin is widely used as an emulsifier in food industry.

Saponification

A combination of a fatty acid and a cation forms soap and the process is called saponification. The number of milligrams of Potassium hydroxide required to saponify 1 gram of fat or oil is called saponification value or saponification number.

Iodine Number

To determine the extent of unsaturated fatty acids present in fats and oils iodine number is used. It is defined as number or grams of iodine absorbed by 100 grams of fat.

Rancidity

Oxidation of fats results in odor and flavour changer. This is called Rancidity. These changes are accelerated on exposure to air. Oxygen acts on double bonds of fatty acids to form Feroxider. Peroxidation occurs rapidly in fats that have high proportion of unsaturated fatty acids.

FUNCTIONS

Energy

One gram of fat when oxidized gives 9 k. cals of energy. It is more than twice of carbohydrate and protein. A normal healthy person has about 85,000 K cals of energy as adipose tissue.

Satiety Value

Fatty foods reduce gastric motility and remain longer time in the stomach. So a feeling of satiety is created and hunger sensations are delayed.

Palatability

Fats impart a special flavour to the diet and increases the palatability.

Insulation and Padding

The subcutaneous layer of fat is an effective insulator and also pads the sensitive internal organs against physical injuries. It prevent the loss of heat from the body in cold weather. But in obese people excessive layers of subcutaneous fat creates discomfort by interfering heat loss.

Carriers of Vitamins

Dietary fat is a carrier of vitamins A, D, E and K. Fat is essential for vitamin A absorption.

ESSENTIAL FATTY ACIDS

Linoleic, Linolenic and arachidonic acids are the essential fatty acids. Linoleic acid is converted to arachidonic acid in the body. Arachidonic acid acts as a precursor of prostaglandins. Prostaglandins appear to stimulate smooth muscle contraction, regulate blood pressure, transmit nerve impulse and inhibit gastric secretions and lipolysis.

Phospholipids

All cells in the body possess phospholipids. Brian, nervous tissue and liver are rich in phospholipids. Body can synthesize phospholipid's for its use.

Cholesterol

Cholesterol is synthesised by the liver and is present in almost all the body tissues. The concentration is high in liver, adrenal, brain and nervous tissues.

Digestion and Absorption of Fats

Fats reduce the gastric motility and hence a diet containing more fat is retained in stomach for longer time. Almost all the dietary fats are triglycerides. Cholesterol esters and phospholipids are only a small fraction. Fats that are liquids at body temperature are hydrolysed fast. Fats are hydrolysed in small intestine. Though gastric juice has lipase its action is not important because the PH in stomach does not favouring its action.

When the chyme enters duodenum a hormone enterogastrone is released which stimulates pancreas. The presence of fat in chyme stimulates the secretion of cholecy stokinin from intestinal wall which in turn initiates the contraction of gallbladder. Bile is pumped into small intestine. Bile neutralises the acid chyme and provides optimum PH for the action of pancreatic Lipose and emulsifies the fats there by increasing the surface areas and lowers the surface tension so that the enzyme can reach the fine fat droplet easily. The triglycerides are hydrolysed by lipare by removing on and fatty acid at a time and finally a monoglyceride is obtained. Cholesteril esters are hydrolysed to cholesterol and fatty acids by cholesterol esterase. Finally fatty acids, glycerol, monoglycerides, diglycerides, triglycerides, cholesterol and phospholipids are presented for absorptions. These mix up with bile salts to form micelles. Micelles are water soluble particles that can penetrate through the mucous membrane. The micelles release the lipids at the brush border and again combine with bile salts. Fatty acids that have Twelve or less number of carbon atoms are absorbed into portal circulation. They are sued in the liver or released to other tissues. Fatty acids with fourteen or more carbons are re-synthesised to triglycerides and are extruded into lymph circulation. There newly formed fats have a lipoprotein envelope made of phospholipids and a little protein which are called chylomicrons. These can penetrate through the lipoprotein membrane of the epithelial cell and enter the lymph circulation. The following figure 3.2 gives a summary of digestion, absorption and transportation of fats.

METABOLISM

The normal triglyceride level in fasting state is below 140 mg per 100 ml. The concentration increases after meal because the chylomicrons and very low density lipoproteins enter the circulation. These levels increase during lipolysis and increase with lipogenesis. The triglyceride levels tend to increase with age which is not desirable. Cholesterol and triglycerides do not exist in free state in blood. They combine with proteins to form lipoproteins.

LOW DENSITY LIPOPROTEINS

This can be divided into very low density lipoproteins and low density lipoproteins. Very low density lipoproteins have a high proportion of triglycerides when compared to the protein fraction. Low density lipoproteins have a high proportion of cholesterol when compared to triglyceride fraction. The concentration of low density lipoproteins increases with age and consumption of saturated fats.

HIGH DENSITY LIPOPROTEINS

High density lipoproteins have about 50 percent protein and 20 percent cholesterol in it. It has been found that these have a protective effect and reduces the risk of coronary heart disease. Concentration of lipoproteins in human plasma is given in Table 3.3

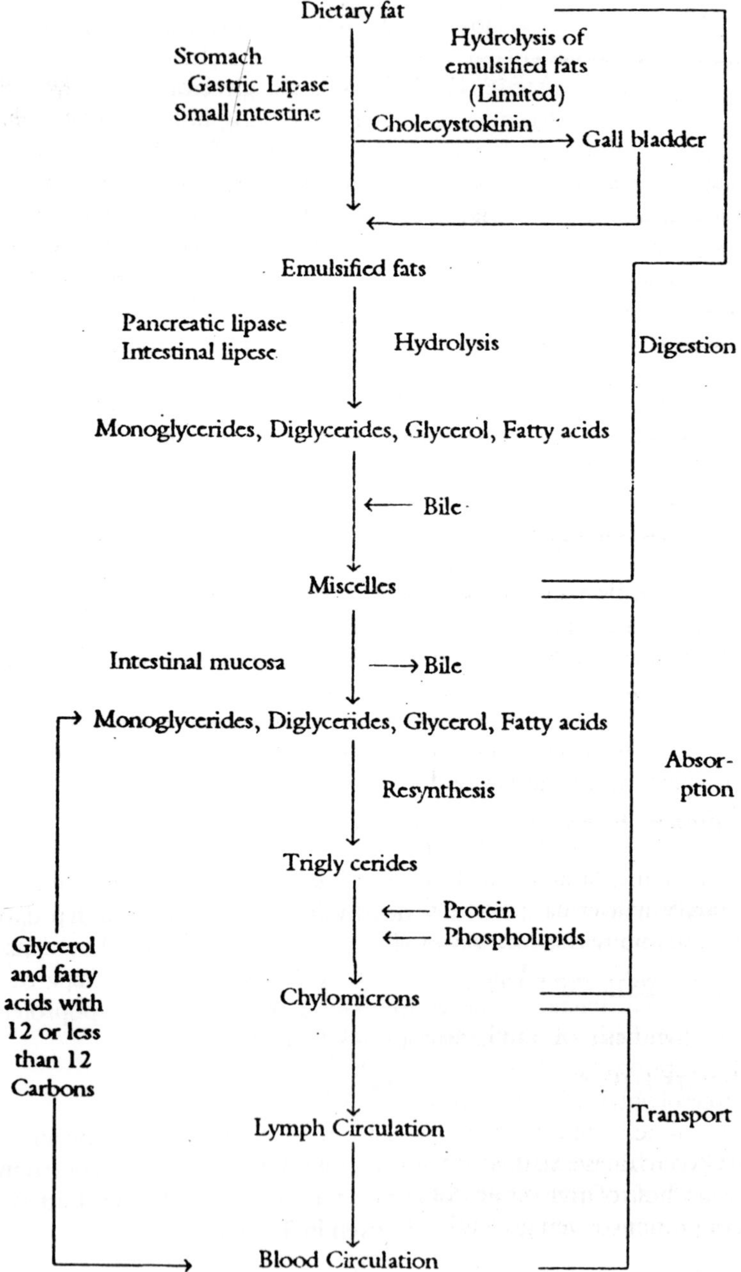

Fig. 3.2 : Summary of Digestion, Absorption and Transportation of Fats

Table 3.3 : Concentration of Lipoproteins in Human Plasma

(Percent Composition)

	Chylomicrons	*Lipoproteins*		
		Very low Density	Low Density	High Density
Proteins	2	9	21	45
Triglycerides	85	50	10	8
Cholesterol	5	23	46	19
Phospholipids	8	18	23	27

ADIPOSE TISSUE

Adipose tissue synthesises, stores and releases fats. It is a unique tissue with cells having less water when compared to other cells. The size of the cell increases with fat depot and water content decreases. The cells of the adipose tissue has enzymes that can bring about lipolysis or lipogenesis. Lipolysis occurs when the energy needs of the body are not met with the diet and lipogenesis occur when there is excess energy supply regardless the energy source whether carbohydrate, protein or fat. The number of adipose cells in the body remain same during the life they only increase in size with fat deposit.

THE LIVER

Liver is the key organ in fat metabolism. It increases or decreases the length of the fatty acids depending on their need to the body. It hydrolyses the triglycerides. It can re-synthesize triglycerides from fatty acids, glucose or other carbon skeletons donated by amino acids. It controls the lipid content of the blood by addition or removal. Particularly liver has complete control over blood cholesterol content and total body cholesterol content.

SYNTHESIS OF FATS

Synthesis of Triglycerides need α- glycerophosphate. This α–glycerophosphate is obtained from Embden Meyerh of path way Glycerol obtained from fat hydrolysis in intestinal mucosa combines with Adenosine Triphosphate to form α–glycerophosphate in the presence of Glycerokinase. So this forms the second source of α-glycerophosphate for synthesis of triglycerides Adipose tissue does not have any glycerokinase so it cannot convert glycerol to glycerophosphate. The hydrolysis of fats and synthesis of acetyl COA provide the fatty acids necessary for Triglyceride synthesis. Synthesis of fats from acetyl COA needs NADPH which is obtained from Glycolytic pathway. Free fatty acids are first converted to fatty acyl COA and attached to glycerophosphate step wise to form friglycerides.

OXIDATION OF FATTY ACIDS

All cells in our body except of central nervous system and Red blood cells can yield energy by oxidizing fatty acids. Brian cells can utilize ketone bodies derived from fat and amino acids source. The oxidation of fatty acids occurs in mitochondria. This oxidation occurs at the carbon at beta position from carboxyl group. So it is called oxidation for which ATP is needed. The result is a fatty acid and acetyl coenzyme A. This acetyl coenzyme A can enter Krebs cycle to give energy, carbondioxide and water or utilised for synthesis of fatty acids and other compounds.

KETOGENESIS

Two acetyl coenzyme A molecules combine to form aceto acyl coenzyme A in the liver. The aceto acyl coenzyme A in turn yield energy but the liver cannot utilize these ketone bodies as it lacks the enzymes for their oxidation. During starvation or decreased carbohydrate metabolism these ketone body production is increased for beyond the ability of the tissues to oxidize thus these ketone bodies accumulate in the body causing a disturbance in acid base balance. These are strong acids and combine with the available base and are excreted (Ketone uria). This reduces the base reserve in the body and leads to acidosis. Acetone is volatice so it is excreted by lungs. This condition is observed in diabetes due to lack of insulin for the metabolism of carbohydrates. It should be treated immediately if not coma and death follows.

CHOLESTEROL

Cholesterol is synthesised mainly in liver and intestines. Acetyl coenzyme A from any source is the precurs of for its synthesis. This cholesterol is independent to dietary cholesterol. Only liver has the capacity to convert it by enzyme action to bile acids. This rate is limited. So any excess supply should be problematic. Bile has both bile acids and cholesterol which are excreted from the intestines. The steps involved in the biosynthesis of cholesterol from acetyl COA are as in figure 3.4 structure of cholesterol is given in Figure 3.3

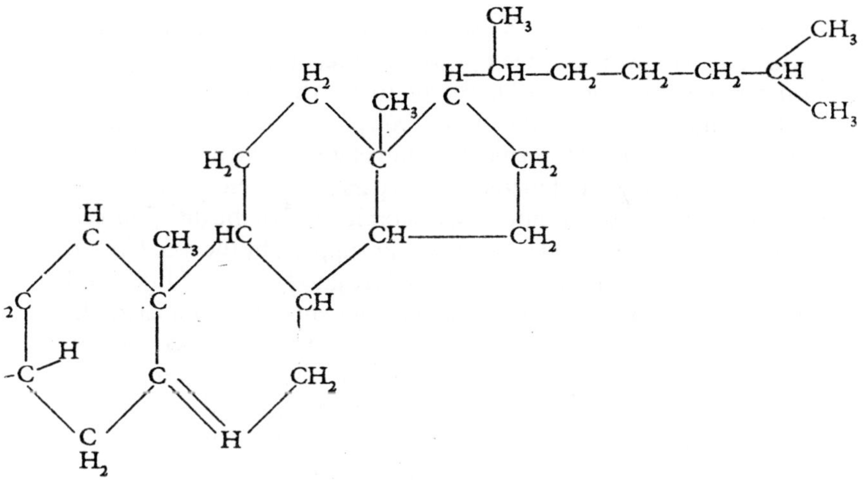

Fig. 3.3 Sturcture of Cholesterol

Acetyl COA

↓

Aceto acetyl COA

↓

Bhydroxy methyl glutary COA

↓

Mevalonic acid

↓

β, δ, dihydroxy methyl valeric acid

↓

3 iso pentonyl pyrophosphate

↓

Geranyl pyrophosphate

↓

Farnesyl pyrophosphate

↓

Squalene

↓

Lanosterol

↓

Cholesterol

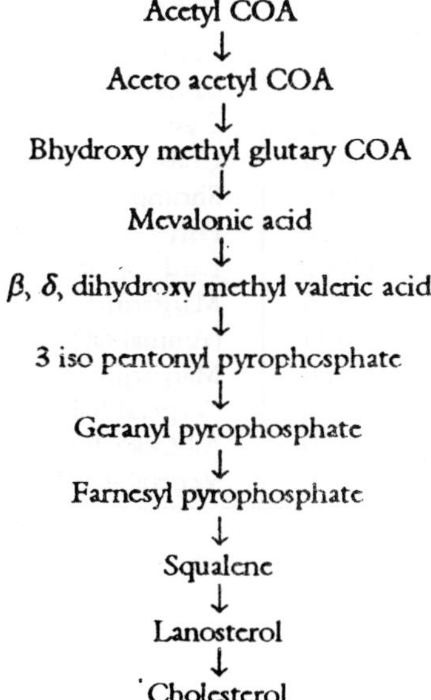

Fig. 3.4 : Bio Synthesis of Cholesterol from Acetyl COA

DIETARY FAT

Dietary fat includes both visible and invisible fat of the diet. Visible fats include oils, hydrogenated oils, shortening, butter ghee margarine, salad dressing etc. The invisible fats are those which are present in the foods but not visible like fats in meat, Fish, poultry, milk cream, cheese, eggs etc. the amount of fat in meat depend of various factors like the cut, trimming, drippings, and method of preparation. These when used in small amounts also contribute to the calorific value of the diet. Linoleic acid is an essential fatty acid which has to be supplied by the diet. Cotton seed oil, sunflower oil, corn oil and soy oil are good sources. Cholesterol is another important factor. Cholesterol is present only in animal foods. Egg yolk, kidney, brain liver, and sweet bread (thymus) are rich sources. Milk, cream, butter ghee cheese and meat also contribute to the cholesterol content of the diet. Hyper cholestremia is found to associated myocardial in fraction, coronary event, ischemic etc. is many cases. So the intake of total fat especially saturated fat should be cut down and it an be substituted with poly unsaturated fatty acids. The total amount of energy from fats should not exceed 10-20 percent of total energy intake. Table 3.4 gives the amount of cholesterol in some foods.

Table 3.4 : Cholesterol Content of Some Foods

Food stuff	*mg per 100 g.*	*Food stuff*	*mg per 100 g.*
Egg yolk	1500	Mutton	65
Whole egg	550	Chicken	60
Egg white	0	Oyster	>200
Butter	250	Crab	125
Cheese	100	Shrimp	125
Milk	10	Fish	75
Brain	>2000	Lard	95
Kidney	375	Margarine	
Liver	300	(Animal fat)	65
Thymus	250	Margarine	
Heart	150	(Vegetable fat)	0
Pork	70	All foods from	
Beef	70	Vegetable origin	0

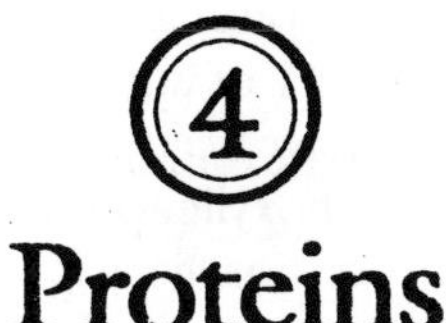

Proteins

Mulder in 1838 described certain organic substance which is the most important of all known substances in the organic kingdom. It was named as protein. The word protein was derived from the Greek word 'Protos' which means 'First Place'. Protein now means a nitrogenous constituent of protoplasm of all plant and animal tissues. Protein is necessary for innumerable functions in the body primarily for synthesis of all body tissues.

COMPOSITION

Proteins are made up of Aminoacids as units in various proportions and arrangements. The possess carbon, hydrogen, oxygen nitrogen and in few sulphur. Some proteins have phosphorus, small amounts of iron, copper etc. The presence of Nitrogen makes protein different from carbohydrates and fats. Protein on average have 16 per cent nitrogen. Protein molecular are larger than carbohydrate and lipid molecules and form colloidal solutions.

STRUCTURE

Protein are made up of Aminoacids. Aminoacids are organic compounds with Amino group (NH_2) and acid or caboxyl group. The structure of an amino acid can be represented as

$$\begin{array}{l} R\text{—}\,CH\text{—}COOH \\ \quad\;\;\; | \\ \quad\;\; NH_2 \end{array}$$

R is the carbon chain it may be straight chain, or branched chain; an aromatic or hetero cyclic ring structure or a sulphur grouping. Amino acids with one amino and one carboxyl groups and one amino group are acid in reaction and those with two amino groups and one carboxyl group are basic in reaction. These amino acids are linked to each other by peptide linkage i.e. amino group of one amino acid is linked to carboxyl group of other by removal of water molecule. The amino acids naturally occurring in proteins have been classified under the following heads **1**. Mono amino mono carboxylic acids **2**. Mono amino dicarboxylic acids **3**. Diamino mono carboxylic acids **4**. Sulphur containing amino acids and **5**. Aromatic amino acids Heterocyclic amino acids as shown in the Table 4.1.

Table 4.1 Classification of Amino Acids

1.	Mono amino mono carboxylic acids	a) Glycine b) Alanine c) Valine d) Levcine e) Isoleucine f) Nor leucine g) Serine h) Threonine
2.	Mono amino di carboxylic acids	a) Aspartic acid b) Glutamic acid
3.	Diamino-Mono Carboxylic acids	a) Arginine b) Lysine
4.	Sulphur containing amino acids	a) Cysteine b) Methinine c) Cystine
5.	Aromatic amino acids and Hetero cyclic amino acids	a) Phenylanine b) Tyrosine c) Try ptophan d) Histidine e) Proline f) Hydro proline

The Structure of these amino acids are given in figure 4.1 below:

1. Mono amino mono carboxylic acids : (Aliphatic amino acids)		
a) Glycine (Gly)	Amino acetic acid	$H{-}CH(NH_2){-}COOH$
b) Alanine (Ala)	α Amino propionic acid	$CH_3{-}CH(NH_2){-}COOH$
c) Valine (Val)	α amino isovaleric acid	$(CH_3)_2CH{-}C(NH_2)(H){-}COOH$
d) Leucine (Lev)	α amino isocaproic acid	$H_3C{-}C(H)(CH_3){-}CH_2{-}C(H)(NH_2){-}COOH$
e) Isoleucine (Ile)	α amino, β methyl (Valeric acid)	$H_3C{-}CH_2{-}C(H)(CH_3){-}C(H)(NH_2){-}COOH$
f) Serine (Ser)	amino, hydroxy propionic acid	$CH_2(OH){-}CH(NH_2){-}COOH$
g) Threonine (Thr)	α amino, β hydroxy butyric acid	$CH_3{-}CH(OH){-}CH(NH_2){-}COOH$
2. Mono amino dicarboxylic acids : (Acidic amino acids)		
a) Aspartic acid (ASP)	α amino succinic acid	$HOOCCH_2{-}CH(NH_2){-}COOH$
b) Glutamic acid (Glu)	α amino Glutaric acid	$HOOCCH_2CH_2{-}CH(NH_2){-}COOH$

3. Diamino Monocarboxylic acids

a) Arginine (Arg) — α amino δ guanidino-n-valeric acid

$$(NH_2)_2C{-}NH{-}CH_2{-}CH_2{-}CH_2{-}C(H)(NH_2){-}COOH$$

b) Lysine (Lys) — α E diamino caproic acid

$$CH_2(NH_2){-}CH_2{-}CH_2{-}CH_2{-}CH(NH_2){-}COOH$$

4. Sulphur containing amino acids

a) Cysteine (Cys) — α amino β mercapto -propionic acid

$$HS{-}CH_2{-}CH(NH_2){-}COOH$$

b) Methionine (Met) — α amino γ methylthio -n-butyric acid

$$H_3C{-}S{-}CH_2{-}CH(NH_2){-}COOH$$

c) Cystine

$$COOH{-}CH(NH_2){-}CH_2{-}S{-}S{-}CH_2{-}CH(NH_2){-}COOH$$

5. Aromatic and heterocyctic amino acids

a) Phenyl alamine (Phe) — α amino β phenyl propioniacid

$$H_5C_6{-}CH_2{-}CH(NH_2){-}COOH$$

b) Tyrosine (Tyr) — p-hydroxy phenyl alanine

$$HO{-}H_5C_6{-}CH_2{-}CH(NH_2){-}COOH$$

c) Tryptophane (Trp) — α amino, β indole propionic acid

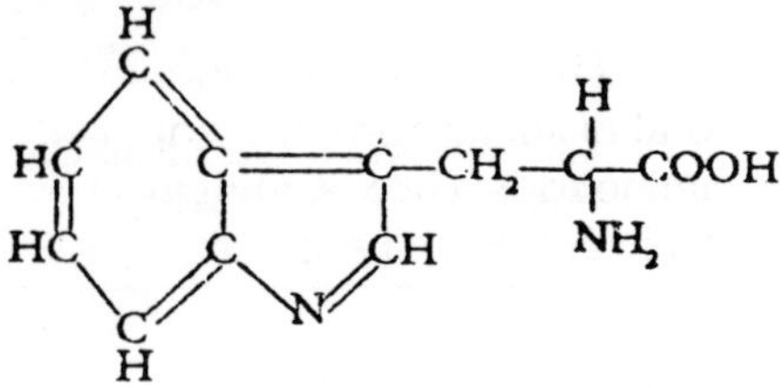

H
C
HC C = C—CH_2—C(H)—COOH
HC C CH NH_2
N
C
H

d) Histidine (His)	α amino β imidazole propionic acid	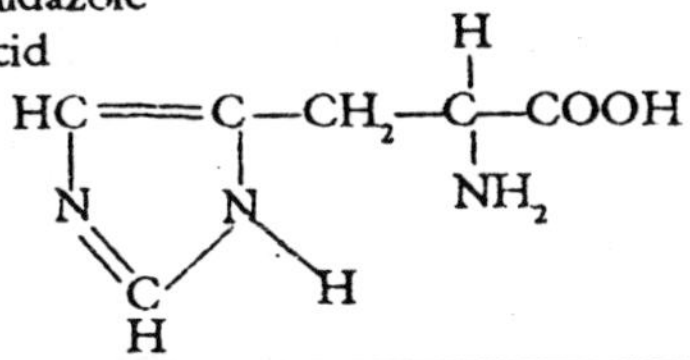 HC=C–CH_2–C(H)(NH$_2$)–COOH; ring: HC–N=CH–NH–C
e) Proline (Pro)	Pyrrolidine 2 carboxylic acid	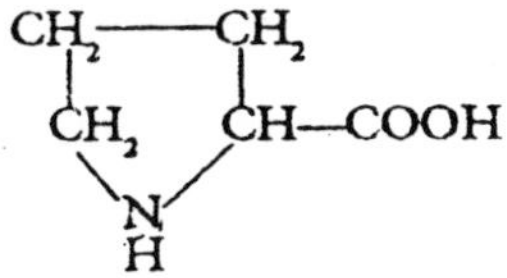 CH_2–CH_2–CH_2–CH(COOH)–NH (ring)

Fig. 4.1 : Structures of Aminoacids

Amino acids are classified into three groups depending on their reaction in solution 1. Neutral 2. Acidic and 3. Basic Aspartic acid and Glutamic acid are acidic aminoacids. But their amides asparagine and glutamine are neutral on account of the additional amide group. Arginine, lysine and Histidine are basic amino acids. The rest are rental amino acids.

Proteins consist of chains of amino acids joined to each other by the peptide linkages. The amino group of one amino acid is attached to carboxyl group of other amino by removal of water as shown in the figure. The PRIMARY STRUCTURE of protein molecule is deter-

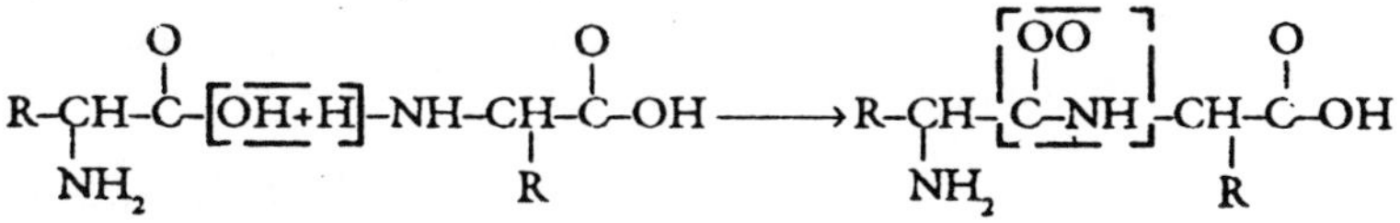

$$\text{R-}\underset{NH_2}{\text{CH}}\text{-}\overset{O}{\overset{\|}{C}}\text{-}\boxed{\text{OH+H}}\text{-NH-}\underset{R}{\text{CH}}\text{-}\overset{O}{\overset{\|}{C}}\text{-OH} \longrightarrow \text{R-}\underset{NH_2}{\text{CH}}\text{-}\boxed{\overset{O}{\overset{\|}{C}}\text{-NH}}\text{-}\underset{R}{\text{CH}}\text{-}\overset{O}{\overset{\|}{C}}\text{-OH}$$

Removal of water — Peptide linkage

Fig. 4.2 : The amino group of one amino acid is linked to the carboxyl group of another aminoacid by removal of water.

mined by the chain of amino acids. The chains vary with the number and kind of amino acids, the length of the chain and repetition of different amino acids. The SECONDARY STRUCTURE of the Protein depends on hydrogen and sulphur bonds that occur between amino acids in the chain, which are not adjacent. The TERTIARY STRUCTURE of protein is the manner in which the amino acid chains are bound to give shape and characteristics. Some protein molecules are complexes of more than one polypeptide chain. Each chain in the molecule is called monomer. The compound structure is called oligomer. This type of complexity determines its QUARTERNARY STRUCTURE.

CLASSIFICATION OF PROTEINS

Proteins are classified in a number of ways like physical and chemical properties, physical shape and nutritional properties.

Physical and Chemical Properties

According to this classification proteins are divided into

1. Simple Proteins
2. Conjugated Proteins and
3. Derived Proteins.

1. Simple Proteins

These on hydrolysis by acids, alkalies or enzymes yield only amino acids or their derivatives.

a) **Albumins** : These are soluble in water and are heat coagulable. They are precipitated from solution by saturating with ammonium sulphate. Ex : Egg albumin, lactalbumin, Serum albumin etc.

b) **Globulins** : There are insoluble in water but soluble in neutral salt solutions. They are heat coagulable and can be precipitated by half saturation with ammonium sulphate. These are present alongwith albumins.

c) **Glutelins** : These are not soluble in neutral solvents, but are soluble in dilute acids and alkalies.

   Ex : Wheat protein

d) **Prolamines** : These are soluble in 70 – 80 percent alcohol.

   Ex : Proteins in wheat (gliadin), maize (Zein), barley etc.

e) **Sclero Proteins or Albuminoids or Fibrous Proteins** : They are characteristic of the skeletal structures of animals and external protective tissues. They are insoluble in almost all solvents. They are present in skin, hair, horns and hoof containing amino acids rich in sulphur.

f) **Histones** : They are soluble in water, dilute acids and salt solutions but insoluble in very dilute ammonia. On hydrolysis theyyield several amino acids, among which the basic ones like arginine are predominant.

Ex. : Nucleic acids and hemoglobin.

g) **Protamines** : These are strongly basic proteins. They are simplest proteins with very low molecular weight, soluble in water not coagulable by heat and on hydrolysis yield large amounts of basic amino acids like Arginine. There occur in sperm.

2. Conjugated Proteins

The Proteins in this group are combined with a non-protein group called the Prosthetic group.

a) **Nucleoproteins** : These are compounds of proteins with nucleic acid.

b) **Glyco Proteins** : These are protein molecules with a carbohydrate group. *Ex* : Mucin.

c) **Phospho Proteins** : These are proteins with phosphorus. *Ex* : Casein of milk and vitelline of egg yolk.

d) **Chromo Proteins** : The Prosthetic group is a coloured compound. *Ex* : Hemoglobin.

e) **Lipo Proteins** : Proteins in combination with phospholipids. These occur in blood serum, egg yolk, milk etc.

f) **Metallo Proteins** : Proteins in combination with metals like Iron, Copper, Zinc, Magnesium etc.

3. Derived Proteins

These are products of denaturation or of partial digestion of proteins.

i) Primary Protein Derivatives

These are derivatives of the protein molecules due to hydrolytic changes which involve only slight alterations.

a) *Proteins* : There are insoluble products formed as a incipient action of very dilute acids or enzymes.

b) *Meta Proteins* : On treatment with acid or alkali, the corresponding acid or alkali meta protein is formed which is insoluble in neutral solvents.

c) *Coagulated Proteins* : There are denatured insoluble proteins which are formed to the action of heat or action of alcohol on protein.

ii) Secondary Protein Derivative

The products formed due to the partial digestion or protein are called secondary protein derivatives.

a) *Proteoses* : There are soluble in water but cannot be coagulated by heat. There can be precipitated by saturating with Ammonium sulphate.

b) *Peptones* : These are soluble in water but cannot be coagulated by heat or precipitated by Ammonium sulphate.

c) *Peptides* : There have two or more amino acids. These form as a result of hydrolytic cleavage of peptones.

NUTRITIONAL PROPERTIES

The classical investigation of Dr. William C. Rose and co-workers during 1930–36 showed that out of 20 amino acids 10 are essential for growth and maintainence of good health in rats. They fed the rats on diets containing pure amino acids instead of protein. They were successful. Then they omitted one amino acid at a time from the mixture and studies the growth. Thus they found that 10 amino acids are essential for the growth of rats and called them essential or indispensable amino acids. While others were called non-essential amino acids or dispensable amino acids. The essential amino acids cannot be synthesised in the body and has to be supplied through diet. It can be defined as one which is necessary for the growth and health of a growing animal and which cannot be synthesised in adequate amounts in the body and must, therefore be supplied by the protein in the diet. Classification of amino acids is given in Table 4.2.

Based on the amino acid proportion proteins are classified into complete proteins, partially complete proteins and incomplete proteins. A complete protein have a good proportion of essential amino acids to promote the normal growth rate and to maintain the body. A complete protein is also referred as high biological value protein. Usually Animal proteins like proteins in egg, milk, meat, fishes are referred as High

Table 4.2 : Nutritional Classification of Amino Acids

Essential amino acids	*Semi essential amino acids*	*Non-essential amino acids*
Histidine	Arginine	Glutamicacid
Lysine	Tyrosine	Aspartic acid
Tryptophan	Cystine	Hydroxyproline
Phenyl alanine	Glycine	Alanine
Methionine	Serine	Proline
Threonine		
Leucine		
Iroleucine		
Valine		

biological value proteins. Partially complete protein lacks sufficient amounts of some essential amino acids. There proteins can maintain life. Incomplete proteins completely lack one or more essential amino acids and cannot even maintain life.

FUNCTIONS OF PROTEIN

Protein constitute the Chief matter of our body. The function of dietary protein is 1. Replacement of endogenous loss of body proteins due to wear and tear. 2. Formation of new tissues during growth period. 3. Synthesis of enzymes, blood, hormones etc. which are proteins in nature. The blue print .for synthesis of all the body proteins lies with Nucleoproteins. The resistance of the body to the disease depends on immunoproteins, all enzymes are proteins, Actin and myosin are contractile proteins of muscle, Hormonal proteins control metabolic processes, hemoglobin, lipoproteins, Retinal binding protein etc. are proteins. Proteins yield energy equal to that of carbohydrates. Proteins give 4 k cals of energy on an average. When the body is not supplied with sufficient amounts of carbohydrate and fat for energy purposes through diet protein which is meant for tissue building is used for obtaining energy. In case if the protein supply is also not ensured through diet first fat reserves of the body are used and tissue break down follows.

DIGESTION AND ABSORPTION PROTEIN

During digestion the proteins are hydrolysed to amino acids which can be absorbed and utilized easily. Salire has no proteolytic enzymes. So, Protein digestion does not start in mouth. Chewing increases the surface area of the food. Protein hydrolysis occurs in stomach, duodenum and jejunum. Proteases and peptidases act on proteins to split them into smaller fragments. The enzymes needed for protein digestion are secreted in Zymogen form. These are activated when needed. Each enzyme is highly specific in its function that is it attacks only the type of peptide linkage. Pepsinogen secreted in stomach is activated to pepsin by Hydrochloric acid. Then pepsin acts on the peptide linkages where phenylalanine or tyrosine furnishes the amino group. Trypsinogen secreted by pancreas is activated to trypsin by enterokinase. This Trypsin splits the peptide chain where lysine or arginine provides the carboxyl group. Chymotrysinogen of pancreas is a activated to chymotrypsin by trypsin acts on peptide chains where tryptophan, methionine, tyrosine or phenylalanine furnishes the Carboxyl group. Carboxyl peptidase an pancreatic secretion splits peptide linkage next to a terminal carboxyl group. Aminopeptidase splits the peptide linkage next to a terminal aminogroup. The rate of hydrolysis is directly proportional to the rate of absorption so that excess of aminoacids may not be present in intestines.

Some foods contain enzyme inhibitors. Soyabean has trypsin inhibitor. This is inactivated by heating. So cooking of Soyabeans improves digestibility of its protein. During heating the cross linkages of proteins split thereby increasing the digestibility. On the other hand prolonged heating may create new linkages and the protein may become unavoidable for digestion.

NUTRITIVE VALUE OF PROTEINS

Knowing the aminoacid make up on the protein would help us to interpret nutritional differences. But the suitability of the particular protein to meet the protein requirements of the body can be assessed by experiments on animals or human beings. There are various methods of evaluating the quality of protein. Protein efficiency ratio (PER), Net protein ratio (NPR), Net protein utilisation (NPU), Digestibility coefficient (DC), Biological value (BV), and chemical score are some of them.

PROTEIN EFFICIENCY RATIO (PER)

Osborne, Mendel and Ferry in 1919 developed this method. This method is based on growth of young rats. A 10 per cent of test protein diet with all other dietary essentials is fed to the rats for four weeks. The Gain in body weight and protein intake of rats is recorded. Then the protein efficiency ratio is calculated using the following formula:

$$PER = \frac{\text{Gain in body weight in grams}}{\text{Protein in take in grams}} = \frac{\text{gain in weight per gram}}{\text{of protein consumed.}}$$

NET PROTEIN RATIO (NPR)

This is a modified PER method developed by Bender and Doell in 1957. In this method two groups of weaning rats, one on 10 per cent test protein diet and other on non protein diet are fed for 10 days. Then the loss in weight of control group is added to the gain in weight of test group and is divided by the quantity of protein consumed by the test group which gives the Net protein ratio.

$$NPR = \frac{\text{Gain in Weight (g) of the test group + loss in weight (g) of non protein group}}{\text{Protein in take (g)}}$$

The values of NPR correlate closely with NPU values.

DIGESTIBILITY COEFFICIENT (DC)

It is the percentage of protein available for absorption from its total intake. When animal is fed on Nitrogen free diet some amount of Nitrogen is lost from the body through feces. This is called endogenous fecal Nitrogen. When Protein food is given feces consist of endogenous Nitrogen and Nitrogen lost from digestion of protein. So to find the Nitrogen lost in digestion endogenous nitrogen should be determined. Then Digestibility coefficient is calculated using the following formula

$$\text{Digestibility Coefficient} = 100 \times \frac{\text{Nitrogen intake} - (\text{Nitrogen in feces} - \text{Endogenous fecal Nitrogen}}{\text{Nitrogen intake}}$$

If Food nitrogen intake is I_n, Total fecal Nitrogen is F_n and Endogenous fecal nitrogen is F_e

$$\text{Digestibility Coefficient} = 100 \times \frac{I_n - (F_n - F_e)}{I_n}$$

$F_n - F_e$ is food nitrogen lost in digestion.

BIOLOGICAL VALUE (BV)

This method measures the amount of dietary proteins utilised by the animal to meet the protein needs of its body. In this method two groups of 28 day old rats are fed on two different diets. One on protein free diet and other on 10 per cent test protein. Rats are kept in metabolic cages and fed for 10 days. Food intake is recorded. The urine, feces are collected and analysed for Nitrogen. The Dietary Nitrogen is also estimated. From these records the following calculations are made :

Nitrogen Digested = Nitrogen intake (I_n) — Nitrogen in feces on Protein diet (F_n) + Nitrogen in feces on Protein free diet (F_e)

i.e. Nitrogen digested = $I_n - (F_n - F_e)$

Nitrogen lost in metabolism = Nitrogen in urine (U_n) on protein diet — Nitrogen in urine (U_e) on Protein free diet

$$\text{Biological Value (BV)} = \frac{100 \times \text{Nitrogen digested} - \text{Nitrogen lost in metabolism}}{\text{Nitrogen digested}}$$

$$= \frac{I_n - (F_n - F_e) - (U_n - U_e)}{I_n - (F_n - F_e)} \times 100$$

NET PROTEIN UTILISATION (NPU)

Two groups of albino rats of 28 day old are used and fed in the same way as for Biological value. Net protein utilisation is a product of digestibility coefficient and biological divided by 100.

$$\text{NPU} = \frac{\text{Digestability Coefficient} \times \text{Biological value}}{100}$$

CHEMICAL SCORE :

Egg protein contain all essential amino acids in adequate amounts and is called a high biological value protein. The Chemical score is the ratio between the content of the most limiting amino acid in the test protein to the content of the amino acid in egg protein expressed as percentage. For example chemical score of milk proteins is 65 and that of gelatin and Maize protein Zein are O. Table 4.3 gives the amounts of essential amino acids in common foods.

Table 4.3 : Essential Amino Acids in Common Foods

Name of the foodstuff	Approx. total N g/100 gms.	Argi-nine	Histi-dine	Lysine	Trypto-phan	Phenyl-alanine	Tyro-sine	Methio-nine	Cys-tine	Threo-nine	Leu-cine	Isoleu-cine	Valine
		mg. per gm N											
(1)	(2)	(3)	(4)	(5)	(6)	(7)	(8)	(9)	(10)	(11)	(12)	(13)	(14)
CEREAL GRAINS AND PRODUCTS													
BAJRA	1.86	300	140	190	110	290	200	150	110	240	750	26	330
BARLEY	1.84	300	180	230	100	310	180	100	100	200	420	240	310
ITALLIAN MILLET	1.97	220	130	140	060	420	—	180	100	190	1040	480	430
JOWAR	1.66	240	160	150	070	300	180	100	090	210	880	270	340
MAIZE (dry)	1.78	290	160	200	040	290	240	120	100	280	720	240	300
PANIVA RAGU	2.00	290	110	190	050	310	—	160	—	150	760	410	410
RAGI	1.17	300	130	220	100	310	220	210	140	240	690	400	480
RICE paraboiled, milled	1.02	640	190	220	070	350	300	220	100	290	560	310	460
RICE, raw, milled	1.09	480	130	230	080	280	290	150	090	230	500	300	380
SAMAI	1.23	250	120	110	060	330	—	180	090	190	760	370	350
VARAGU	1.33	270	120	150	050	430	—	180	110	200	650	360	410
WHEAT, whole	1.89	290	130	170	070	280	180	090	140	180	410	220	280

(Contd.)

Table 4.3 : (Contd.)

Name of the foodstuff	Approx. total N g/100 gms.	Arginine	Histidine	Lysine	Tryptophan	Phenylalanine	Tyrosine	Methionine	Cystine	Threonine	Leucine	Isoleucine	Valine
		mg. per gm N											
(1)	(2)	(3)	(4)	(5)	(6)	(7)	(8)	(9)	(10)	(11)	(12)	(13)	(14)
WHEAT flour, refined	1.76	190	120	110	060	290	130	090	140	150	400	220	240
WHEAT, germ	4.67	460	,0	380	070	230	190	110	100	260	410	240	300
<u>PULSES AND LEGUMES</u>													
BENGAL GRAM (whole)	2.74	570	160	440	050	360	180	080	080	220	580	320	310
BLACK GRAM dhal	3.84	520	170	400	070	310	140	090	080	220	500	340	310
COW PEA	3.86	420	200	430	070	320	230	090	080	230	480	270	310
FIELD BEAN	3.98	530	180	500	030	330	—	040	080	250	550	360	310
GREEN GRAM, whole	3.84	500	170	460	060	350	100	080	060	200	510	350	320
HORSE GRAM	3.52	530	190	520	070	380	—	070	130	230	540	370	390
KHESARI DHAL	4.51	490	160	470	050	260	—	030	070	140	410	410	250
LENTIL	4.02	540	160	440	060	270	200	050	070	220	470	270	310
MOTH BEANS	3.78	—	210	340	040	280	—	060	030	—	420	310	200
PEAS	1.15	570	130	400	060	250	220	060	080	240	380	290	290
PEAS (dry)	3.15	570	130	440	060	280	170	05C	070	240	430	280	300

(Contd.)

Table 4.3 : (Contd.)

Name of the foodstuff	Approx. total N g/100 gms.	Argi-nine	Histi-dine	Lysine	Trypto-phan	Phenyl-alanine	Tyro-sine	Methio-nine	Cys-tine	Threo-nine	Leu-cine	Isoleu-cine	Valine
		mg. per gm N											
(1)	(2)	(3)	(4)	(5)	(6)	(7)	(8)	(9)	(10)	(11)	(12)	(13)	(14)
RAJMAH	3.66	370	180	460	060	340	100	060	040	270	470	300	330
REDGRAM DHAL	3.57	360	250	480	040	460	130	060	060	200	450	250	260
SOYABEAN	6.91	450	150	400	080	300	210	080	100	240	480	320	320
LEAFY VEGETABLES													
AGATHI	1.34	360	120	250	100	380	—	090	090	300	560	390	430
AMARNATH, gangeticus tender	0.64	240	130	250	070	180	190	070	040	140	370	290	280
BATHUA LEAVES	0.59	—	—	750	020	110	—	050	—	170	410	440	290
BEET GREENS	0.54	180	090	210	060	190	150	050	060	200	300	180	210
BOTTLE GOURD LEAVES	0.37	280	140	300	—	310	—	090	070	220	410	260	040
BRUSSELS SPROUTS	0.75	390	140	340	080	230	—	060	040	270	340	310	300

(Contd.)

Table 4.3 : (Contd.)

Name of the foodstuff	Approx. total N g/100 gms.	Arginine	Histidine	Lysine	Tryptophan	Phenylalanine	Tyrosine	Methionine	Cystine	Threonine	Leucine	Isoleucine	Valine
		mg. per gm N											
(1)	(2)	(3)	(4)	(5)	(6)	(7)	(8)	(9)	(10)	(11)	(12)	(13)	(14)
LEAFY VEGETABLES													
BRUSSELS SPROUTS	0.75	390	140	340	080	230	—	060	040	270	340	310	300
CABBAGE	0.29	450	130	240	070	200	120	060	070	220	340	230	260
CARROT LEAVES	0.82	270	120	280	090	410	—	110	—	280	440	280	340
CELERY LEAVES	0.13	250	090	150	080	280	—	140	—	210	430	240	300
COLOCASIA LEAVES	1.09	250	130	260	040	180	—	060	—	150	360	310	280
DRUMSTICK LEAVES	1.07	380	140	320	100	290	—	110	130	250	460	280	350
FENUGREEK LEAVES	0.70	350	110	300	080	300	—	090	—	200	390	330	320
GOGO	0.27	310	090	400	040	200	—	070	—	210	440	320	240
KNOL-KHOL GREENS	0.56	—	—	540	370	160	—	050	—	130	500	330	310
PUMPKIN LEAVES	0.74	430	100	340	080	340	310	110	060	310	630	310	360
SAFFLOWER LEAVES	0.40	—	—	610	030	160	—	060	—	170	700	540	410

(Contd.)

Table 4.3 : (Contd.)

Name of the foodstuff	Approx. total N g/100 gms.	Argi-nine	Histi-dine	Lysine	Trypto-phan	Phenyl-alanine	Tyro-sine	Methio-nine	Cys-tine	Threo-nine	Leu-cine	Isoleu-cine	Valine
		mg. per gm N											
(1)	(2)	(3)	(4)	(5)	(6)	(7)	(8)	(9)	(10)	(11)	(12)	(13)	(14)
LEAFY VEGETABLES													
SPINACH	0.32	350	140	400	400	330	310	110	080	290	530	300	350
TAMARIND LEAVES, tender	0.92	370	140	300		390	220	080	060	290	580	330	360
TURNIP GREENS	0.64	300	120	320	080	260	220	080	070	240	410	240	280
ROOTS AND TUBERS													
BEET ROOT	0.27	320	100	410	060	210	170	070	120	250	330	200	230
CARROT	0.14	250	090	230	040	210	140	070	060	210	310	230	310
COLOCASIA	0.48	470	110	300	110	320	230	080	160	280	510	270	380
ONION	0.19	170	070	290	090	180	—	070	—	090	170	090	140
POTATO	0.26	330	100	320	100	270	170	090	050	220	380	270	310
RADISH	0.11	700	160	270	020	270	—	050	—	230	420	300	390
SWEET POTATO	0.19	280	090	260	110	270	150	100	030	280	360	290	380
TAPIOCA	0.12	580	110	290	080	180	100	050	090	200	300	250	240
TURNIP	0.08	250	070	230	080	180	—	050	010	210	340	220	230
YAM (ordinary)	0.22	480	120	280	070	300	200	100	—	220	400	230	290

(Contd.)

Table 4.3 : (Contd.)

Name of the foodstuff	Approx. total N g/100 gms.	Arginine	Histidine	Lysine	Tryptophan	Phenylalanine	Tyrosine	Methionine	Cystine	Threonine	Leucine	Isoleucine	Valine
		mg. per gm N											
(1)	(2)	(3)	(4)	(5)	(6)	(7)	(8)	(9)	(10)	(11)	(12)	(13)	(14)
OTHER VEGETABLES													
ASH GOURD	0.06	190	040	070	030	160	—	060	—	190	380	350	310
BITTER GOURD	0.26	270	080	210	040	240	—	150	—	250	420	370	370
BOTTLE GOURD	0.03	100	040	350	030	140	—	030	—	170	350	320	230
BRINJAL	0.22	210	130	330	060	250	240	070	030	230	380	270	320
CAULIFLOWER	0.42	290	120	360	090	230	—	100	—	260	440	300	350
CUCUMBER	0.06	470	090	270	050	140	—	060	—	160	260	190	210
FRENCH BEANS	0.27	280	150	360	090	260	210	080	060	250	430	280	340
JACK, tender	0.42	120	060	300	080	480	—	090	090	360	500	450	550
JACK FRUIT seed	1.06	—	—	360	070	260	—	050	060	270	330	300	410
LADIES FINGERS	0.30	230	110	210	040	140	270	080	060	140	240	150	190
PLANTAIN, green	0.22	260	280	350	040	280	—	040	—	170	340	320	280
PUMPKIN	0.2	230	100	270	070	210	—	050	—	170	330	230	300
TOMATO, green	0.30	190	050	160	020	150	—	050	—	190	210	420	270

(Contd.)

Table 4.3 : (Contd.)

Name of the foodstuff	Approx. total N g/100 gms.	Arginine	Histidine	Lysine	Tryptophan	Phenylalanine	Tyrosine	Methionine	Cystine	Threonine	Leucine	Isoleucine	Valine
		mg. per gm N											
(1)	(2)	(3)	(4)	(5)	(6)	(7)	(8)	(9)	(10)	(11)	(12)	(13)	(14)
NUTS AND OILSEEDS													
ALMOND	3.33	660	140	160	050	300	180	100	050	170	450	250	310
CASHEW NUT	3.39	650	130	290	110	270	—	090	—	200	510	320	360
COCONUT, dry	1.09	850	130	240	070	280	170	100	080	180	430	240	320
GINGELLY SEEDS	2.93	750	170	170	080	370	230	180	120	230	500	250	290
GROUND NUT	4.05	690	140	230	060	310	240	060	080	170	400	240	280
LINSEED	3.25	560	120	230	100	270	180	100	120	210	360	310	320
NIGER SEED	3.82	660	140	230	—	300	—	090	100	210	380	250	320
PISTACHIO NUT	3.17	590	140	320	060	320	190	080	110	200	550	300	370
PIYAL SEEDS	3.04	1230	170	240	070	330	—	100	—	200	740	350	410
SUNFLOWER SEEDS	3.17	500	150	230	090	280	120	120	090	230	400	270	320
WALNUT	2.50	770	120	100	060	260	—	080	—	170	470	240	280
FRUITS													
APPLE	0.03	170	120	370	060	160	090	050	080	230	390	220	250
APRICOT	0.16	080	100	180	—	100	080	030	—	130	180	110	150

(Contd.)

Table 4.3 : (Contd.)

Name of the foodstuff	Approx. total N g/100 gms.	Argi-nine	Histi-dine	Lysine	Trypto-phan	Phenyl-alanine	Tyro-sine	Methio-nine	Cys-tine	Threo-nine	Leu-cine	Isoleu-cine	Valine
		mg. per gm N											
(1)	(2)	(3)	(4)	(5)	(6)	(7)	(8)	(9)	(10)	(11)	(12)	(13)	(14)
FRUITS													
AVOCADO PEAR	0.27	210	110	310	060	220	140	090	—	180	340	210	290
BANANA	0.19	360	370	270	070	260	160	080	170	190	320	250	260
DATES	0.40	150	050	190	—	170	050	050	120	180	260	150	220
FIGS	0.21	140	090	250	050	150	270	050	100	200	270	190	240
GRAPES	0.08	460	230	140	030	130	110	210	100	170	130	050	170
GUAVA COUNTRY	0.14	—	—	190	060	—	—	060	—	—	—	—	—
MANGO RIPE	0.10	—	—	830	130	—	—	070	—	—	—	—	—
PAPAYA	0.10	—	—	400	130	—	—	030	—	—	—	—	—
PEACHES	0.19	130	130	230	030	140	160	240	070	210	220	100	310
STRAW BERRY	0.11	270	120	250	070	180	210	010	050	190	320	140	180
OTHER FLESH FOODS													
BEEF	3.60	410	200	540	070	260	220	160	080	280	510	320	330
EGG, hen	2.13	400	150	440	090	360	250	210	140	320	520	410	450
FOWL	4.14	350	160	500	060	250	210	160	080	250	460	330	320
MUTTON	2.96	430	170	510	080	250	210	150	080	290	480	310	320
PORK	2.99	410	190	570	090	280	230	180	080	310	520	340	360

(Contd.)

Table 4.3 : (Contd.)

Name of the foodstuff	Approx. total N g/100 gms.	Arginine	Histidine	Lysine	Tryptophan	Phenylalanine	Tyrosine	Methionine	Cystine	Threonine	Leucine	Isoleucine	Valine
		mg. per gm N											
(1)	(2)	(3)	(4)	(5)	(6)	(7)	(8)	(9)	(10)	(11)	(12)	(13)	(14)
MILK AND MILK PRODUCTS													
MILK, buffalo's	0.69	200	130	490	090	270	—	170	090	300	640	330	380
MILK, cow's	0.51	220	170	500	090	320	300	160	050	280	600	340	400
MILK, goat's	0.53	210	180	470	080	240	200	110	—	350	560	250	340
MILK, human	0.18	250	170	420	110	230	230	100	110	290	520	330	310
CURD	0.50	200	160	480	080	330	370	170	060	310	680	320	470
CHEESE	3.86	240	200	520	080	350	340	180	040	260	640	360	480
WHOLE MILK POWDER	4.13	220	180	490	090	310	300	170	050	280	630	360	420
YEAST, dried (Brewers)	6.32	310	160	570	—	300	200	100	060	350	500	370	460

METABOLISM

Metabolism of proteins is metabolism of amino acids. The non-essential amino acids synthesised in the liver are also released into circulation. All amino acids reach the amino acid pool in the body. The synthesis and breakdown of tissue proteins takes place constantly. The liver rapidly removes the amino acids from circulation and synthesises numerous proteins and non nitrogenous substances like creatine. The loss and gain of proteins in the body are equal and is known as dynamic equilibrium. The amino acid pool includes dietary source and tissue breakdown. Fig. 4.3 gives different aspects of Protein Metabolism.

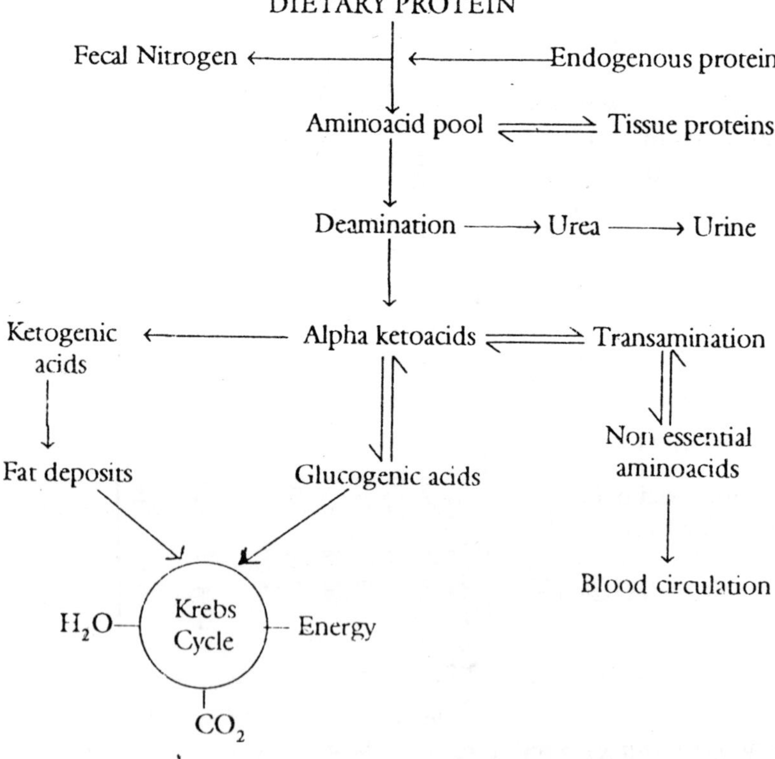

Fig. 4.3 : Protein Metabolism

DEAMINATION

Deamination occurs in liver and kidney. Due to the action of oxidative enzymes amino acids give keto acid and Ammonia.

$$\underset{\text{Amino acid}}{R{-}\overset{\overset{\displaystyle NH_2}{|}}{CH}{-}COOH} + \tfrac{1}{2}O_2 \longrightarrow \underset{\text{Keto acid}}{R\,COCOOH} + \underset{\text{Ammonia}}{NH_3}$$

The Keto acids are completely oxidised to yield energy, carbondioxide and water. Some amino acids are Glucogenic i.e. they can be synthesised to Glucose after deamination and some are ketogenic i.e. they can be synthesised to fat. Most of the ammonia obtained from deamination is synthesised to urea. Some of the ammonia is used in the formation of creatine and other non-protein mitrogenous substances. About 10 to 18 grams of Ammonia is produced in a adult human being with about 60 to 100 grams of Amino acids. Ammonia is toxic so it is converted to urea, Aspertic acid, glutamic acid, glutamine etc. Glutamic acid, glutamine, non essential amino acids, carbonyl phosphate and urea form by fixing ammonia.

TRANSAMINATION

It is a process of transfer of amino group from one amino acid to keto acid from other amino acid. Liver has transaminases which act as catalysts in transamination.

$$\text{Glutamic acid} + \text{keto acid} \xrightarrow{\text{Transaminase}} \alpha\,\text{ketoglutaric acid} + \text{Amino acid}$$

Glutamate oxalo acetale transminase (GOT) and Glutamate pyruvate transaminase (GPT) are present abundantly.

$$\text{Glutamic acid} + \text{Oxaloacetic acid} \xrightarrow{\text{Transaminase}} \alpha\text{ keto glutaric acid} + \text{Aspartic acid}$$

$$\text{Glutamic acid} + \text{Pyruvic acid} \xrightarrow{\text{Transaminase}} \alpha\text{ keto glutaric acid} + \text{Alanine}$$

DISPOSAL OF AMMONIA

9 to 18 grams of ammonia is produced in adult human when the oxidation of amino acid is about 50 to 100g. Normal range of ammonia in normal adult blood is 40 to 70 mg per 100 ml. Ammonia is toxic to

tissues so it is rapidly converted into other compounds. The compounds formed by fixing ammonia are

1. Formation of glutamic acid from keto glutaric acid.
2. Formation of glutamine;
3. Formation of non-essential amino acids,
4. Formation of carbamyl phosphate, and
5. Formation of urea.

UREA SYNTHESIS

One nitrogen atom of carbamyl phosphate and one from amino group of aspartic acid are used in urea formation. Here aspartic acid donates its amino group without undergoing deamination. Liver is the main place of urea synthesis. 70 per cent of ammonia formed in the body is converted into urea and is excreted out. Figure 4.4 shows the synthesis of urea.

1) $NH_3 + CO_2 + ATP + H_2O \longrightarrow$ Carbamyl phosphate (Ornithine)

2) Ornithine + Carbamyl phosphate $\longrightarrow$ Citrulline

3) Citrulline + Aspartic acid $\longrightarrow$ argino succinic acid

4) Argino succinic acid $\xrightarrow{\text{argino succinase}}$ Arginine + Fumaric acid

5) Arginine + $H_2O \xrightarrow{\text{arginase}}$ Ornithine + urea

Fig. 4.4 : Steps involved in urea synthesis.

The fumaric acid formed in step 4 can be converted to malic acid and from that to oxaloacetate in the citric acid cycle. The oxaloacetate on animation forms aspartic acid again. In the final step of urea synthesis the enzyme arginase hydrolyzes arginine to form urea and ornithine. Ornithine formed in this step reenters into step 2. This cycle is also called Krebs — Henseleitt urea cycle. Which is shown in Fig. 4.5. Normal blood urea level is 15 to 40 mg/100 ml. The urea formed is excreted by kidney. The urea clearance value is about 75ml/min when urine formation is 2.0 ml./min. or more. When urine formation rate is less than 2.0ml/min urea clearance falls to about 55ml/min which is called standard clearance.

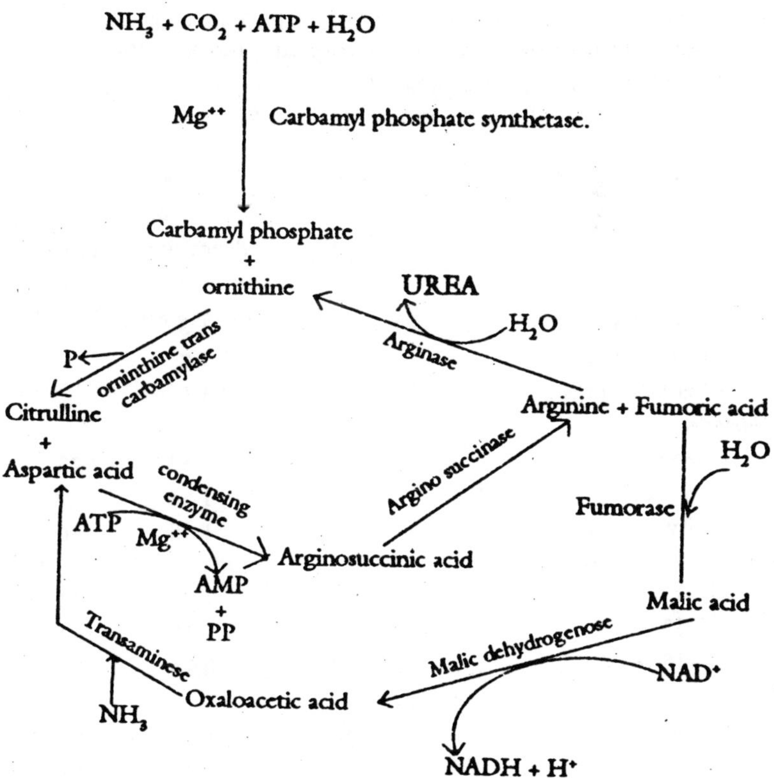

Fig. 4.5 : Synthesis of Urea
(Krebs-Henseleitt Urea Cycle)

RECOMMENDED ALLOWANCES OF PROTEINS

Table 4.4 gives the recommended daily allowance of proteins for Indians in different age groups.

PROTEIN CALORIE MALNUTRITION

This term includes kurashiorkar and marasmus which are widely prevalent in underdeveloped and developing countries. Kwashiorkar occurs in children shortly after weaning, usually between the ages 1 and 4. The following are the signs and symptoms of kwashiorkar.

Table 4.4 : Recommended Daily Allowance of Proteins for Indians

Age Group	*Body Weight* (Kg)	*Protein Allowance* g/kg/day	g/day
Infants			
Birth to 3 months		1.3	
4 to 9 months		1.8	
10 to 12 months		1.5	
Children			
1—3 years	12	1.83	22
4—6 years	19	1.56	29
7—9 years	26	1.35	36
Males			
10—12 years	34	1.24	43
13—15 years	47	1.10	52
16—18 years	57	0.94	53
Females			
10—12 years	37	1.17	43
13—15 years	46	0.95	43
16—18 years	50	0.88	44
Adults			
Man	55	1.00	55
Woman	45	1.00	45
Pregnancy			
4—9 months			+14
Lactation			
Parturition to 6 months			+25
7 to 12 months			+15

Anemia

Anemia is invariably present in children suffering with kwashiorkar. Anemia is due to deficiencies of iron and folic acid. The condition may be aggravated if parasitic infections are present.

Edema

Edema occurs first in the feet, lower legs and then thighs, hands and face. Edema is due to the lowered serum albumin levels, high sodium and low potassium levels in the blood.

Gastrointestinal Tract

Loss of appetite and vomiting are common and diarrhoea is present in most cases.

Growth Failure

Length of the body would be less than normal body weight inspite of edema will be low. These symptoms are because of protein deficiency.

Liver

Slightly enlarged and fatty infiltration is common.

Mental Changes

In severe cases children will be listless and so no interest on the happenings around.

Moon face

The face becomes round which is called moon face.

Muscle Wasting

Muscle wasting is a constant symptom and is more evident on fore arm inspite of edema.

Skin and Hair Changes

Buttocks, back of thighs and axile show trazy pavement dermatosis. Hair becomes rough, thin and crinky.

Serum Albumin

The normal serum albumin content is 3.5 to 4g/100ml. In kwashiorkar the serum albumin level goes low ranging from 0.7 to 2.4g/100ml. This is a reliable index of the extent of disease and rate of recovery

The treatment of kwashiorkar is to provide easily digestible diet rich in proteins, calories, vitamins, minerals, etc. Fat is introduced usually in the 2nd week of the treatment. The diet usually consists of skimmed milk powder, cereals, sugar, and ripe banana. Cooked vegetables are also given. The calorie intake should range from 125 to 150 k cals/kg. body weight. This can be achieved by adding sugar to the diet. Good quality protein should be provided for which skimmed milk powder is used usually. 3 to 5g/kg. body weight provides marked recovery. Anemia can be cured by administering iron and folic acid supplements. Potassium chloride and magnesium chloride should be added to the diet daily in the amounts of 3.5g and 0.75g respectively. Vitamin A deficiency is common which can be cured by giving a oral dose of 50,000 IU.

Maramus occurs due to diets deficient in both proteins and calories. It is seen in weaned infants of about 1 year age. Growth retardation and wasting of muscles is seen in marasmus. The arms are thin and skin is loose. Loss of weight is more marked than height. Subcutaneous fat is practically absent. The skin is dry and dehydration is present. Anemia may be present serum albumin is slightly low. The treatment is similar to kwashiorkar.

5

Fat Soluble Vitamins

Funk in 1912 proposed the name vitamine for the unknown substances of foods that are essential for growth of animals. The studies on these substances were known from sixteenth century itself but no specific name was given to these factors. Jacques Cartier in 1535 observed that scurvy could be cured by administering a decoction of pine needles. In 1564 Rousseus reported citrus fruits cured scurvy in dutch seamen and James Lancaster in 1591 observed that lemons cure scurvy. Rickets is a known disease with unknown reason in 1650. But cod-liver oil was known to be curative. It is only in 1918 Mellanby was able to produce rickets experimentally in dogs and cured by administering cod-liver oil. In 1919 Huldschinsky cured rickets in children by exposing them to ultraviolet light. In 1922 Mcollum showed that the rickets curative agent in cod-liver oil was different from vitamin A. Steenbock and Hess in 1924 independently showed that the foods exposed to ultraviolet light have antirachitic property. It is only in 1931 Angus was able to crystalise vitamin D_2 that is calciferol. It took another five years for Windaus to isolate vitamin D_3. Dumas in 1871 observed that the health is not maintained in people who were given purified mineral, water, carbohydrate, protein and fat food. Lunin also reported the same in 1880. Addition of Milk in these peoples diet restored them to normal. Eijkman observed that people who take polished rice in their diet suffered from Beriberi and addition of rice polishings cured their health.

Grijns in 1901 tried to isolate the beriberi causative factor from rice polishings but couldn't do it. These protective substances were called as accessory factors by Hopkins in 1911. Funk in the same year isolated a crystalline substance from rice polishings which can cure or prevent polyneuritis. It was chemically an amine and was vital for life so he called it "vitamine". Further developments in chemistry of vitamins showed that only few are amines so 'e' from the word 'vitamine' is dropped and is called only 'vitamin'.

DEFINITION

Vitamins are a group of potent organic compounds other than Carbohydrate, protein and fat, but are necessary in minute amounts and are necessary for maintenance, growth and reproduction. These cannot be synthesized by the organism.

The vitamins are broadly divided into two groups fat soluble and water soluble. Within the classes the vitamins differ widely in their properties, functions and distribution. About 15 vitamins are isolated in pure state from natural foods.

(a) Fat soluble vitamins

1. Vitamin A
2. Vitamin D
3. Vitamin E
4. Vitamin K

(b) Water soluble vitamins

I Vitamin B Complex

1. Vitamin B_1 or thiamin
2. Riboflavin
3. Niacin and Niacinamide
4. Pyridoxine or vitamin B_6
5. Pantothenic acid
6. Folic acid
7. Biotin
8. Choline
9. Para amino Benzoic acid

10. Inositol
11. Vitamin B_{12} or Cobalamine
12. Lipoic acid.

II Vitamin c or ascorbic acid

III Vitamin P or Bioflavanoids

IV Carbitine and taurine.

FAT SOLUBLE VITAMINS

VITAMIN A

HISTORY

Vitamin A occurs only in foods of animal origin. Mc collum is credited with the discovery of this vitamin. He along with Davis of Wisconsin university and Osborne and Mendel of Yale university in 1913 independently discovered the fat soluble factor in butter was essential for growth of rats on synthetic diets. Steenbock in 1919 discovered the vitamin A activity of carotenoids. These carotenoids are found in plants. These carotenoids and carotenes are converted to vitamin A in the body. So, these are referred as precursors of vitamin A or Pro vitamin A. In 1930 Moore found that when carotene is fed to vitamin A deficient rats vitamin A was found in the liver. Karrer in 1931 determined the structure of Vitamin A. Kuhn and Morris synthesised vitamin A in 1937. Holmes and corbet in the same year obtained the crystalline form of vitamin A.

SOURCES

The ultimate source of all vitamin A is carotene. It is synthesized by plants. These carotenoids are dark red crystalline compounds that give deep yellow colouration to plants. Deep green plants are also rich in carotenoids but the colour is masked with chlorophyll. Fish, Animals as well as humans consume plant carotene which is converted to vitamin A and is stored in Liver. Carnivorus animals derive the preformed vitamin A from the livers of their victims. Carotene or vitamin A content of various foods is given in Table 5.1.

CHEMISTRY:

The general term 'vitamin A' includes all compounds which have vitamin A activity. The nomenclature is as follows.

Table 5.1 : Carotene or Vitamin A Content of Some Foods

Food Stuff	*Carotene* Mg	*Food Stuff*	*Carotene* Mg
CEREALS		**NUTS AND OIL SEEDS**	
Bajra	132	Cashew nut	60
Maize dry	90	Gingelly seeds	60
Wheat Whole	64	Mustard seeds	162
PULSES		Pistachionut	144
Bengal gram whole	189	**CONDIMENTS AND SPICES**	
Bengal gram dal	129	Chillies Dry	345
Green gram Whole	94	Chillies green	175
Lentils	270	Cloves	253
Red gram dal	132	Coriander	942
LEAFY VEGETABLES		Cumin seeds	522
Agathi	5,400	Mace	3027
Amaranthus tender	5,520	Pepper	1080
Beet greens	5,862	Tamarind pulp	60
Celery leaves	3,990	**FRUITS**	
Curry leaves	7,560	Apricots fresh	2160
Drumstick leaves	6,780	Banana ripe	78
Gogu	2,898	Figs	162
Mint	1,620	Jack fruit	175
Radish leaves	5,295	Mango ripe	2743
Spinach	5,580	Musk melon	169
ROOTS AND TUBERS		Orange	1104
Carrot	1,890	Papaya ripe	666
Potato	24	Plum	166
Yam	260	Raspberry	1248
OTHER VEGETABLES		Tomato ripe	351
Bittergourd	126	**MILK AND MILK PRODUCTS**	
Cluster beans	198	Milk, buffalos	160
Drumstick	110	Milk, cows	174
Kovai	156	Curd, Cows milk	102
Onion stolks	595	Chane, Cows milk	366
MEAT AND POULTRY		Cheese	273
Beef muscle	18 Mg Vit. A	Whole Milk Powder	1400
Egg, duck	540 Mg Carotene 360 Mg Vit. A	**FATS**	
Egg, hen	600 Mg Carotene 360 Mg Vit. A	Butter	3200
Liver Sheep	6690 Mg Vit. A	Ghee (Cow)	2000
Mutton	9 Mg. Vit. A	Ghee (buffalo)	900
		Hydrogenated oil	2500

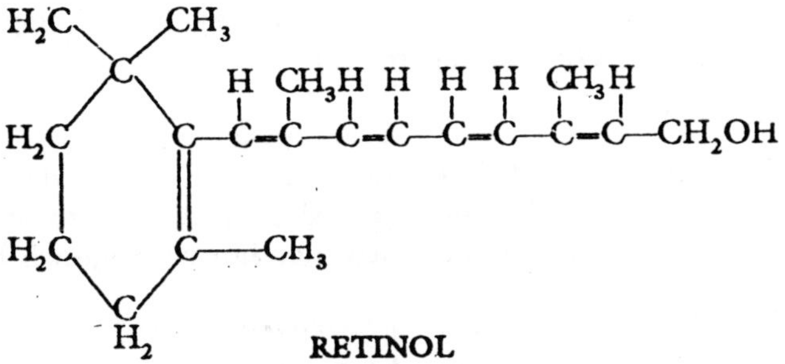

RETINOL

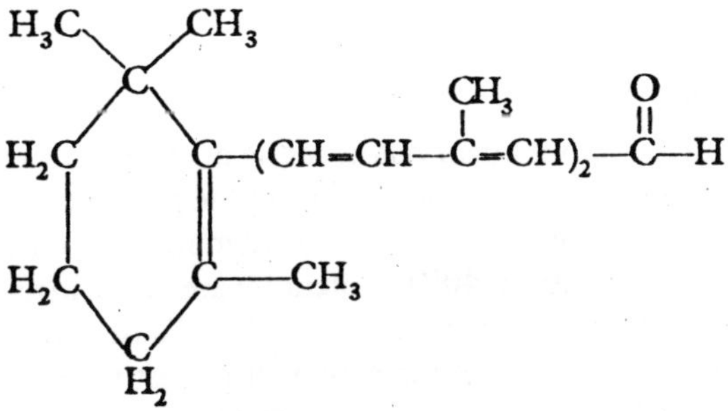

RETINOL DEHYDE

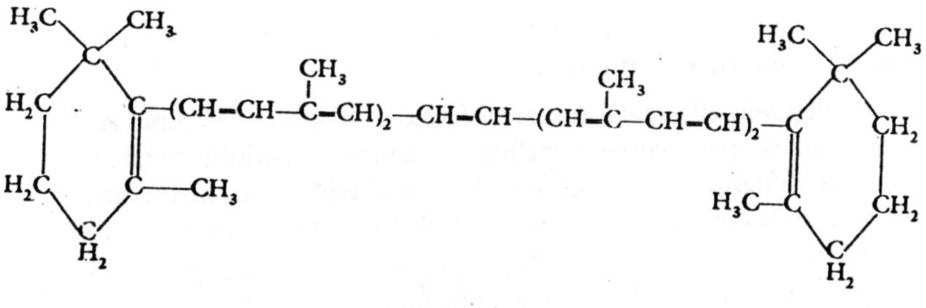

β-CAROTENE

Fig. 5.1 : Various Forms of Vitamin A

Retionol

Vitamin A has a characteristic ring structure called the β ionone ring attached to a long hydrocarbon chain ending in an alcohol group and is chemically known as Retinol. This vitamin A alcohol is found in

Mammals and is abundant in liver oils of salt water fish. Its emphirical formula is C_{20} H_{29} OH. (see Figure 5.1)

Retinaldehyde

This is the aldehyde form of vitamin A. This is combined with the protein opsin in the retina and forms Rhodopsin, a photo sensitive pigment. Retinaldehyde has the structure as shown in Figure 5.1

Retinoic Acid

This is active form of vitamin A (retinol) which has local therapeutic action. It cannot be converted to retionol and cannot take part in visual cycle.

Carotene

Vegetable foods contain yellow pigments called carotenoids some of which are converted to vitamin A during the process of absorption in small intestine. Carotene is precursor of vitamin A in our body so it is called provitamin A. About 400 Carotenoids are found in nature. Alpha, beta, and gama isomers of carotene are widely distributed in foods and gives vitamin A effectively. β carotene is the most plentiful in human foods and resembles two retinol molecules joined together (See figure). It has a empirical formula C_{40} H_{56} and gives two molecules of vitamin A on hydrolysis.

$$C_{40}H_{56} + 2H_2O \longrightarrow 2C_{20}H_{29}OH$$

Alpha and gama carotenes possess only one β ionone rings and can give rise to only one vitamin A molecule.

Collectively all these forms are referred as vitamin A. Vitamin A in its pure form is a pale yellow crystalline substance. It is soluble in fat and fat solvents. Vitamin A is unstable to light and acid. It can be oxidized rapidly. It is relatively stable to heat and alkali. Ordinary cooking does not destroy vitamin A. But over cooking, exposure to high temperatures in presence of Air and ultraviolet radiations rapidly destroys this vitamin.

MEASUREMENT OF VITAMIN A

Vitamin A is measure din International units. One International unit of vitamin A is 0.3 micrograms of Retinol.

1 micro gram - 1 millionth of a gram
- 10–6 of a gram
- 1 thousandth of a milligram

1 IU	=	0.3 µg Retinol
1 IU	=	0.6 g Beta Carotene
1 IU	=	1.2 g carotenoids.

In 1967 FAO/WHO proposed that Vitamin A value of foods be stated as equivalent weight of Retinol.

1 Retinol equivalent	=	1 microgram Retinol
	=	6 microgram carotene
	=	12 microgram carotenoids
	=	3.33 IU Retinol
	=	10 IU β-Carotene and other carotenoids

METABOLISM AND FUNCTIONS

Preformed vitamin A in food is hydrolysed to retionol by pancreatic and intestinal enzymes. Vitamin A is absorbed along with fat in small intestine. The absorption is poor in case of diarrhoea and oral administration of paraffin. Water miscible forms of vitamin A are absorbed independently of fat absorption. After absorption retinol is esterified and incorporated to chylomicrons for transport through lymph and reaches the liver for storage. Carotenes are first reduced to retinaldehyde and then to retinol in the intestinal mucosa. Absorption of Vitamin A is facilitated by bile. Diet very low in fat and obstruction of bile duct impairs vitamin A absorption.

Hydrolysis and re-esterification of retinyl esters occur in liver and stored in association with lipid droplets. From this store retinol is released bound to a specific transport protein present in plasma called retinol binding Protein (RBP). A halo retinol binding protein. RBP is synthesised in liver and probably Zinc accelerates its synthesis.

PLASMA VITAMIN A

The Plasma values fluctuate markedly depending on season and diet. In healthy persons plasma vitamin A is 50 - 90 micro grams per 100 ml. In deficiency state vitamin A in plasma levels falls below 25 micrograms per 100 ml.

STORAGE

Vitamin A in liver is stored in the form of retinyl esters. A healthy well nourished person has 60-100 micrograms of retinol per every gram of liver. ie about 120,000 micrograms of retinol. This amounts to 90 percent of body's store othe r10 percent is stored in kidney, lungs, adrenal glands and adipose tissue. There reserves are sufficient for several months.

FUNCTIONS

On the Retina

The retina contains two kinds of light receptors, rods for vision in dim light and cones for vision in bright light and for colour vision. Rods produce a photosensitive pigment Rhodopsin or visual purple and cones produce Iodopsin or visual violet. In both these pigments the proteins are different but the retinal dehyde is the prosthetic group. When light strikes the pigments they are split into the respective proteins and retinaldehyde. Regeneration of rhodopsin occurs in dark. During this cycle some retinaldehyde is last. So, there must be a continuous supply of vitamin A from blood. The visual cycle and the role of vitamin A is shown in Figure 5.2.

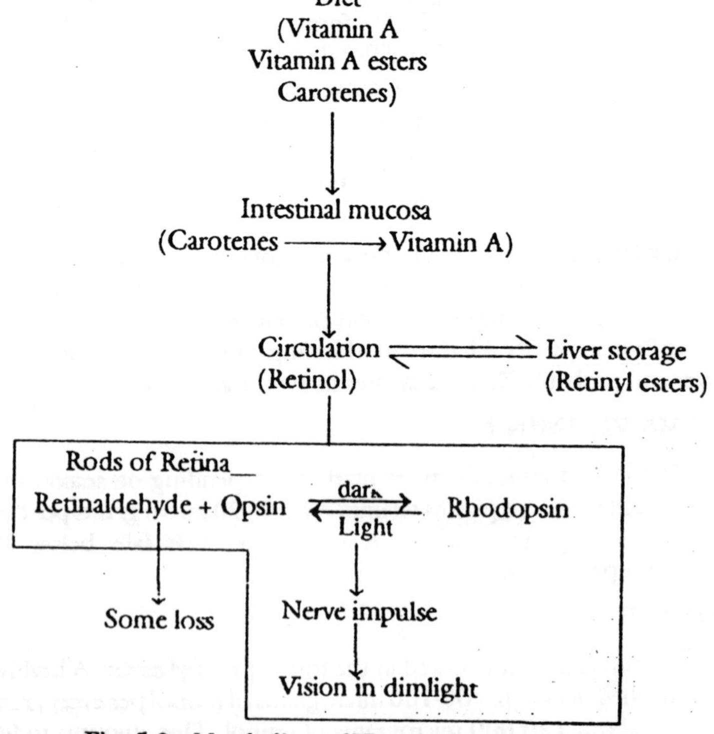

Fig. 5.2 : Metabolism of Vitamin A in Visual Cycle

Epithelial Tissues

Vitamin A is required for a healthy epithelium whether it is covering the body extremely or lining internally. Vitamin A is essential for the integrity of the mucous secreting cells of epithelial tissue. This effects the synthesis of mucoproteins and mucopolysaccharides. These secretions maintains the integrity of epithelium especially of eyes, mouth, gastrointestinal tract and urino genital tract. These membranes protect against bacterial infection. Vitamin A is therefore credited with anti-infective action.

Bone

Vitamin A is concerned with osteoblastic activity and takes part in the formation of bony matrix.

DAILY ALLOWANCES

Vitamin A requirements can be expressed as

1. Total vitamin A requirements
2. Total β - carotene requirements or
3. Combined requirements of vitamin A derived from animal foods and vegetable foods.

In the last case it is assumed that one half of vitamin A is retinol and one half is β-carotene. The vitamin a requirements are given in Table 5.2

Table 5.2 : Recommended Dietary Allowance of Vitamin A

Group		*Vitamin A*	
		Retinol (mg)	β-Carotene (mg)
Man		600	2,400
Woman	Normal	600	2,400
	Pregnancy	600	2,400
	Lactation	950	3,800
Infants	0—6 months	400	1,200
	6—12 months	350	1,200
Children	1—3 years	400	1,600
	4—6 years	400	1,600
	7—9 years	600	2,400
Boys and Girls	10—12 years	600	2,400
	13—15 years	600	2,400
	16—18 years	600	2,400

ASSAY METHODS

Biological assay methods are based on the growth of rats fed on vitamin A deficient diets or cure of vitamin A deficiency in rats. It can also be done by measuring the blue colour developed in chloroform solution with antimony chloride at 620 mu in a colorimeter.

DEFICIENCY

Vitamin A deficiency occur when the intake is poor, malabsorption, habitual intake of paraffin, low fat diet, steatorrhoea, biliary obstruction, cirrhosis and damage of liver. Low protein diets reduces the synthesis of retinol binding protein and aggravates the problem.

The important deficiency states due to lack of vitamin A are :

(i) Night blindness

(ii) Xerosis of conjunctiva

(iii) Xerosis of cornea

(iv) Bitot spots

(v) Keratomalacia

(vi) Follicular hyperkeratosis.

i) Night Blindness

This is also called Nyctalopia. In this condition the individual would be unable to see in dim light, especially on coming into darkness from a bright light. In dimlight rhodopsin in the rods is converted to chemical energy. With vitamin A deficiency rhodopsin is not formed so the person cannot see in dimlight. In early stages difficulty in reading or identifying objects in dimlight is experienced. In advanced stages one cannot see in dimlight.

ii) Xerosis of Conjunctival or Conjunctival Xerosis

Xeros means dry. In this condition the conjunctiva becomes dry and lusterless. The glistening transparent appearance is lost. Due to keratinisation of epithelial cells the conjunctiva becomes thickened, wrinkled and pigmented. Due to pigmentation conjunctiva appears to be smoky.

iii) Xerosis of Cornea or Corneal Xerosis

When the dryness spreads to cornea it becomes dull, hazy and lusterless. Cornea becomes insensitive to touch. This is due to the keratinisation of corneal epithelium.

iv) Bitot Spot's

Glistening white or greyish plagues of desquamated thickened conjunctival epithelium usually triangular in shape firmly adherent to conjunctive are described as bitotspots. These are localized elevated areas frequently bilateral on the temporal side of the conjunctiva.

v) Keratomalacta

When conjunctival xerosis and corneal xerosis are not treated it may develop into a condition known as keratomalacia. Cornea becomes dull and vascularization takes place at the periphery. Necrosis leading to ulceration and bacterial invasions bring about destruction of cornea and vision is lost.

vi) Follicular Hyperkeratosis

The skin becomes dry and scaley. A rough sensation is felt when the ski is touched. Skin becomes dry and papules of varying sizes arise. This condition is also called phrynoderma. This condition can be cured by administering essential fatty acids and B complex vitamins.

CHANGES IN MUCUS MEMBRANES

Mucus membranes respiratory tract become rough and dry which results in stasis and bacterial infection. Mucus membrane of alimentary canal becomes thick and dry which results in diminished digestive juice secretion which ultimately causes impaired absorption, liability to infections and diarrhoea. Vaginitis, urinary tract infection and stone formation results a change in mucus membranes of urino genital tract.

TREATMENT

Adequate protein intake aids in formation of retinol binding protein. A balanced diet containing milk, vegetables, and fruits supply adequate amount of vitamin A.

Prophylactic measures to combat vitamin A deficiency include

1. A tea spoon full of cod-liver oil daily
2. Feeding children with atleast 30gms of green vegetables daily
3. Addition of 4ml of Red palm oil for school children diet daily

4. In severe cases children should be given 1,00,000 IU vitamin A every 6 months, etc.

But prophylaxis is not periodic administration of vitamin A the people should be educated about the importance of vitamin A consum ing spinach - a cheaply available food, sprouted cereals and pulses, etc., should be encouraged.

HYPERVITAMINOSIS

Hypervitaminosis is observed with massive intake A. Liver of polar bear has 13,000 - 18,000 IU/gm consumption of this liver or consumption of 100-150ml of halibut liver oil produces hypervitaminosis. Whose symptoms are irritability, drowsiness, headache and vomiting. Loss of appetite, weight loss, cracking of lips, dry skin, itching and hair loss follows. Later enlargement of liver, spleen, subcutaneous swelling, pain in joints and bones, high serum calcium and tenderness in long bones is observed. When the excessive intakes are stopped these symptoms disappear gradually.

VITAMIN D

HISTORY

Cod liver oil was recommended to cure rickets by Mellanby in 1919. Mc. Collun and coworkers in 1922 established that the antirachitic vitamin was different from vitamin A. They reported that cod-liver oil in which vitamin A was destroyed still retained anti rachitic property. In 1924 Hess and Steencock independently found that foods exposed to ultra violet light have antirachitic property. Subsequently in 1930 Angus, Reerick, Van Wijk, Windaus and other isolated vitamin D in crystalline form.

SOURCES

1. **Food** : The natural sources of vitamin D are egg yolk, milk and butter. It is assumed that animal foods contain vitamin D. A vegetarian diet is devoid of this vitamin unless milk is added to it. The vitamin D content of foods depend on the exposure of fowls and milch animals to sunlight. Vitamin D is found plentiful in liver.
2. **Sunlight** : Exposure of skin to sunlight brings about systhesis of Vitamin D from 7 -dehydrocholesterol.

Liver oils form a best source of vitamin D of therapeutic purposes.

CHEMISTRY

There are many substances which possess antirachitic property. Of those only vitamin D_2 and D_3 are important. Vitamin D_2 is also called Ergocalciferol or calciferol or viosterol and vitamin D_3 is called cholecalciferol. Vitamin D_2 and D_3 are formed from the provitamins ergosterol of plants and 7- dehydrocholesterol found in skin. Structurally ergosterol and 7- dehydrocholesterol have similar nucleus but dissimilar side chains. The conversion of ergosterol and 7 dehydrocholesterol to vitamin D_2 and D_3 results in opening of ring B which results in one more unsaturated linkage. The structural forms of ergo sterol, calciferol, 7-dehydrocholesterol and cholecalciferol are given in the Figure 5.3. Pure vitamin D is white odorless crystalline substance which is stable to heat, alkali, and oxidation. It is insoluble in water but is soluble in fat and fat solvents.

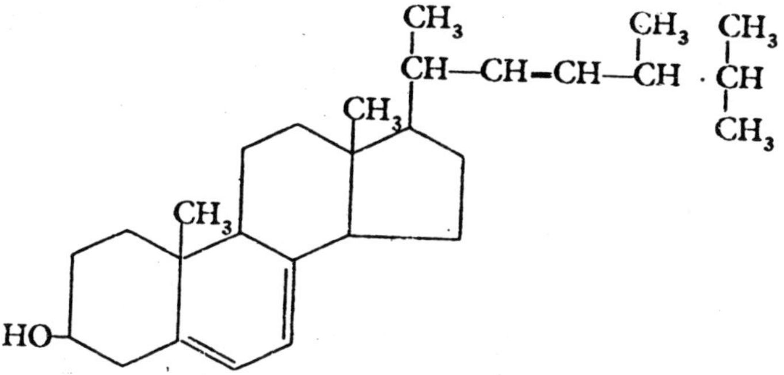

CH_3 CH_3 CH_3

CH—CH=CH—CH · CH

CH_3 CH_3 CH_3

HO

ERGO STEROL

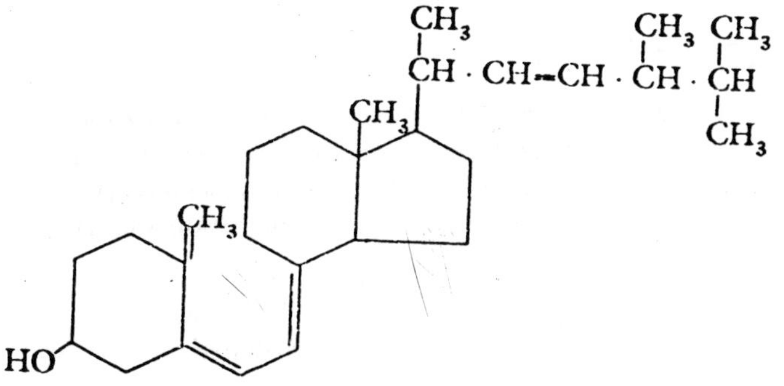

CH_3 CH_3 CH_3

CH · CH=CH · CH · CH

CH_3 CH_3 CH_3

HO

CALCIFEROL

(Contd.)

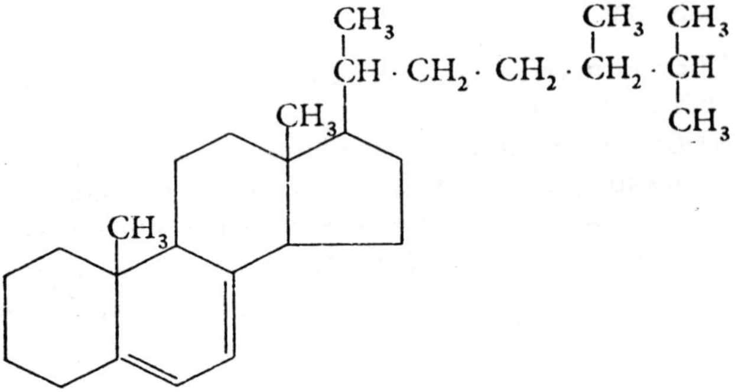

CH$_3$ CH$_3$ CH$_3$
CH · CH$_2$ · CH$_2$ · CH$_2$ · CH
CH$_3$ CH$_3$
CH$_3$

7- DEHYDRO CHOLESTEROL

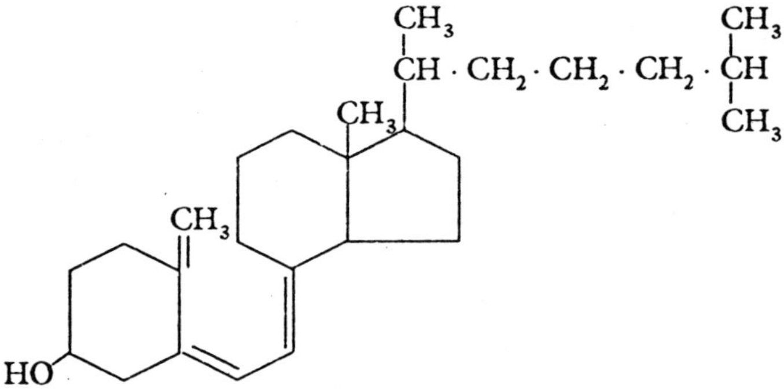

CH$_3$ CH$_3$
CH · CH$_2$ · CH$_2$ · CH$_2$ · CH
CH$_3$ CH$_3$
CH$_3$
HO

CHOLECALCIFEROL

Fig. 5.3 : Structures of Ergosterol, Calciferol, 7-Dehydrocholesterol and Cholecalciferol

METABOLISM AND FUNCTIONS

Dietary vitamin D is absorbed readily from gastro intestinal tract along with fats. It is then transported in chylomicrons through lymph circulation. Any situation which affects the fat absorption effect vitamin D absorption. *Ex* : pancreatitis, sprue etc. Skin also absorbs vitamin D when oil like cod-liver is massaged. Liver skin, brain lungs and bones store vitamin D.

The active form of vitamin D is its dehydroxyderivative. Liver adds one OH at twenty fifth carbon and vitamin D now is called 25- hydroxy vitamin D_3 or 25 hydroxycholecalciferol or simply 25-OH-D_3. The kidney further hydroxylates 25–OH–D_3 to different metabolite forms. One OH is added by the kidney at first carbon now the vitamin D is called 1,25 dehydroxycholecalciferol or 1,25–$(OH)_2D_3$. This form is said to be the active form of vitamin D. The functions of vitamin D are:

1. It promotes absorption of calcium and phosphorus by the intestines by stimulating the synthesis of a specific calcium binding protein by intestinal epithelium.
2. It facilitates normal functioning of parathormone.
3. It increase renal excretion of phosphate
4. It promotes mineralization of bone by its action on calcium and phosphorus metabolism
5. It exerts antirachitic property.
6. It helps in increase in citrate content in bones and blood.

DAILY REQUIREMENTS

In tropical countries with plenty of sunlight, smaller amounts of vitamin D through diet is sufficient. The nutrition expert group, India recommended a daily supply of 200 IU.

ASSAY METHODS

Chemical methods and biological methods are available for the assay of vitamin D.

CHEMICAL METHOD

In this method vitamin D is separated by column chromatography and then estimated colorimetrically. This method can be used for pure vitamin D.

BIOLOGICAL METHODS

Biological methods are accurate even for the assay of very small amounts of vitamin D. There are three methods.

a. Growth method
b. Boneash method
c. Line test

a) Growth method

Graded amounts of vitamin D and unknown are given to vitamin

D deficient rats. By comparing the growth rates of the two groups the vitamin D potency can be calculated.

b) Bone Ash Method

Graded amounts of standard vitamin D and unknown are given to vitamin D deficient rates. The ash content of tibia is determined. The increase in ash content is proportional to vitamin D content.

c) Line Test

Graded amounts of standard vitamin D and unknown food are given to vitamin D deficient rates. The proximate end of the tibia or distal end of ulnae are taken cleaned and longitudinal medium section is made. This section is dipped in 2% aqueous silvernitrate for one minute and washed with water. Newly deposited calcium phosphate is converted to silver phosphate which is seen as black line and the width of this line is the index of cure effected by vitamin D.

DEFICIENCY OF VITAMIN D

Deficiency of vitamin D leads to inadequate absorption of calcium and phosphorus from the intestinal track which ultimately results in faulty mineralisation of bones and tooth. The bones thus cannot withstand the stress of weight and skeletal malformations occur. Deficiency of vitamin D causes rickets, delayed and malformed teeth in children, osteomalacia in adults and osteoporosis in old age. See sketch 5.1.

Rickets

Rickets was first described by Glisson in 1650. The disease occurs in infants whose diets are deficient in vitamin D and who grow in dark, overcrowded areas of large cities where sunshine cannot penetrate. Dark skinned infants are more susceptible when compared to children of white race. Premature infants are also more susceptible than full term infants as the growth rate and calcification impose additional demand of vitamin D.

Fully developed rickets prevent the following signs and symptoms.

Head

Delayed closure of the frontanelles, softening of the skull (craniotabes) and bossing of fore head due to thickening of frontal and parietal eminences makes the head appear some what enlarge, elongated and flattened on the vertex with box like appearance.

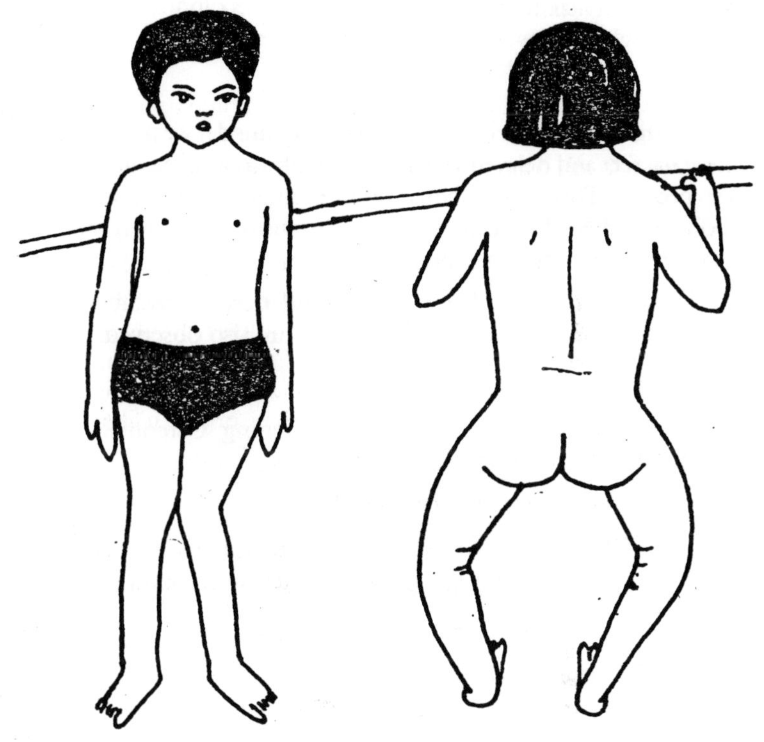

Sketch 5.1 : Knock Knees and Bow Legs

Chest

The costochondral junctions enlarge and appear as beaded junctions (Rachitic rosary) and chest sinks in at the line of junction of the ribs and cartilages so that abroad groove called 'Harrison's sulcus' is formed. The sternum may be depressed or with a prominent lateral depression of ribs causes pigeon breast appearance.

Enlargement of wrist, knee and ankle joints

The enlargement and cupping of the epiphyses cause a characteristic swelling appearance. This may not be visible in fat babies.

Deformities of Long Bones

The Osteoblast proliferation does not take place normally and so is the mineralization of bone. The cartilage cells do not degenerate and the long bones becomes soft and bulky. The bone mineral may be reabsorbed and makes the bone soft. These bones cannot withstand the stress of weight so bowlegs or knock knees develop.

Muscles

There is generalized hypotonia and muscle weakness. It may present flat feet and delayed walking. Pot belly or protuberant abdomen is also present. This is a combined result of muscle hypotonia, excessive carbohydrate diet which causes gaseous distension and down ward push of liver and spleen due to thorax deformity.

Dentition is delayed, restlessness and nervous irritability, high serum phosphatase and low serum calcium are also observed.

Osteomalacia

Osteomalacia literally means bone softening. Osteomalacia is the adult counterpart of rickets. It occurs due to

1. Interference with fat absorption
2. Steatorrohea
3. Lack of dietary intake of vitamin D or sunlight
4. Impaired hydroxylation by liver or kidney
5. Excessive demand in pregnancy.
6. Excessiver excretion in milk during lactation

The biochemical changes in blood are same as those of rickets. The mineral content of the bone decreases due to lack of calcium phosphate deposition. This process goes all over the body but spine, legs, thorax and pelvis are worst effected. Skeletal pain, tenderness of bones and multiple fractures also takes place. If serum calcium goes below 7.5mg/100ml tetany results. Tetany is characterised by muscle twitchings, cramps and convulsions. Spontaneous fractures may occur independent of pseudofractures known as looser's bones. There losers bones are characteristic of osteomalacia. The differences between osteomalacia and osteoporosis are given in table 5.3 Treatment for osteomalacia and Rickets both is administering massive does of vitamin D at intervals and in case of mild cases daily administration of small doses is sufficient.

Osteoporosis

Osteoporosis is the disease of bone frequently seen in old people. Hormonal deficiency and vitamin D deficiency are the causes for

Table 5.3 : The differences between Osteomalacia and Osteoporosis

	Clinical features	*Osteonalecia*	*Osteoporosis*
1.	Skeletal pain	Persistent	Associated with fracture
2.	Fracture	Occasional	Very Common
3.	Fracture healing	Delayed	Normal
4.	Deformity	Common	Absent
5.	Histology	Increase in Osteoid tissue	Bone quantity reduced
6.	Density of bone	Wide spread loss	Irregular loss
7.	Loosers zones	Diagnostic	Absent
8.	Serum Calcium and phosphate	Low	Normal
9.	Serum alkaline phosphate	High	Normal
10.	Urinary calcium	Low	Normal or High
11.	Response to Vitamin D treatment	Dramatic	Nil

osteoporosis. It occurs frequently in women after menopause. Failure in sex hormone production may be one of the reason for osteoporosis. High fecal excretion of calcium and low absorption are observed in some patients. Severe bone pain is reported which is relived by immobilization. Fractures occur die to brittle bones which heal off normally.

Hypervitaminosis

Excessive intakes of vitamin D produces symptoms like hypotonia, anorexia, irritability, polydipsia, polyuria, vomiting nocturia, diarrhoea and weight loss. With continued intakes in excessive amounts renal damage and calcification of soft tissues like heart, blood vessels, bronchi, stomach, etc., occur.

VITAMIN E

HISTORY

Mattill and Conklin in 1920 reported the inter relationship between food factors and reproduction. In 1922 Evans and Bishop established that fat soluble factor was essential for reproduction in rats.

They named that factor as X which was subsequently renamed as Vitamin E. In 1936 Evans and coworkers isolated two different compounds that possess vitamin E activity. They are α and β tocopherols. Tocopherol is a Greek word where 'tocos' means 'birth', 'phero' means 'to bear' and 'ol' means 'alcohol'. Fernoholtz in 1937 and Evans and coworkers in 1939 elucidated the structure of tocopherol.

SOURCES

Tocopherols are not synthesised in the body. The principal sources of vitamin-E in diet are vegetable oils, cereals, poultry, meat and fish. Hydrogenated fats, whole grains, dark green leafy vegetables nuts and legumes are fair sources. Human milk has more vitamin E than cow milk and is sufficient for infants.

CHEMISTRY

Of the α, β and r tocopherols alpha tocopherol is the most potent. β and r tocopherols have 30 and 15 percent activity as tocopherol. The structure of vitamin E is shown in figure. 5.4.

The double ring structure is called chromane ring. The tocopherol is 5,7,8 trimethyl derivative. β Tocopherol and game tocopherol has 2 methyl groups in 5—8 and 7—8 positions respectively Tocopherols are soluble in fats and fat solvents. They readily oxidize and act as anti oxidants and protect other vitamins like vitamin A form oxidation. High temperatures and acids do not affect the stability of vitamin E. But in alkanemedium the vitamin activity is destroyed.

METABOLISM AND FUNCTIONS

Absorption of vitamin A is facilitated by the presence of fat and bilesalts. This vitamin is not excreted to any extent. The absorbed vitamin

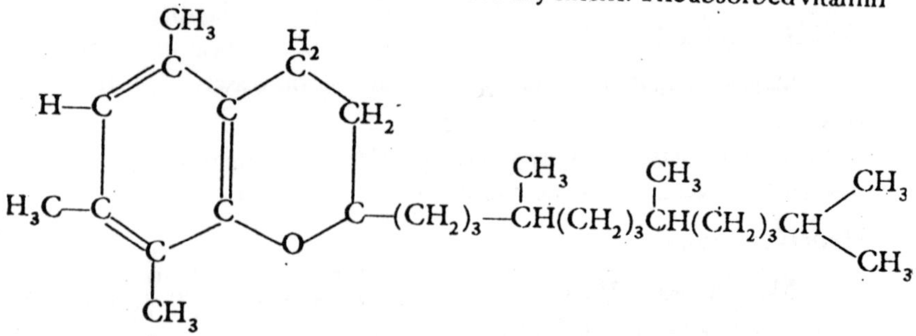

CH_3 H_2 C C H—C C CH_2 CH_3 CH_3 CH_3 H_3C—C C C—$(CH_2)_3$—$CH(CH_2)_3CH(CH_2)_3CH$ C O CH_3 CH_3

Fig. 5.4 : Structure of α- Tocopherol

E is carried with the chylomicrons into lymph circulation and is stored mainly in liver. Skeletal muscles, body fat and visceral organs also store this vitamin. Vitamin E has a special role in productive physiology. If deficiency of this vitamin occurs in males the result is sterility and in case of females ovulation, conception and implantation occurs normally but the fetus dies in utero and resorption occur. The change in males is irreversible.

The metabolic role of vitamin E is not completely understood. Vitamin E acts as anti oxidant, prevents accumulation free radicals, toxic. Oxidation products, prevents hemolysis and cell membrane destruction. Vitamin E is present in all cell membranes that contain polyunsaturated fathy acids which can be destroyed by oxidation. Thus vitamin E maintains the integrity of cell membrane. Vitamin E has a sparing action on other vitamins like A and C by protecting them from oxidation. Incorporation of Pyramidines into nucleicacids especially in synthesis of heme is one of the other proposed function of vitamin E.

DAILY REQUIREMENTS

No clear basis exists for recommended daily allowances of this vitamin. Vitamin E deficiency is extremely rare it may be assumed that diets commonly consumed by normal healthy individuals provide adequate amounts of vitamin E.

ASSAY METHODS

Emerson–Evans resorption gestation method is the biological assay method. In this the amount of substance required to support gestation in a vitamin E deficient pregnant rat is estimated. In chemical method the amount of vitamin E is estimated for reducing Ferric Chloride to ferrous chloride.

DEFICIENCY

Vitamin E deficiency is extremely rare. In severe deficiency muscular dystrophy and erythrocyte hemolysis may occur. In animal studies irreversible testicular degeneration in male rats, intrautero death and resorption of fetus in female rats and Necrosis of liver also observed.

Hypervitaminosis

Mega doses of Vitamin E appears non-toxic. Most adults appear to tolerate doses as high as 100 to 1000 IU per day. However continuous intake of such doses may cause muscle weakness, nausea, fatigue, elevated serum triglycerides, reduced serum thyroid hormones and impaired blood coagulation as large doses of vitamin E decrease vitamin K activity and inhibit prothrombin formation.

VITAMIN K

HISTORY

The existence of vitamin K was first suggested by Dr. Dam and his associates working in copenhagen. They found that chicks fed on purified diet containing all vitamins known at that time developed hemorrhagic condition. They called it coagulations vitamin later it was called vitamin K. Dam and Kareer in 1939 isolated pure vitamin K_1 and Doisy and coworkers isolated vitamin K_2.

SOURCES

Green leafy vegetables, cereals, legumes, milk, eggs, meat, fish and other vegetables are good sources of vitamin K. It can be synthesized by the microorganisms in gastrointestinal tract of higher animals including Man. It also occurs in putrid fish meal.

CHEMISTRY

Vitamin K has a number of related compounds called quinones. Vitamin K_1 was isolated from vegetable sources and it is also called phylloquinone. Vitamin K_2 was isolated from putrid fish meal and it is also called Menaquinone. Vitamin K_3 also called Menadione is a synthetic product and it is two to three times potent as natural vitamin. Vitamin K_3 is slightly water soluble but it must be converted to vitamin K_2 in liver. Natural vitamin K is fat soluble, resistant to heat but easily destroyed by acids, alkalies, light and oxidizing agents.

METABOLISM AND FUNCTIONS

Vitamin K is fat soluble vitamin so it is readily absorbed along with fats in presence of bilesalts. It is not stored in the body so constant supply is needed. Fifty percent of the recommended daily allowance is obtained by the bacterial synthesis in our Gastro intestinal tract. Feces has vitamin K but this is bacterial in origin. Vitamin K is not excreted through urine.

Vitamin K is required for the formation of proconversion, plasma thromboplastin component, stuart factor and prothrombin. These are synthesized by liver in inactive form. These can be activated by the conversion of Glutamic residues to carboxyl glutamic acid which requires vitamin K. This carboxyl glutamic acid helps in chelating calcium form protein-calcium-phospholipid interaction. A similar reaction in osteocalcin of bone matrix helps in mineralization of bone. A high prothrombin - level indicates good coagulating ability of blood where as a low prothrombin level indicates slow clotting. The absence of vitamin K in diet or ingestion of vitamin K antagonists like warfarin sodium, coumarin compounds inhibits the vitamin K activity.

DAILY REQUIREMENTS

On account of intestinal synthesis no allowance is to be supplied normally if there is not liver damage. 1 to 2 mg per kilogram body weight is assumed as safe and adequate. The lower amount is based on assumption that half of recommended daily allowance is synthesized in the body and the upper value is calculated assuming the entire RDA to be supplied through diet.

ASSAY METHODS

Colorimetric methods, Fluorimetric methods, spectrophotometric methods and biological methods are available for the assay of vitamin K.

DEFICIENCY

Deficiency of Vitamin K does not normally occur as it is available form intestinal abacterial syntheses. Deficiency of vitamin K occurs in (i) deficiency production by bacteria in gastro intestinal tract (ii) deficient vitamin K absorption. In new born infants especially premature infants the intestinal flora is not yet established so the production of vitamin K is low. Prolonged use of antibiotics prevent the growth of intestinal flare so also the production is lowered. In case of diarrhoea and biliary obstruction vitamin K absorption is impaired causing vitamin K deficiency. Manifestation in all these cases if delayed prothrombin time and hemorrhagic tendency.

Hypervitaminosis

Vitamin K does not produce any toxic effect in doses 10-20 mg which is used in treatment of patients with liver or intestinal disorders. However long term use of excessive amounts of vitamin may alter liver function. Especially infants liver capacity is limited for glucuronide formation which is essential for bilirubin conjugation and vitmain K excretion. In case of excessive intkae of vitamin K in infants the unconjugated bilirubin level increases which is called kernicterus and may also increase the breakdown of red blood cells.

Water Soluble Vitamins

B- COMPLEX GROUP

THIAMIN

HISTORY

Takaki, a Japanese medical officer, observed a serious disease affecting nerves in the people who had polished rice as their staple food. During 1878-1883 he compared the diets of two groups of navy personnel serving two sailing vessels and found that people who had received meat, milk and vegetables along with rice are not as much affected as people who had polished rice only as staple food. He believed that protein made all the difference. Eijkman a Dutch Physician in 1897 produced Beri Beri in fowls that is similar to the one of human beings by feeding polished rice and demonstrated that the situation can be cured by adding rice polishings to the diet. Jansen and Donath in 1926 isolated vitamin B from rice polishings. Windans and co-workers in 1931 isolated vitamin B from yeast and established its empirical formula.

SOURCES

Thiamin is widely distribute in many foods. Rice polishings, dried yeast and wheat germ are rich sources. Whole cereals, legumes, oil seeds, nuts, and liver are good sources. Meat, fish, eggs, and milk are fair sources of thiamin. Table 6.1 gives thiamin content in different foods.

Table 6.1 : Thiamin Content of Some Food Stuffs

Food Stuff	*Thiamin* mg/100g	*Food Stuff*	*Thiamin* mg/100g
Cereals and Cereal Products :		Peas dry	0.47
Bajra	0.33	Red gram dal	0.45
Barley	0.47	Soya bean	0.73
Italian millet	0.59	**Nuts and Oil Seeds :**	
Jowar	0.37	Almonds	0.24
Maize (dry)	0.42	Cashewnuts	0.63
Maize (Tender)	0.11	Gingelly seeds	1.01
Ragi	0.42	Ground nut	0.90
Rice paraboiled milled	0.21	Mustard seeds	0.65
Rice Raw Milled	0.06	Pistachio	0.67
Rice flakes	0.21	Sunflower seeds	0.85
Rice puffed	0.21	**Flesh Foods :**	
Semolina	0.12	Hens egg	0.10
Vermicelli	0.19	Sheep liver	0.36
Bread brown	0.21	Mutton	0.18
Bread white	0.07	Pork muscle	0.54
Wheat flour whole	0.49	**Milk and Milk Products :**	
Wheat flour refined	0.12	Buffalo milk	0.04
Pulses and Legumes :		Cows milk	0.05
Bengal gram dal	0.48	Khoa (Whole cow milk)	0.23
Black gram dal	0.42	Skimmed milk powder (Cow's milk)	0.45
Cowpea	0.51		
Green gram dal	0.47	Whole milk powder (Cow's milk)	0.31
Horse gram	0.42		

CHEMISTRY

Thiamin is available commercially as thiamin hydro chloride which has a thiazole and a pyramidine nucleus. It has a emhirical formula $C_{12} H_{17} N_4 OSCI. HCL$. It is a white crystalline powder with faint yeast like odor and salty nut like taste. Thiamin is soluble in water and stable until 120°C in acid medium. It is destroyed in alkaline or neutral medium. The structure of thiamin is given in figure 6.1.

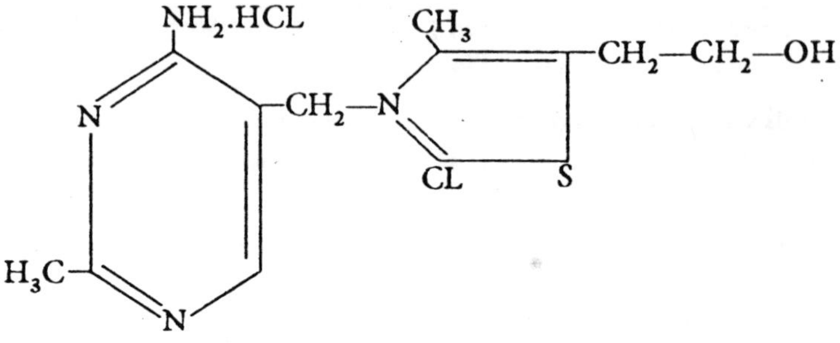

Fig. 6.1 : Thiamin Chloride Sturcture

METABOLISM AND FUNCTIONS

Thiamin whether free or bound as thiamin pyrophosphate or protein phosphate complex it is readily absorbed from duodenum and jejunum. After absorption thiamine is converted to thiamin pyrophosphate (TPP) in the presence of thiamin kinase and ATP.

This thiamin pyrophosphate acts as a co-enzyme in a number of enzyme systems. Foods such as fish, shrimp and raw animal tissues contain thiaminase and enzyme which splits the thiamin molecule and in activates it. Cooking destroys this enzyme. Tannings present in tea, betelnuts etc. act as thiamin antagonists. Less than 50 mg of thiamine is stored in our body. Of this liver, kidney, muscles and brain have a little higher concentration than blood. 80% of the thiamin stored is thiamin pyrophosphate 10% is thiamin triphosphate and remainder as free thiamin and thiamin monophosphate. Excess thiamin is excreted in urine.

Firstly thiamin pyrophosphate plays a critical role in oxidative decarboxylation of pyruvic acid which inturn forms acetyl coenzyme and enters the Krebs cycle. Secondly thiamin is essential in oxidative decarboxylation of - keto glutarilacid to succinic acid. Thirdly TPP also functions as coenzyme in transketolase system associated with the direct oxidative path way of glucose metabolism. In addition thiamin in some way influence the action in nerve conduction.

DAILY REQUIREMENTS

Thiamin is necessary for carbohydrate metabolism and thus the thiamin requirement is proportional to the carbohydrate intake. Since carbohydrates supply most of the energy the thiamin requirement is based on calorie intake. About 0.35mg of thiamin per 1000 k cals is recommended. Thiamin requirement is increased in the following conditions 1. increased metabolic rate 2. pregnancy and lactation and 3. metabolism of carbohydrate. Thiamin requirements are given in Table 6.2 as thiamin is excreted in human milk more thiamin is required by lactating mothers.

Table 6.2 : Recommended Dietary intake of Thiamin

	Group	*Thiamin* mg
Man	Sedentary work	1.2
	Moderate work	1.4
	Heavy work	1.6
Woman	Sedentary work	0.9
	Moderate work	1.1
	Heavy work	1.2
	Pregnancy (Second half)	+0.2
	Lactation	
	0–6 months	+0.3
	6–12 months	+0.2
Infants	0–6 months	55 Mg/Kg
	6–12 months	50 Mg/Kg
Children	1–3 years	0.6
	4–6 years	0.9
	7–9 years	1.0
Boys	10–12 years	1.1
Girls	10–12 years	1.0
Boys	13–15 years	1.2
Girls	13–15 years	1.0
Boys	16–18 years	1.3
Girls	16–18 years	1.0

ASSAY METHODS

Physicochemical methods, biological methods and micro biological methods are available for thiamin assay.

I. Physio Chemical Methods

(a) Thiochrome method

This method was first described by Jansen in 1936. Several workers modified this method. This method is highly sensitive and can be applied for assay of thiamin in both animal tissues and food stuffs. In this method the sample is hydrolysed with phosphatase and proteolytic enzymes to obtain thiamin from thiamin pyrophosphate and protein bound thiamin. This thiamin is then oxidized with fatassium ferricyanide in alkaline medium to obtain thiochrome sitis extract with isobutanol to determine the fluorescence in a fluorimeter.

(b) Colormetric method

Thiamin reacts with diazotized P-amino aceto phenone to give a red colour which can be measured photemetrically. This method is less specific than thiochrome method.

II. Biological Methods:

Cure of Polyneuritis in Pigeons or rats

Pigeons or rats are fed on thiamin deficient diet until they develop paralysis and convulsion. Then they are fed with minimum quantities of thiamin until they recover and the total amount of vitamin fed is determined.

III Micro Biological Methods

Employing experimental animals is expansive than employing micro organisms. Micro organisms whose growth requires thiamin like lactobacillus - L- viridescens or yeast are cultured on agar plates or nutrient broth which contain all other nutrients except thiamin. They are separated two groups and for one unknown substance and a graded amount of the vitamin for the other are added. The growth of the standard and unknown are compared by measuring the size and number of colonies.

DEFICIENCY

Severe thiamin deficiency is rare. Deficiency of thiamin is usually associated with low calorie intake and other factors of vitamin B complex. Deficiency of Thiamin may be due to (1) low in take (2) poor absorption and (3) excessive demand. Deficiency of Thiamin Occur (a) where highly refined cereals form the staple food (b) Patients with diseases of Gastrointestinal tract (c) Alcoholics where the intake of food is low (d) increased metabolic rate like fever, hyperthyroidism (e) pregnancy and lactation. Clinically thiamin deficiency is of 3 types :

1) In fantile Beri Beri
2) Dry Beri Beri
3) Wet Beri Beri

Infantile Beri Beri

Infantile beri beri occurs in the first few months of life if the mother has thiamin deficiency due to consumption of over refined cereals as staple food and poor thiamin content in breast milk. The onset of the disease is sudden and may be of two types. (i) Cardiovascular type (ii) neuritic type.

(i) Cardiovascular Type

This type is usually found infant around 3 months age. The infant may present the classic symptoms of congestive heart failure, tachycardia, dysponoa, enlargement of heart, tender and enlarged liver, edema and oliguria. Cyanosis and pulmonary edema may also be present in some cases and death occurs in few hours.

ii) Neuritic Type

The Classic symptoms of dry beri beri may not be found in children but irritability, apathy, drowsiness and coma may occur due to rise in intra cranial pressure and death follows. In case of infantile beri beri thiamin therapy gives a dramatic response.

Dry Beri Beri

In Dry beri beri involvement of the peripheral nerves of legs and arms is seen. Bilateral and symmetrical tingling, numbness and burning of hands and feet are observed fatigue, lack of interest, emotional instability, anger, fear, anorexie, weight loss are also found in the first stage. In the second stage tenderness and wasting of calf muscle, food drop, wrist drop, sluggish knee and ankle jerks are seen the muscle degeneration may be so pronounced that co-ordination is not possible and the characteristic high stepping gait results. Thiamin therapy gives a dramatic response and if untreated death follows.

Wet Beri Beri

Edema is the important feature of wet beri beri. Palpitation, breathlessness, tender calf muscle, scanty urine, rapid pulse, engorged neck veins, enlarged heart and finally heart failure occurs. This form is a medical emergency and if treatment is not prompt death occurs. Intravenous and intramuscular thiamin produce dramatic response along with other supportive measures.

HYPERVITAMINOSIS

Toxicity due to excess intake of thiamin have not been reported. Since the excess vitamin is readily excreted through the kidney there is no benefit of taking in megadoses for a normal healthy person.

RIBOFLAVIN

Synonyms : Vitamin B_2, Lactoflavin.

HISTORY

In 1897 a yellow green pigment in milk was discovered. Later than pigment was found in liver, yeast, heart and egg white this pigment was given a name flavin. In 1926 Gold Berger found a substance in yeast which cures pellegra. Unlike thiamin this substance withstood autoclaving also. So it was given a name as vitamin B_2. It was discovered that vitamin B_2 molecule consists a group similar to ribose sugar also this vitamin is given a prefix 'Ribo' and the second part was flavin which represents the source of the vitamin. Thus the name Riboflavin was coined. Warburg and Christian in 1932 isolated an yellow enzyme from yeast. Subsequently in 1933 pure vitamin was isolated and synthesized.

SOURCES

Milk, liver, kidney, heart, eggs, yeast, milk, meat, fish, whose cereals and millets, legumes and green leafs vegetables are good sources of riboflavin. Milled cereals, roots, tubers, and other vegetables are fair sources. The Riboflavin content of some foods is given in Table 6.3.

CHEMISTRY

Riboflavin is 6,7 dimethyl 9 (D- ribityl 5 phosphate) isoalloxazine. The empirical formula is $C_{17} H_{20} N_4 O_6$. It structure is shown in Figure 6.2 In pure state the vitamin is bitter to taste, orange-yellow, odor less compound whose crystals are needle shaped. It is slightly soluble in water (12 mg per 100 ml at 25°C and 230 mg per 100 ml at 100°C) and ethyl alcohol. It is stable in acid medium. It is rapidly destroyed in alkaline medium and bright light. It is stable to heat and oxidizing agents.

Table 6.3 : Riboflavin Content of Some Food Stuffs

Food Stuff	*Riboflavin* mg/100g
Cereals and Cereal Products :	
Bajra	0.25
Barley	0.20
Italian millet	0.11
Jowar	0.13
Maize Tender	0.18
Ragi	0.19
Rice Praboiled hand pounded	0.12
Rice raw hand pounded	0.16
Rice raw milled	0.06
Rice flakes	0.05
Wheat whole	0.17
Pulses and Legumes :	
Bengal gram Dal	0.18
Black gram dal	0.20
Cowpea	0.20
Green gram dal	0.21
Horsegram	0.21
Peas (Dry)	0.19
Red gram dal	0.19
Soyabean	0.39
Leafy Vegetables :	
Amarnath tender	0.30
Beet greens	0.56
Brussels sprouts	0.16
Cabbage	0.09
Carrot leaves	0.37
Curry leaves	0.21
Fenugreek leaves	0.31
Gogu	0.39
Mint	0.26
Radish leaves	0.47
Spinach	0.26
Other Vegetables	
Beans scarlet	0.19
Brinjal	0.11
Cauliflower	0.10
Nuts and Oil Seeds :	
Almonds	0.57
Cashewnut	0.19
Gingellyseeds	0.34
Mustard seeds	0.26
Pistachio	0.28
Wal nut	0.40
Flesh Foods :	
Eggs hen	0.40
Egg duck	0.26
Fowl	0.14
Liversheep	1.70
Mutton	0.14
Pork muscle	0.09
Milk and Milk Products :	
Buffalo milk	0.10
Cows milk	0.19
Curds (Cow's milk)	0.16
Khoa (Whole Cow's milk)	0.41
Skimmed milk powder	1.64

Ordinary cooking loss accounts to 20% only.

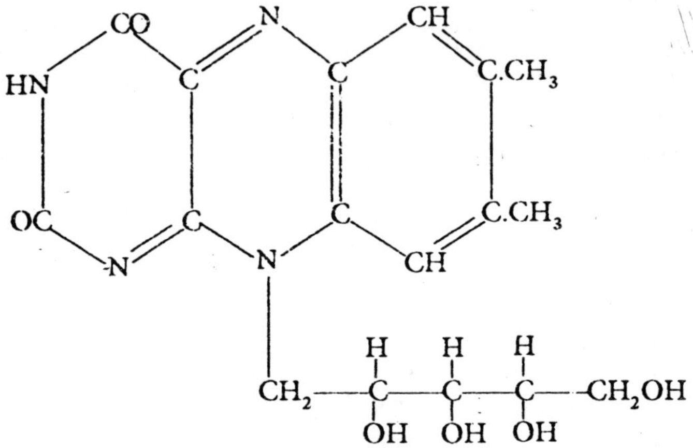

Fig. 6.2 : Riboflavin

METABOLISM AND FUNCTIONS

Riboflavin is readily absorbed form small intestine and is phosphorylated in the intestinal wall. Then it is passed to all tissues in the form of co-enzyme or flavoprotein. Riboflavin exists in animal tissues and yeast in the form of nucleotides in combination with enzymes. The two nucleotides are Riboflavin mononucleotide (FMN) and Riboflavin adenine dinucleotide (FAD). There two nucleotides are part of enzymes or act as coenzymes and act as hydrogen acceptors, and play an important role in the metabolism of carbohydrates proteins and fats. The retina contains riboflavin which helps in the stimulation of optic nerve.

DAILY REQUIREMENTS

The daily requirement of Riboflavin is 1.6 mg per day. An intake below 1.1 mg per day cannot maintain the body reserve Hyper thyrodism, fevers, stress conditions like injury or surgery and malabsorption increase the requirement. The recommended dietary allowance are given in Table 6.4.

ASSAY METHODS

Riboflavin assay can be done by physico chemical methods,

Table 6.4 : Recommended Dietary intake of Riboflavin

	Group	*Riboflavin* mg
Man	Sedentary work	1.4
	Moderate work	1.7
	Heavy work	2.0
Woman	Sedentary work	1.1
	Moderate work	1.3
	Heavy work	1.8
	Pregnancy (Second half)	+0.2
	Lactation:	
	0–6 months	+0.3
	6–12 months	+0.2
Infants	0–6 months	65 Mg/Kg
	6–12 months	60 Mg/Kg
Children	1–3 years	0.7
	4–6 years	1.0
	7–9 years	1.2
Boys	10–12 years	1.3
Girls	10–12 years	1.2
Boys	13–15 years	1.6
Girls	13–15 years	1.2
Boys	16–18 years	1.6
Girls	16–18 years	1.2

Biological method and Micro biological method.

Physico chemical methods: Riboflavin was first extracted by dilute acids then it is treated with potassium permanganate and hydrogen peroxide and removing the pigments. Then the fluorescence of the extract is estimated by treating with sodium hydeosulphite at 80°c or exposing to bright light.

BIOLOGICAL METHOD

A group of rats are fed on riboflavin free diet until deficiency symptoms are visible. Then they are divided in two groups. One group is fed with graded amount of pure riboflavin added to the diet and other is given varying amounts of test food. The growth response is then compared and the riboflavin content of food can be calculated.

MICROBIOLOGICAL METHOD

In this method lactobacillus casei are used. The lactic acid produced by the organism is measured by titration. In this method also graded amounts and unknown amounts of vitamin are used.

DEFICIENCY

Deficiency of riboflavin cause:

1) Oral and facial lesions
2) Ocular lesions and
3) Scrotal and vulval lesions

1) Oral and Facial Lesions

Sebrell and Butler studied a group of human subjects who were kept on low riboflavin diet for 4 months. They presented greasy dermatitis around the nose, cheilosis, glossitis increased vascularisation of cornea and atrophic lingual papillae.

2) Ocular Lesions

Blurring of vision, itching, watering, soreness, proliferation and engorgement of bulbar conjuctival capillaries of lumber plexus are the signs of riboflavin deficiency in eye. These can be cured by administering riboflavin.

3) Scrotal and Vulval Lesions

These are observed in the subjects suffering with pellergra 12 out of 15 subjects fed on riboflavin deficient diets showed these signs which are cured by administering riboflavin.

HYPERVITAMINOSIS

No toxicity in human beings is reported. Death in rats occurred when 560 mg/kg in traperitoneal dose was given. But in human beings oral doses of 5 to 10 mg per day are given and no toxic symptoms were seen.

NIACIN

Synonyms : Nicotinic acid, Nicotinamide

HISTORY

Nicotinic acid was synthesized as early as 1867 by oxidizing nicotine, an alkaloid of tobacco. The physiological activity of nicotine and nicotinic acid are entirely different. Gold Berger of US public health service studied the etiology of pellergra and concluded that it is similar to black tongue in dogs and can be cured by administering dried yeast or liver. He defined this factor as heat stable vitamin of B and named vitamin B_2. Elvenjem and his co-workers in 1937 isolated nicotinic acid from liver and proved to effectiveness as a curative agent for black tongue in dogs. Later in 1937 spices et al, Foutsetal and Smith, et al., independently reported that Nicotinic acid cures pellegra in human beings. Cowgill suggested the name niacin to this vitamin to avoid association with nicotine of tobacco.

SOURCES

The general sources of vitamin B complex contain his vitamin. Dried yeast, rice polishings, liver and peanut, are good sources. Tryptophan in essential amino acid is converted to nicotinic acid in the presence of vitamin B_6. About 60 mg of tryptophan yield 1 mg niacin. Milk and eggs are good sources of tryptophan. Important sources of niacin are given in Table 6.5

CHEMISTRY

Nicotinic acid and niacinamide have equal biological activity. Niacin is the common name for both the forms. Nicotinic acid is a pyridine beta carboxylic acid with an empirical formula $C_6H_5O_2N$. Niacinamide is formed by addition of $NH^2{}_2$ radical to nicotinic acid. These two forms are white bitter compounds slightly soluble in water i.e. 1 mg in 60 ml water at 25°C. The It is stable to heat, acid, alkali, light, oxidation and autoclaving. The chemical structures of nicotinic acid and nicotinamide are given in the Figure 6.3.

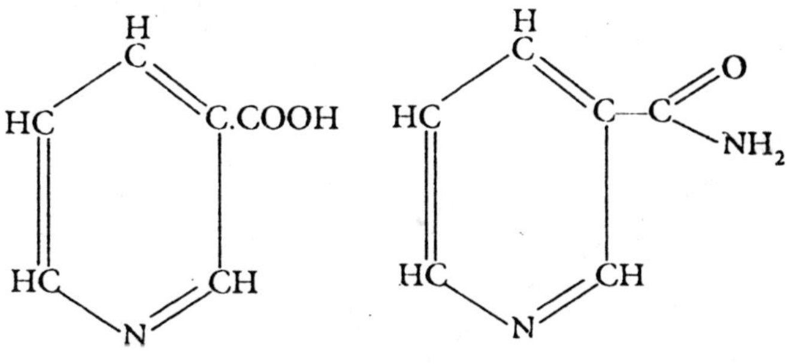

Fig. 6.3 : Nicotinic Acid and Nicotinamide

Table 6.5 : Niacin Content of Some Foods

Food Stuff	Niacin mg/100g	Food Stuff	Niacin mg/100g
Cereals :		***Other Vegetables***	
Bajra	2.3	Ashgourd	0.4
Barley	5.4	Bitter gaurd	0.5
Jowar	3.1	Brinjal	0.9
Maize dry	1.8	Cauliflower	1.0
Ragi	1.1	Cluster beans	0.6
Rice hand pounded	4.0	Peas	0.8
Rice paraboiled milled	3.8	Pumpkin	0.5
Rice raw milled	1.9	***Roots and tubers***	
Rice flaker	4.0	Beat root	0.4
Rice puffed	4.1	Carrot	0.6
Semolina	1.6	Colocasia	0.4
Vermicelli	1.8	Onion	0.5
Whole wheat	5.5	Potato	1.2
Wheat flour whole	4.3	Radish white	0.5
Wheat flour refined	2.4	Sweet potato	0.7
Pulses and Legumes :		**Nuts and Oil Seeds :**	
Bengal gram Dal	2.4	Almonds	4.4
Black gram dal	2.0	Cashewnuts	1.2
Green gram dal	2.4	coconut dry	3.0
Horse gram	1.5	Gingelly seeds	4.4
Peas	3.4	Ground nuts	19.9
Red gram dal	3.9	Mustard seeds	4.0
Soyabean	3.2	**Fish and Other Flesh Foods :**	
Yeast (Dried) :		Cat fish	2.5
Brewers	40.0	Crab (muscle)	3.1
Food	27.0	Fish meal	5.3
Leafy Vegetables :		Hilsa	2.8
Amarnath tender	1.2	Pomfrets white	2.6
Coriander	0.8	Prawn	4.8
Curry leaves	2.3	Ribbon fish	2.1
Fenugreek leaves	0.8	Sardine	2.6
Gogu	1.1	Shark	2.5
Lettuce	0.5	Liver sheep	17.6
Mint	1.0	Mutton muscle	6.8
Spinach	0.5	Pork muscle	2.8
Tamarind leaves tender	4.1		

METABOLISM AND FUNCTIONS

Nicotinic acid and nicotinamide are readily observed from the small intestine through the portal vein in the general circulation. It is changed to NAD and NADP in the tissues. Excess of niacin is excreted in the urine as N-methyl nicotinamide and N methyl 6 pyridoe 3 carboxynamide. Niacinamide is a component of NAD and NADP which are hydrogen acceptors and are involved in many enzyme reaction. Some of them are tabulated in Table 6.6.

Nicotinic acid is essential for normal functioning of the skin, intestinal tract and nervous system. Deficiency of nicotinic acid produce lesions in these tissues.

Table 6.6 : NAD(P) — Dependent Dehydrogenases

Enzyme	*Co-enzyme*	*Reaction*		
Alcohol dehy-drogenese	NAD zn	Alcohols	⟶	Aldehydes
Aldehyde dehydro-genose	NAD	Aldehydes	⟶	Acids
Glucose dehydro-genose	NAD (NADP)	Glucose	⟶	Gluconate
Glucose 6 P dehy-drogenose	NADP	Glucose	⟶	Gluconate 6 phosphate
Gluconate 6 P dehydrogenose	NADP	Gluconate 6 P	⟶	Ribulose 5P + CO_2
L Glucomate dehy-drogenose	NAD, NADP+Zn	Glucomate	⟶	Ketoglutarate+ NH_3
L Glycerophosphate dehydrogenose	NAD	Glycerophosphate	⟶	Dehydroxy acetone P
Glyceraldehyde 3P dehydrogenose	NAD SH	Glyceraldehyde 3P	⟶	dephosphogly-cerate
Hydroxybutyrate dehydrogenose	NAD	Hydroxybutarate	⟶	Acetoacetate
Hydroxysteroid dehydrogenose	NAD, NADP	Hydroxysteroid	⟶	Ketosteroid
Isocitrate dehydro-genose	NAD, NADP	Isocitrate	⟶	Ketoglutarate
Lactate dehydro-genose	NAD, (NADP)	Lactate	⟶	Pyruvate
Malate dehydro-genose	NAD (NADP)	Malate	⟶	Oxaloacetate

DAILY REQUIREMENTS

The FAO/ WHO expert group on vitamin requirements recommended 6.6 mg niacin equivalent for every 1000 k cals for a normal healthy person. The Nutrition expert group of ICMR India also adopted this recommendation. Table 6.7 shows the dietary niacin requirements in various age groups.

Table 6.7 : Recommended Dietary Intake of Niacin

	Group	*Niacin* mg
Man	Sedentary work	16
	Moderate work	18
	Heavy work	21
Woman	Sedentary work	12
	Moderate work	14
	Heavy work	16
	Pregnancy (Second half)	+2
	Lactation:	
	0–6 months	+4
	6–12 months	+3
Infants	0–6 months	710 Mg/Kg
	6–12 months	650 Mg/Kg
Children	1–3 years	8
	4–6 years	11
	7–9 years	13
Boys	10–12 years	15
Girls	10–12 years	13
Boys	13–15 years	16
Girls	13–15 years	14
Boys	16–18 years	17
Girls	16–18 years	14

ASSAY METHODS

Chemical, biological and microbiological methods are available for the assay of niacin.

CHEMICAL METHOD

This method is used for the assay of niacin in foods, urine and tissues. First niacin and its derivatives are extracted using dilute acid at 80°C. Niacinamide is then hydrolyseal to niacin and other interfering substances and pigments are removed using lead acetate. To this cyanogen bromide and aniline are added in neutral pH and aqueous medium. The colour developed is then noted.

BIOLOGICAL METHOD

Mostly chicks are used in this method. Different levels standard niacin and unknown foods are given to niacin deficient chicks and their growth rates are compared.

MICROBIOLOGICAL METHOD

Lactobacillus arabinoses is used in this method. Known amounts of standard Niacin is fed and the growth of the organism is assessed by titrating the amount of lactic acid produced with sodium hydroxide.

DEFICIENCY

Nicotinic acid deficiency causes pellegra. This disease involves skin, gastrointestinal tract and nervous system. Early symptoms are fatigue, restlessness, headache, backache, anorexia weight loss, sore tongue, mouth and throat and glossitis of gastrointestinal tract. Nausea and vomiting are seen after severe diarrhoea. A characteristic symmetric dermatitis especially on exposed surface of the body are seen. Sunshine and exposure to heat aggravate the problem. Dizziness, confusion, poor memory, dementie and irritability are seen as the severity increases. The disease is characterized by classic 'D's. They are Dermatitis, Diarrhoea, Dementia and finally death.

HYPERVITAMINOSIS

There is no possibility of any excess niacin in the body which is derived from dietary source. The excess is always excreted in urine. Nicotinic acid as synthetic product even when taken in dose of recommended allowance causes burning, itching, tingling and flushing which are transient and harmless (lasts for few seconds to a minute) may alarm the patient. The Blood pressure, pulse rates and body temperature remain normal. Nicotinamide on the other hand does not present these symptoms and can be used in treatment of pellagra (100 mg divided into four doses per day orally or 50 mg twice a day intramuscularly).

PYRIDOXIN

Synonyms : Vitamin B_6, Rat anti dermatitis factor, Adermin, rat acordynia factor, Pyridoxal.

HISTORY

Gyorgy in 1934 reported that vitamin B_2 has two factors riboflavin and factor B_6 which prevents acordynia (skin lesions) in rats. In 1938 Kerseztesy and stevens, Gyorgy, Lepkosky, Kuhn and Wndt, Itiba and Miti five groups of workers independently isolated this factor in its pure form. Kuhn and Wendt and Kerseztesy et al in 1939 synthesised it independently in Germany and USA respectively. The chemical structure was identified by Harris and Folkers.

SOURCES

Rice polishings, wheat germ, dried yeast, liver, whole cereals, legumes, oil seeds, eggs, milk, meat, fish and green leafy vegetables are good sources of pyridoxin.

CHEMISTRY

Vitamin B_6 has a group of related pyridines. They are pyridoxine, pyridoxal and pyridoxamine. Pyridoxine has a pyridine nucleus, two primary alcoholic groups and one phenolic hydroxyl group. Pyridoxal has an aldehyde group in place of one primary alcoholic group. Pyridoxamine has a primary amine side chain in place of primary alcoholic group. The structures of pyridoxin, pyridoxal and pyridoxamine are given in Figure 6.4.

Pyridoxin is readily soluble in water and relatively stable to heat and acids. It is destroyed in alkaline medium and is sensitive to heat.

METABOLISM AND FUNCTIONS

Pyridoxin is readily absorbed from intestines. It can also be absorbed through skin. There is no appreciable storage in the body so it has to be supplied daily. Excess of Vitamin is excreted in urine as it is a water soluble vitamin. The active form of pyridoxin is the co-enzyme pyridoxal phosphate which can be formed from pyridoxin, pyridoxal and pyridoxamine.

Pyridoxal phosphate is essential for growth and its deficiency produce degeneration of nerves and microcytic anemia. Pyridoxal

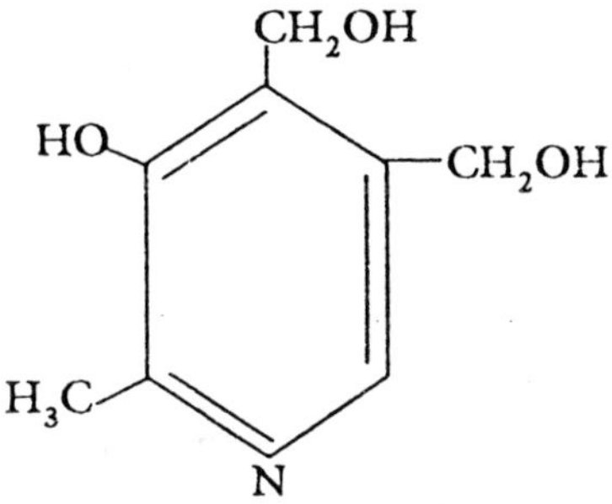

CH_2OH HO CH_2OH H_3C N

PYRIDOXIN

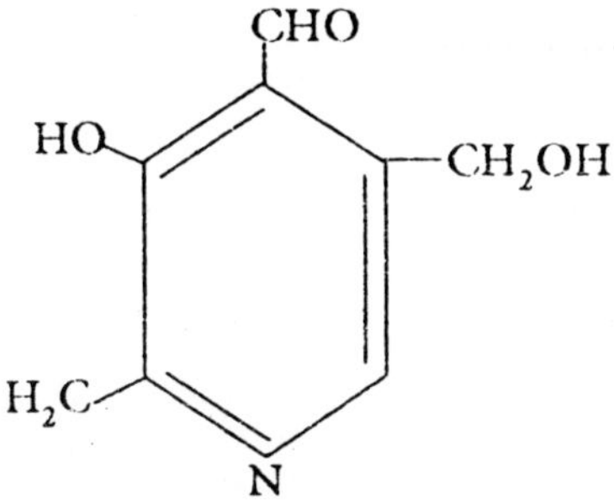

CHO HO CH_2OH H_2C N

PYRIDOXIN

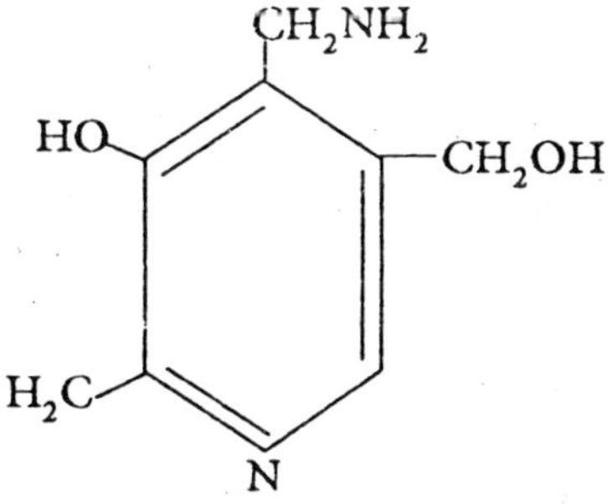

CH_2NH_2 HO CH_2OH H_2C N

PYRIDOXAMINE

Fig. 6.4 : Pyridoxin, Pyridoxal and Pyridoxamine Structures

phosphate act in several enzyme systems like transaminase system, aminocecid decarboxylase system, conversion of tryptophan to niacin, catabolism of threonine, serine and homoserine, converting D aminoacids to Amino acids, Porphyrin synthesis, formation of neurohormones, co-enzyme A synthesis etc. The deficiency of pyridoxal phosphate produced hypercholes terolemia and Oxaluria in experimental animals.

DAILY REQUIREMENTS

The recommended dietary allowances are given in Table 6.8. An average Indian diet supplies a minimum of 3.5 mg of vitamin B_6 daily.

ASSAY METHODS

The general methods employed for other B complex Vitamins are applicable to this method.

Table 6.8 : Recommended Dietary Allowances of Pyridoxin

	Group	Pyridoxine mg
Man	Sedentary work Moderate work Heavy work	2.0
Woman	Sedentary work Moderate work Heavy work	2.0
	Pregnancy (Second half)	+2.5
	Lactation:	
	0–6 months 6–12 months	2.0
Infants	0–6 months	0.1
	6–12 months	0.4
Children	1–3 years	0.9
	4–6 years	0.9
	7–9 years	1.6
Boys Girls	10–12 years 10–12 years	1.6
Boys Girls	13–15 years 13–15 years	2.0
Boys Girls	16–18 years 16–18 years	2.0

DEFICIENCY

Usually the deficiency of Vitamin B_6.is associated with deficiency of Vitamin B complex. Specific deficiency is produced in human beings and the symptoms were anorexia, nausea, hyperpigmentation, seborhoea, restlessness, lethargy and pellegra like changes in skin. Microcytic hypochromic anemia may be developed as pyridoxin as a decarboxylase is required in synthesis of Heme. Homocystinuria and cystathionuria occur due to impaired metabolism of methionine.

HYPERVITAMINOSIS

Pyridoxine in doses of 50—200 mg taken daily over two months did not produce any ill effects. Extremely high doses upto 6 g. daily may produce progressive sensory unsteadiness of gait and distal limb impairment These changes are reversible by stopping the intake of pyridoxin.

PANTOTHENIC ACID

Synonyms : Filterate factor, chick anti dermatitis factor.

HISTORY

Pantothenic acid derives its name from Greek word 'Pantothen' which means 'Everywhere'. It is also called filterate factor because when Riboflavin and Niacin were absorbed on fullers earths Pantothenic acid passed into the filterate. Absence of this factor produced human pellagra factor or chick antidermatitis factor. Pantothenic acid was isolated in 1938 by Dr. R. J. Williams and associates and was synthesized in 1940 by workers of Merck and Company.

SOURCES

This Vitamin is distributed throughout all animal tissues especially liver, kidneys, spleen, heart and adrenals. Egg yolk, yeast, rice polishings, wheal germ, legumes, peanut, leafy vegetables and milk are good sources.

CHEMISTRY

Pantothenic acid is α r dihydroxy β, β dimethyl-butyryl-β-alanide. It is a pseudopeptide formed by combination of a butyric acid derivative with alanine. It is a pale yellow coloured viscous oil, soluble in water. It can be cystalised as a potassium Orsodium or calcium salt. Commercially pantothenic acid is available as calcium panto thenate. Which when dissolved in water is slight sweet and stable. It destroys rapidly in acid or alkaline medium. It is heat resistant and can withstand autoclaving at 120°C for 30 minutes in a neutral solution. The structure of pantothenic acid is given in Figure 6.5.

$$\begin{array}{ccccccccccccc} H_2 & & CH_3 & & OH & & O & & H & & H_2 & & H_2 \\ | & & | & & | & & \| & & | & & | & & | \\ C & - & C & - & C & - & C & - & N & - & C & - & C - COOH \\ | & & | & & | & & & & & & & & \\ OH & & CH_3 & & H & & & & & & & & \end{array}$$

Fig. 6.5 : Pantothenic Acid Structure

METABOLISM AND FUNCTIONS

Pantothenic acid is mainly absorbed from intestines. Excess vitamin is excreted through urine. The urinary excretion is 3 mg a day. It is a component of a very important co-enzyme called co-enzyme A. Coenzyme A is a complex molecule consisting of a sulfur compound, aldenine, ribose, phosphoric acid and pantothenic acid. It is concerned with acetylation reactions. It plays a important role in metabolism of amino acids, synthesis of fatty acids and cholesterol, and formation of steroids. Liver kidney, brain, adrenal and heart are metabolically active and possess high concentrations of co-enzyme A.

DAILY REQUIREMENTS

The exact daily requirements are not known.

ASSAY METHODS

Physico-Chemical, biological and microbiological methods are available and these are similar to other B complex vitamins.

DEFICIENCY

Due to widespread occurrence of this vitamin in nature there is no clear cut demonstration of deficiency is reported. By feeding pantothenic acid antagonists to human beings (Volunteers) and the following symptoms were observed. Qnorexia, indigestion, abdominal pain, peripheral neuritis, insomnia, burning sensation of feet, respiratory infections and irritability.

HYPERVITAMINOSIS

No toxic effects are recorded either in human beings or animals even after giving excessive doses for prolonged periods. It may be because the vitamin is water soluble and excess is excreted in urine.

BIOTIN

Synonyms : Vitamin H, Anti egg white injury factor

HISTORY

In 1927, Boas reported that rats fed on a diet with raw egg white as protein source developed dermatitis, loss of fur especially around eyes, rapid weight los , paralysis of hind legs muscular incoordination and eventual cyanosis and death. The factor was called 'Anti egg white injury factor'. Gyorgy in 1931 gave this factor a name vitamin Hant or vitamin H where 'Hant' mean 'skin'. Kogl and Tonnis in 1936 isolated this factor from egg yolk. Later in 1940 Gyorgy et al identified that this vitamin is identical with a growth factor for yeast i.e. Biotin. The substance in raw egg white was identified as a glycoprotein that binds this biotin and makes it unavailable. It is called avidin which means hungry albumin. Cooking in activates this property.

SOURCES

Dry yeast, liver, milk, eggs, rice polishings, wheat germ, peanut, soyabean, oilseeds and nuts are good sources.

CHEMISTRY

Du Vigncand and colleagues, Gyorgy elucidated the chemistry and functions of Biotin. Harris et al synthesised this vitamin in 1943 44. The structure of Biotin is given in Fig. 6.6. Biotin is sparingly soluble in cold water and soluble in hot water. It is stable to heat, light and acids. It is slightly labile to alkalies and oxidizing agents. It is stable to autoclaving at 120°C for 30 min. in aqueous medium and neutral pH.

```
              O
              ||
              C
           /     \
        HN         NH
        |          |
        HC         NH
        |          |
       H2C         CH.CH2CH2CH2CH2COOH
           \     /
              S
```

Fig. 6.6 : Biotin

METABOLISM AND FUNCTIONS

Biotin is readily absorbed from intestines through portal vein into the circulation. This vitamin is synthesised by intestinal flora. Biotin is excreted in feces and urine.

Biotin acts as co-enzyme in several metabolic functions mainly involved in CO_2 transfer. It catalyses the conversion of acetyl COA to malonyl COA. It acts as co enzyme in the conversion of propionic acid to succinic acid. It catalyses conversion of pyruvate to oxaloacetate.

Biotin also catalyses the conversion of methyl crotonyl COA to omethyl glutaconyl COA. It is essential in the formation purines which are essential constituents of DNA and RNA. Biotin deficiency causes hyper keratosis, a canthosis and edema. Its deficiency causes paralysis of hind legs in experimental animals.

DAILY REQUIREMENTS

Recommended dietary allowance for biotin are not established as this vitamin is synthesised by intestinal flora also. About 100 to 300 micrograms of biotin is estimated as adequate allowance.

ASSAY METHODS

The usual methods used for the assay of other B complex vitamins can be used.

DEFICIENCY

Biotin deficiency does not occur in persons consuming normal diets. Induced deficiency is demonstrated when large amount of Raw egg white is consumed (about 60 egg whites) daily for a period of 10 weeks. From the third week scaly desqualmation, lassitude, muscle pain, hyperesthesia, pallor, anorexia and nausea were observed. All these abnormalities were cured within 5 days when 150 mg biotin is given daily.

HYPERVITAMINOSIS

Crystalline biotin when administered 1gm/kg body weight did not produce any harmful effect in experimental animals. It may be assumed that 200-300 mg of biotin can be administered parenterals to human beings for therapevtic purposes.

FOLIC ACID

Synonyms : Liver - casei factor, vitamin B, streptococcus Lactis R (SLR) factor, vitamin B_c, Norite eluate factor, Pteroylglutamic acid, folicin, factor U_1 Citrovorum factor.

HISTORY

Folic acid was known since 1933. It has several names as mentioned above. There names are given by different people for its curative effect in different deficiency states in man, monkey chick, guinea pig, rat and as growth promoting factor in micro organisms. Dr. Lucy wills described wills factor which cures tropical macrocytic anemia, factor essential for monkeys factor M, unknown factor required for chick growth as factor U, anti anemia factor for chicks as vitamin B_c, α-casei factor (Noriteeluate factor) essential for growth of L. Casei, and SLR factor essential for growth of many microorganisms. Shell, Mitchell and Williams reported the presence of this factor in leaves i.e. folic so it is called Folic acid. This vitamin is obtained in pure crystalline form and was also synthesized by the workers of lederle laboratories. Folic acid contains a pteridyl group and glutamic acid, so it is called pteroylglutamic acid also. It is essential for leuconostoc citrovorum so its is also called citrovorum factor.

SOURCES

Liver, yeast leafy vegetables, wheat germ, whole cereals and legumes are very good sources. Folic acid content of different foods is given in Table 6.9.

CHEMISTRY

Pure folic acid is bright yellow crystalline compound slightly soluble in water and is stable in PH5 and above even when heated up to 100°c. It is oxidised in acid medium and is sensitive to light. The structure of folic acid is given in Figure 6.7. It has pteridine group linked para-aminobenzoic acid to α-glutamic acid.

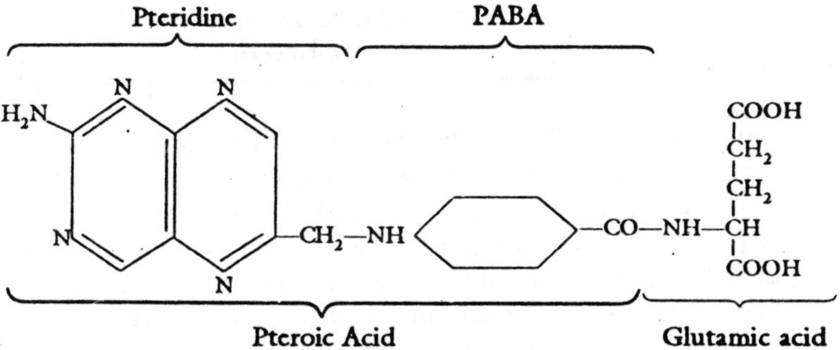

Fig. 6.7 : Folic Acid (Pteroyl Glutamic Acid or PGA) Structure

METABOLISM AND FUNCTIONS

Folic acid is readily absorbed from the intestine through portal vein to reach the general circulation. Folacin is stored principally in liver and

Table 6.9 : Free Folic Acid Content of Some Food Stuffs

Food Stuff	*Folic Acid* mg/100g	*Food Stuff*	*Folic Acid* mg/100g
Cereals and Cereal Products :		*Other Vegetables*	
Bajra	14.7	Cluster beans	50.0
Italian millet	4.2	Cucumber	12.6
Jowar	14.0	French beans	15.5
Maize dry	14.0	Kovai	18.0
Ragi	5.2	Ladies fingers	25.3
Rice raw milled	4.1	Snake gourd	7.5
Rice paraboiled milled	8.9	**Nuts and Oil Seeds :**	
Whole wheat	14.2	Conconut dry	15.3
Pulses and Legumes :		Gringelly seeds	51.0
Bengal gram Dal	32.0	Ground nut	16.0
Black gram dal	24.0	**Flesh Foods :**	
Cowpea	69.0	Ducks egg	80.0
Green gram dal	24.5	Hens egg	70.3
Peas	4.6	Fowl	3.2
Red gram dal	19.0	Liver goat	61.2
Soya bean	8.7	Liver sheep	65.6
Leafy Vegetables :		Mutton	1.0
Amarnath tender	41.0	**Milk and Milk Products :**	
Cabbage	13.3	Buffalo's milk	3.3
Curry leaves	23.5	Cow's milk	5.6
Mint	9.7	Curd	3.3
Spinach	51.0	**Miscellaneous :**	
		Dried yeast	150.0

is about 250 mg/100gms. The absorbed folacin undergoes several reactions to form coenzymes known as tetra hydrofolates which are linked to methyl, hydroxymethyl, formyl, and formimino groups. The ability to link up and to donate these single carbon units leads to the synthesis of methionine from homocysteine, formation of choline and synthesis of service etc. Folacin in essential for DNA synthesis. The importance of folacin in protein synthesis is well utilised in cancertherapy. Folacin inhibitors are used to inhibit tumor growth and cell prolifera-tion. Mean folate absorption from food is 50 percent. Table 6.10 shows availability of folates from some foods.

Table 6.10 : Availability of Folates from Some Foods

Food	*Total amount of food supplement (g)*	*Availability (mean %)*
Bengal gram	100	68.8
Green gram	200	55.2
Tomato	1000	37.2
Spinach	200	62.8
Banana	533–700	45.6
Hen's egg	300–500	72.4
Goat liver	100	70.0
Brewer's yeast	20	10.1

Ref: Babu S, Srikantia S G. Availability of folates from some foods Am J Clin Nutr 1976; 29 : 376–79.

DAILY REQUIREMENTS

Folic acid occurs in foods in two forms 1) Tetrahydrofolic acid and its derivatives and 2) folic acid conjugate. The folates represent the first group and the second group is bound. Total folate represents both. In human beings free folates are well absorbed and utilised then conjugate forms. The recommended daily allowances always represent free folate. The recommended dietary allowance of Nutrition expert group ICMR are given in Table 6.11.

Table 6.11 : Recommended Dietary Intakes of Folic Acid

	Group	*Folic Acid* mg
Man		100
Woman		100
	Pregnancy (Second half)	400
	Lactation	150
Children	1–18 years	100
Infants		25

ASSAY METHODS

Microbiological methods are employed usually. Lactobacillus and streptococcus fecalis are used.

DEFICIENCY

Deficiency of folic acid may occur due to deficiency intake Defective absorption or excessive demands. Defective absorption may occur in sprue and excessive demands include pregnancy, lactation, hemolytic anemia, drug therapy and infections. The deficiency of folic acid produces megaloblastic anemia. In which the number of circulating red blood cells decrease, the cells in circulation possess a large nucleus and low hemoglobin content. But the colour of blood is due to lowered leucocyte and platelet levels. Administration of folic acid brings dramatic recovery.

HYPERVITAMINOSIS

Therapeutic use of 5 to 20 mg orally does not produce any toxicity. Even intramuscular doses of 2 to 5 mg can be administered in severe cases of deficiency. These doses are well tolerated. Very highly doses should not be give as there is a danger of crystallization in kidney tubules causing renal injury, because the solubility of folic acid is low. This type of observation is made in experimental animals receiving 50 mg folic acid per kilogram of body weight.

VITAMIN B_{12}

Synonyms : Cobalamin, Cobamide; Antipernicious Anemia factor; Extrinsic factor of castle.

HISTORY

Minot and Murphy in 1926 announced that the fatal disease pernicious Anemia can be cured by giving large amounts of liver. It was only in 1948 two groups of workers Smith and Parker from Great Britain and Ricks etal from U.S.A. independently isolated the active principle. The structure of this factor was identified in 1955 and its synthesis was successful 25 years after isolation. Castle hypothesized that liver has an extrinsic factor which can be absorbed only in the presence of intrinsic factor of gastric secretion. So it was called extrinsic factor of castle. This vitamin has cyanidyl group and cobalt so is the name cobalamin.

SOURCES

Liver, kidney, meat, fish, brain, eggs are good sources. Vegetables does not contain this vitamin. It is exclusively of animal origin. Fresh milk, milk powder and cheese are fair sources. Vitamin B_{12} content in some foods is given in Table 6.12.

Table 6.12 : Vitamin B_{12} Content of Some Foods

Food Stuff	*Vitamin B_{12}* mg/100g
Shrimp	9.0
Egg hen	1.8
Goat meat	2.8
Goat liver	90.4
Sheep liver	91.9
Mutton	2.6
Buffalo milk	0.14
Cow's milk	0.4
Curd, Buffalo's milk	0.10
Curd, Cow's milk	0.13
Skim milk powder	0.83

CHEMISTRY

The structure of cobalamin is shown in the fig. It has a complicated structure with molecular weight of 1355 and empirical formula $C_{63}H_{90}O_{14}N_{14}PCO$. It is a red crystalline substance soluble aspects. It has four pyrrole rings three of which are linked by methylene bridges. The tetrapyrrole ring of cobalamin is called corring ring system. Instead of iron, cobalt atom is present in the centre. OH, NO_2, Cl or SO_4 may replace CN in which case it is called hydroxycobalamin, Nitrotio cobalamin, chloro cobalamin, sulfatocobalamin etc All these have the vitamin activity but it is less than cyanocobalamin.

METABOLISM AND FUNCTIONS

Vitamin B_{12} is unique and large molecule it needs special mechanism for its absorption. Intrinsic factor produced by parietal cells of stomach help in its absorption. This factor is nondialyzable, thermolabile when present in gastric juice. First vitamin B_{12} is separated from its polypeptide linkages with food by gastric acid and enzymes. Then it is bound to intrinsic factor. The complex thus formed bounds to the receptor sites in the ileum in the presence of calcium. Then vitamin B_{12}

is bound to a protein transcobalamin for transport into blood circulation.

Cobalamin is essential in conversion of cysteine into methionine. It acts as a coenzyme after combining with a adenosyl noiety that replaces the - CN group. It is essential for the isomerisation of glutamic acid to threo - methyl aspertare, conversion of methyl malonyl COA to succinyl COA and Ethylene glycol to acetaldehyde etc.

DAILY REQUIREMENTS

The recommended dietary allowances for vitamin B_{12} by different groups are given in Table 6.13.

Table 6.13 : Recommended Dietary Intakes of Vitamin B_{12}

	Group	*Vitamin B_{12}* g
Man		1
Woman		1
	Pregnancy (Second half)	1
	Lactation	1.5
Infants		0.2
Children	1–18 years	0.2–1.0

ASSAY METHODS

Microbiological methods are widely used for the assay of vitamin B_{12}. The growth response of microorganisms to standard vitamin and foodstuff is determined. Usually lactobacillus lactis, lactobacillus leichmanii, E-coli, Euglena Gracillis, and Ochromonas malhamensid are used. Ochrononan has specific requirements so it is advantageous than others.

DEFICIENCY

Deficiency of vitamin B_{12} may be produced due to

1. Lowered or lack of intake
2. Lack of intrinsic factor
3. Diseases like tuberculosis of intestines, sprue, enteritis etc.

The specific manifestations of vitamin B_{12} deficiency are hematological and neurological changes. Hematological changes include macrocytic anemia, megaloblasts in bone narrow and reduction of life span of RBC from 120 days to about 60 days. Neurological changes include degeneration of the lateral and posterior columns of spinalcord, peripheral neuropathy and occasionally mental changes like depression, psychosis and paranoia.

HYPERVITAMINOSIS

High doses such as 1000 g intramuscularly does not have any toxic effects.

CHOLINE

Best and Huntsman in 1934 discovered that choline deficiency produced fatty liver in rats. All living cells has choline a principle content in phospholipids such as phosphatidyl choline (cecithin). These phospholipids are present in nervous tissue and are essential for life processes.

Choline is hydroxyethyl trimethyl ammonium hydroxide. It structure is as follows.

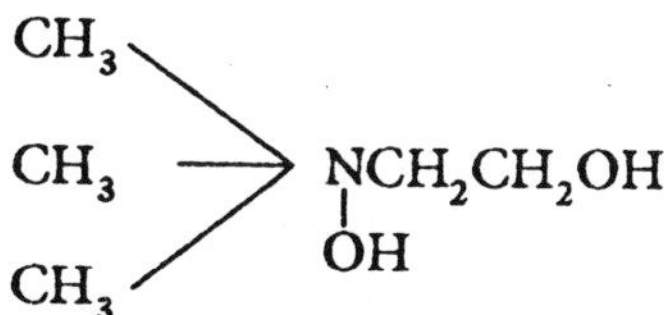

Fig. 6.8 : Structure of Choline

It is a hygroscopic colourless crystalline compound. It is a strong base soluble in water and alcohol. Choline is readily absorbed from the intestines and is converted to phospholipids and is converted to phospholipids and trimethylamine. The later is excreted in urine. Choline requirements are not known and deficiency is not likely to occur. Chemical and microbiological methods are employed in the assay of choline.

PARA AMINO BENZOIC ACID (PABA)

Ansbacher in 1941 reported that para amino benzoic acid is essential for growth in rats. It is an integral part of structure of folic acid. The chemical structure is as follows.

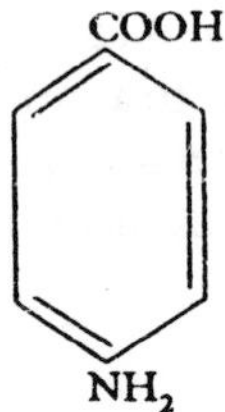

Fig. 6.9 : Structure of PABA

PABA is a crystalline substance soluble in water and alcohol. It is stable to heat in acid and neutral solution. This is absorbed from intestines and partially acetylated in liver. Excess intake of PABA is converted to paraamino hippuric acid which is excreted in urine. It has been reported that paramino benzoic acid inhibits the production of thyroid hormones and oxidative destruction of adrenaline in the tissues. Microbiological methods for assay of PABA are available. The requirements and deficiency of para-aminobenzoic acid are not known.

INOSITOL

Inositol also known as myoinositol or mesoinositol is a water soluble, sweet tasting substances. Inositol occurs in both plant and animal tissues. Inositol is have hydroxy cyclohexane which soluble in water and is stable to heat in neutral, acid and alkaline medium. The structure is as follows.

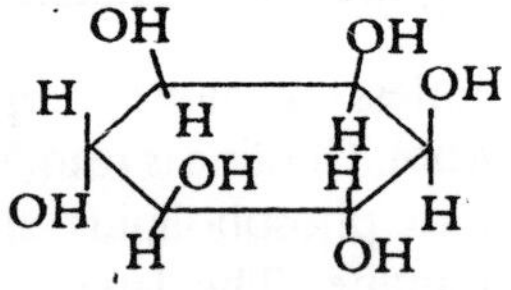

Fig. 6.10 : Structure of Inositol

As inositol is present in both plant and animal tissues deficiency does not occur and actual requirements are not known.

LIPOIC ACID

Reed etal in 1951 isolated lipoic acid, a crystalline compound from processed insoluble liver residues. It is also called thioctic acid and protogen. It is fat soluble and has the following structure :

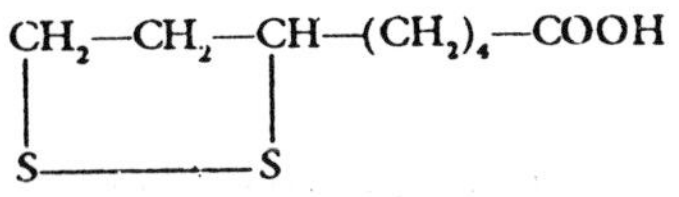

$$\begin{array}{l} CH_2-CH_2-CH-(CH_2)_4-COOH \\ | \qquad\qquad\quad | \\ S\text{————}S \end{array} \qquad \begin{array}{l} CH_2-CH_2-CH-(CH_2)_4-COOH \\ | \qquad\qquad\quad | \\ SH\text{————}SH \end{array}$$

Oxidised form of lipoic acid 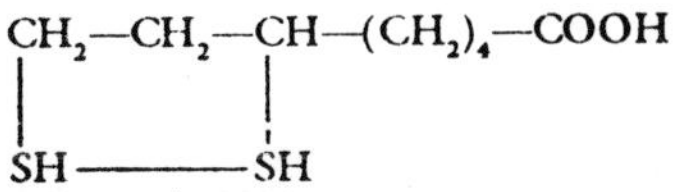 **Reduced form of lipoic acid**

Fig. 6.11 : Structure of Lipoic Acid

Lipoic acid need not be considered as a vitamin because it is not necessary in diet of animals. But a minute quantity in diet claimed to increase the growth rate. It functions in same manner as B complex vitamin do. It acts as a coenzyme along with thiamine pyrophosphate (TPP) in oxidative carboxylation of pyruvic acid.

VITAMIN P OR BIOFLAVANOIDS

In 1936 Szent -gyorgy prepared on a extract from paprika and lemon juice which parents capillary fragility in human beings and named the factor as vitamin P. This vitamin P is renamed as bioflavanoids in 1950. These are nothing but chemical substances comprised primarily of flavine and flavonoid compounds. The exert synergistic effect on vitamin c bioflavanoids are absorbed from intestines through portal vein and passes to the general circulation. Bioflavanoids controls capillary permeability, exerts inhibitory effect on the oxidation of adrenaline. The recommended daily allowance not known. The deficiency of bioflavanoids decrease capillarity resistance, causes petechial bleeding, pain in legs, lassitude and fatigue. Four doses of 200 mg orally did not produce any Toxic symptoms.

VITAMIN C

HISTORY

Scurvy was described as early as 1550 BC in history. In 1757 Dr. James Lind, a British naval surgeon gave the clear description of scurvy and he found that lemons and oranges are curative. Zilva carried much of pioneering work on isolation of vitamins C during 1917 and 1927. In 1928 Szent-Gyorgy isolated a factor from cabbage and adrenaldehd he named it Hexuronic acid which was later found to be identical with vitamin C. In 1932 Waught and King isolated Vitamin C in crystalline from lemon juice. Vitamin C is called Ascorbic acid due to its antiscorbutic properties.

SOURCES

Fresh Green vegetables and fruits are good sources of this vitamin. Dried fruits and vegetables have low values. As this vitamin is found only in fresh foods it is also called "fresh food vitamin" The amount of vitamins C in different food stuffs is given in the Table 6.14.

Table 6.14 : Vitamin C Content of Some Food Stuffs

Food Stuff	*Vitamin C* mg/100g	*Food Stuff*	*Vitamin C* mg/100g
Leafy Vegetables :		Giant Chillies	137
Amarnath tender	99	Knol Khol	85
Cabbage	124	Plantain	24
Coriander	135	**Fruits :**	
Drumstick Leaves	220	Amla	600
Fenu greek leaves	52	Banana	7
Gogu	20	Cashew fruit	180
Mint	27	Cherries	7
Spinach	28	Gawa (Country)	212
Roots and tubers		Lemom Juice	39
Beat root	10	Lemon sweet	45
Onion big	11	Lime	63
Potato	17	Lime Mausambi	50
Radish pink	17	Mango	16
Sweet Potato	24	Musk melon	26
Tapioca	25	Orange	30
Turnip	43	Orange juice	64
Other Vegetables		Papaya	57
Beans Scarlet	27	Pine apple	39
Bitter gourd	88	Pomo granate	16
Cauliflower	56	Seethaphal	37
Cluster beans	49	Tomato	27
Drumstick	120	Zizyphus	76

CHEMISTRY

Ascorbic acid is a white crystalline compound which has structural resemblance with hexoses. It is acidic to taste and is soluble in water. It is stable in acidic solutions and is rapidly destroyed in alkaline solutions, light, heat and oxidative enzymes. Copper and silver ions catalyses oxidation at this vitamin. The structure of vitamin C is as follows.

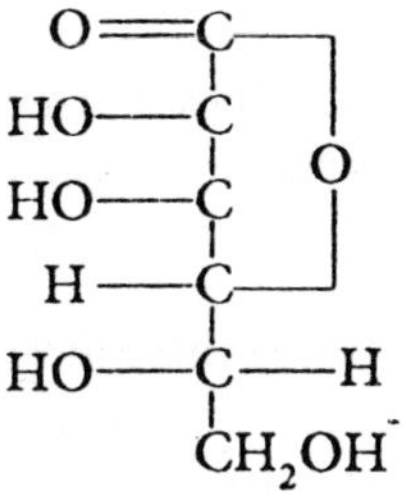

```
 O ══ C ────┐
      │     │
 HO ─ C     │
      │     O
 HO ─ C     │
      │     │
  H ─ C ────┘
      │
 HO ─ C ─ H
      │
      CH2OH
```

Fig. 6.12 : Ascorbic Acid Structure

METABOLISMS AND FUNCTIONS

Ascorbic acid is rapidly absorbed from the intestines. It is not stored in the body so the excess consumed is excreted in urine partly unchanged, partly as the diketogulonic acid and further break down products like oxalic acid. The formation of hydroxy proline from proline requires vitamin C. Hydroxyproline is an important amino acid in collagen. Ascorbic acid helps in the absorption of iron by converting the inorganic ferric iron to ferrous form. Adrenal cortex need this vitamin for its normal function. Vitamin C also helps in the biosynthesis of mucopolysaccharides, micro somal drug metabolism, leucocyte function and synthesis of anti inflammatory steroids by the adrenal gland.

DAILY REQUIREMENTS

As little as 10 mg of Ascorbic acid prevents scurvy. This is the minimum limit. Safe and adequate levels of Ascorbic acid requirement for different age groups is given in Table 6.15.

Table 6.15 : Recommended Dietary Allowances of Vitamin C

	Group	*Vitamin C* mg
Man		40
Woman		40
	Pregnancy (Second half)	40
	Lactation	80
Children	1–18 years	40
Infants		20

ASSAY METHODS

Physico-chemical and biological methods are available for the assay of Vitamin C.

Physico chemical methods are widely used for determining ascorbic acid in foodstuffs and animal tissues.

(a) Dye Method

The vitamin is first extracted using metaphosphoric acid or oxalic acid in order to stabilize the vitamin. Then its reducing action is measured using 2:6 dichlorophenol indophenol. In a modified method excess dye is added and the unreacted due is measured in a colorimeter.

(b) 2:4 Dinitropheny 1 hydrazine Method

Ascorbic acid given red colour with 2 : 4dinitrophenyl hydrazine. This colour is measured photometrically. Biological method is similar to that of B complex vitamins.

DEFICIENCY

Deficiency of ascorbic acid results in defective formation of intercellular substance, irritability, anemia, poor wound healing, joint pains and shortness of breath. These symptoms cannot establish the diagnosis.

SCURVY

In children pain, tenderness and swelling of thigh, loss of weight, fever, diarrhoea, swelling of gums which are tender and hemorrhagic are seen. Enlargement of ends of long bones is also seen as in rickets but tenderness is the distinguishing characteristic. In adults hemorrhagic spots on the skin, swelling, in section and bleeding gums, anemia and tenderness of legs is found. As the disease progresses trivial injury produces excessive bleeding and more hemorshages underneath the skin. 100 to 200 mg of vitamin C administration per day brings dramatic response.

HYPERVITAMINOSIS

Routine sue of large doses of vitamin C may cause gastro intestinal disturbances, destruction of Red blood cells, interference with anticoagulants, excessive absorption of Iron, formation of kidney stones in some persons because of increase in acidity of urine or increase in oxalates excretion which are breakdown products of the vitamin.

7

Macro-Elements

Minerals are those elements that remain as ash when plant or animal tissues are burned. Human body is composed of 65% oxygen, 18% carbon, 10% Hydrogen and 3% nitrogen. This accounts to 96% of body weight. The rest 4% comprises Minerals elements. Many minerals are associated with organic compounds of the body like homoglobin, phosphoproteins etc. Those occurring in appreciable amounts are called Macro elements and those found in minute amounts are called trace elements or micro elements. Calcium, phosphorus, sodium, potassium, sulphur, chlorine, Magnesium and Iron are found in appreciable amounts. Copper, Iodine, Manganese, cobalt, zinc, fluorine, Seleium are found in smaller quantities. Cadmium, boron, arsenic, Aluminium, Lead, Nickel, etc. are found in trace.

Minerals are present in all cells of the body. Soft tissues have higher proportion of potassium while hard tissue like bone has a relatively greater proportion of calcium and phosphorus. Mineral elements like Iron and copper are necessary for hemoglobin formation, Iodine for thyroxine formation, zinc for carbonic anhydrase, etc. Mineral elements regulate body fluid composition permeability of cell membranes, water balance, osmotic pressure, acid base balance, etc. Mineral elements have functional inter relationship between themselves as well as with vitamins. For example calcium and phosphorus are interrelated. Their absorption is dependent on vitamin D vitamin C is essential for Iron absorption.

CALCIUM

A New born baby has about 28 grams of calcium in its body while a adult has about 1200 grams. It institutes 2% of total body weight and 26% of the dry weight of bones and teeth. 99% of calcium is combined as the salts and is present in skeleton. The remaining 15 which is 10 to 12 grams is distributed in sift tissues, in tracellular and extra cellular fluids of the body the important function of calcium are:

1. It is essential for formation of bone and teeth
2. It catalyzes clotting of blood
3. It regulates contraction and relaxation of muscles, including heart muscle.
4. It regulates the permeability of capillary wall.
5. It is essential in synthesis of acetyl choline which is important in transmission of nerve impulsel.
6. It activates a number of enzymes like pancreatic lipase, ATP, etc.

CALCIUM CONTENT OF BLOOD

The serum calcium level is about long per 100 ml calcium is present in plasma but not in the red blood cells. Calcium in plasma occurs in three forms (i) ionised (ii) protein bound and (iii) complexed. About 60 percent of total serum calcium is in ionised form like citrate, phosphate and bicarbonate. Alkalosis reduces the level of ionisable calcium which leads to increased muscle irritability and tetany. On the other hand if the level of ionisable calcium level increases more than 10 mg it results in renal failure and cardiac arrest.

FACTORS REGULATING SERUM CALCIUM LEVEL

Parathyroid

Parathyroid mobilizes calcium and phosphorus from the bone to maintain blood calcium level. In Hyperparathyroidism re-absorption of minerals along with the mater occurs and a condition called osteitis fibrose cystica results. There may be formation of kidney stones without any changes in bone. Lowered intake of Calcium stimulates Parathyroid.

Calcitonin

Calcitonin is a hormone produced by C cells of thyroid gland. It helps in preventing calcium release from bones. Estrogen rises the Calcitonin levels and prevents bone loss. In Postmenopausal women Osteoporosis occurs due to reduction of calcitonin along with estrogen. So in their treatment Calcitonin Therapy is recommended than estrogen therapy.

Hyper Calcium

An increased serum calcium level is seen in Hypervitaminosis D. Large doses of Vitamin D results in excessive absorption of Calcium from the gastro intestinal tract and it also causes mobilization of Calcium from bones.

Hyper activity of the Parathyroid gland causes increased mobilization of Calcium from the bones which results in bending of long bones and compression of vertebrae which inturn reduces the height. When alkalies are given along with milk for treating peptic ulcers systemic alkalosis may occur.

Hyper calcium produces nausea, vomiting, anorexia, constipation associated with Pancreatitis and peptic ulcer. Treatment of hyper calcium is administration of saline and drugs which increase Calcium excretion by preventing kidney re-absorption of Calcium.

Hyper Calcium

Low serum Calcium levels occur in conditions like hypoparathyroidism, Vitamin D deficiency, hypothermia, gastric surgery etc. Retention of Phosphate or failure to acidify urine leads to systemic acidosis and loss of calcium. The motor nerves become over susceptible to stimuli. Particularly face, hands and feet show features of tetany.

Recommended Daily Allowances (RDA)

Nutrition expert group of Indian council for medical research suggested a daily allowance of 1.0 gram in case of growing children, pregnant and lactating women. Others need 0.4 to 0.6 grams of Calcium per day. Table 7.1 shows the Recommended daily allowance of calcium by Indians.

Dietary Sources of Calcium

The Calcium content of some typical foods is shown in Table : 7.2.

The important sources of Calcium are milk and Milk products.

Table 7.1 : Recommended Daily Allowance of Calcium by Indians

Group	Calcium (grams)
Man	0.4 – 0.5
Woman	0.4 – 0.5
Pregnancy	1.0
Lactation	1.0
Infants 0–12 months	0.5 – 0.6
Children:	
1 – 12 years	0.4 – 0.5
13 – 15 years	0.6 – 0.7
16 – 18 years	0.5 – 0.6

Table 7.2 : Calcium Content of Some Typical Food Stuffs

Food Stuff	Calcium mg/100g	Food Stuff	Calcium mg/100g
Cereals and Cereal Products :		*Other Vegetables*	
Barley	26	Beans	50
Italian millet	31	Cho Chomarrow	140
Jowar	25	Field beans	210
Maize Dry	10	Peas	20
Maize Tender	9	**Nuts and Oil Seeds :**	
Ragi	344	Almonds	230
Rice	10	Gingelly seeds	1450
Rice flakes	20	Mustard seeds	490
Wheat flour whole	48	**Fish and Other Sea Foods**	
Pulses and Legumes :		Bacha	520
Bengal gram whole	202	Bombay duck dry	1389
Black gram dal	154	Crab	1370
Green gram whole	124	Herring	429
Horse gram	287	Katla	530
Rajmah	260	Mackeral	429
Soyabean	240	Shark	357
Leafy Vegetables :		**Other Flesh Foods :**	
Amarnath	397	Egg	60
Coriander	184	Mutton	150
Curry leaves	830	Snail (Small)	1321
Fenugreek leaves	395	**Milk and Milk Products :**	
Mint	200	Milk	210
Roots and tubers :		Curd	149
Onion	47	Cheese	790
Potato	10	**Miscellaneous :**	
Sweet Potato	46	Jaggery	80
Tapioca	50	Brewers Yeast	440

Ragi, sesame seeds and green leafy vegetables are also good source of Calcium but the oxalates present may render Calcium inabsorbable. Consumption of small fish with bones would be a good source of Calcium.

Absorption

The absorption and retention of Calcium is dependent on Calcium intake, presence of interfering substances and presence of vitamin D. An acid reaction in gut aids in the absorption of Calcium when bile juice and Pancreatic juice mixes with the chyme the acid medium is lost and solubility of Calcium salts decreases.

Factors Enhancing Calcium Absorption

The 1:1 ratio of Calcium and Phosphorus in the diet aids in Calcium absorption. Vitamin D helps in the formation of vitamin D Calcium Translocates and thus absorption of Calcium is increased. Aminoacids also increases the absorption of Calcium. Lactose of milk ferments in intestines and forms Lactic acid. This Lactic acid, presence of ascorbic acid and acidic medium of aids in stomach solubility and absorption of Calcium.

Factors Interfering Calcium Absorption

Phytic acid is an inorganic form of Phosphorus present in the quterlayers of cereal grains. It binds Calcium to insoluble complexes. If Phytose an enzyme is present it splits phytic acid to inositol and Phosphate so absorption of calcium is not much impaired. Oxalic acid present in some leafy vegetables forms Calcium oxolate with Calcium and impairs Calcium absorption. When large amounts of free falty acids are present in the intestines as in Malabsorption syndrome. They combine with Calcium to form soaps. Which are insoluble. These are excreted in stools.

Loss of Calcium

The unabsorbed Calcium is excreted through the stools. Some amount form the digestive juices, worn out tissues, etc., also add upto the unabsorbed Calcium. About 800 mg per day is excreted in stools. The unutilised fraction from the absorbed Calcium is excreted in urine which accounts to 50-200 mg per day. In Tropical countries considerable losss of Calcium accurs through sweat. When the intake of Calcium is Zero also excretion of calcium takes place. This is called endogenous loss of Calcium which is about 150 to 300 mg per day in adults.

Effect of Calcium Deficiency

Calcium deficiency in children produces decreased growth rate, Negative Calcium balance of calcium from bones Hyperparathyroidism and tetany in children. In adults osteoporosis occurs. It is characterized by decalcification of bones, Fractures, brittle bones, pain and delayed healing of fractures.

Effect of Excess of Calcium

Hyper calcium or increased blood calcium shows excess deposition of calcium in soft tissues and increased calcium excretion. Vomiting, gastro intestinal bleeding, increase in Blood Pressure, Anorexia, indigestion, etc., are also observed in Hyper Calcium Patients.

PHOSPHORUS

Phosphorus accounts for about 1 percent of body weight of this 80-85 percent is in combination with Calcium in insoluble form of bones and teeth. Soft tissues have more phosphorus than Calcium. Organic phosphorus is present in Phospholipids, Nucleoroteins, Hexosephosphates, creative phosphate, ATP, ADP, glycerophosphates etc.

The important functions of Phosphorus are:

1. Phosphorus is very essential for the formation of bone and teeth.
2. Phosphorus forms the linkage in DNA and RNA.
3. It is a constituent of certain co-enzymes.
4. Phospholipids are found in cell membranes and regulates the transport of solutes in and out.
5 In many metabolic processes phosphorylation plays a very important role.
6. Inorganic phosphates in the body act as important constituents in body's buffer system and maintain the neutrality.

Phosphorus Content of Blood

The inorganic phosphorus content of blood is 3 to 4 mg per 100 ml serum and 4 to 5 mg 100 ml serum in children. Usually it goes below 3 mg per 100 ml in Rickets. Phosphorus is widely distributed in foods so deficiency is not observed frequently.

Recommended Daily Allowance

The phosphorus requirement is almost same as calcium. The calcium and phosphorus ratio should be 1:1 in children and 1:2 for adults.

Dietary Sources of Phosphorus

Phosphorus is widely distributed in foods. Milk, eggs, meat fish, peanuts etc. are good sources of phosphorus. While vegetables and fruits are fair sources. The phosphorus content of some foods is given in Table 7.3.

Table 7.3 : Phosphorus Content of Some Foods

Food Stuff	*Phosphorus* mg/100g	*Food Stuff*	*Phosphorus* mg/100g
Cereals and Cereal Products :		Drumstick	110
Barley	215	Peas	130
Italian millet	290	**Nuts and Oil Seeds :**	
Jowar	222	Almonds	490
Ragi	283	Cashewnuts	450
Rice	160	Coconut	240
Wheat	306	Gingelly seeds	570
Pulses and Legumes :		Ground nut	350
Bengal gram	312	Mustard	700
Black gram	385	**Fish and Other Sea Foods :**	
Green gram	405	Bacha	180
Red gram	304	Bombay duck	240
Rajmah	410	Cat fish	230
Leafy Vegetables :		Herring	305
Amarnath	83	Hilsa	280
Coriander	71	Shark	262
Mint	62	**Other Flesh Foods :**	
Roots and Tubers		Egg	220
Beet root	55	Fowl	245
Carrot	530	Goat liver	279
Colocasia	140	Mutton	150
Onion	50	Snail	147
Potato	40	**Milk and Milk Products :**	
Sweet Potato	50	Buffalo's Milk	130
Other Vegetables		Cow's Milk	90
Beans	160	Cheese	520

Absorption

About 70 percent of dietary phosphorus is normally absorbed in the form of inorganic phosphates. Organic forms of phosphorous should be hydrolysed to inorganic forms before absorption. Phosphatase enzyme hydrolyses Phosphorus esters and released free phosphorous. This when combines with calcium forms insoluble calcium phosphate and is not absorbed. The unabsorbed phosphorus is excreted through urine. Almost all foods have phosphorus so deficiency of phosphorus is rare.

MAGNESIUM

Magnesium is the second most abundant intracellular cation in the body. 60-65 percent is present at the surface of the bone, 2 percent in extra cellular fluids and 34 percent in the intracellular space. Normally blood cerium has 2 to 3 mg percent. The functions of Magnesium are:

1. Magnesium acts as activator in several enzymes.
2. Magnesium together with sodium potassium and calcium maintains fluid balance.
3. Magnesium is found in some enzymes like co-carboxylase
4. Magnesium is co-factor for oxidative phosphorylation

Recommended Daily Allowance

Magnesium requirement for different age groups are as follows:

Infants and children	100–150 mg per day
Adolescents -	150–250 mg per day
Adults -	250–350 mg per day

Dietary Sources of Magnesium

Whole grain cereals, dairy products, bananas and leafy vegetables are good sources of magnesium. The Magnesium content of different foods is given in Table 7.4

Absorption

Magnesium is absorbed by active transport. Magnesium competes with calcium for carrier sites. Factors that enhance or inhibit calcium absorption also effect the absorption of magnesium. But vitamin D and parathyroid has no effect. Excretion of Magnesium is under the control

Table 7.4 : Magnesium Content of Different Foods

Food Stuff	*Magnesium* mg/100g	*Food Stuff*	*Magnesium* mg/100g
Cereals and Cereal Products :		***Roots and Tubers***	
Jowar	170	Carrot	17
Maize dry	139	Potato	30
Ragi	137	Pink Radish	196
Rice	90	***Other Vegetables***	
Rice flakes	101	Broad beans	33
Wheat	138	Cauliflower	20
Pulses and Legumes :		Peas	34
Bengal gram	168	Snake gourd	28
Black gram dal	155	Chillies fresh	272
Cowpea	210	**Fruits :**	
Green gram dal	122	Banana	44
Red gram dal	90	Jack fruit	27
Peas dry	100	Jambu fruit	35
Leafy Vegetables :		Mango	270
Amarnath	122	Musk melon	31
Cabbage	30	Water Melon	13
Coriander	31	Papaya	11
Curry Leaves	44	Pine apple	30
		Sapota	26
		Seetaphal	88

of kidneys. Potent diuretics high serum magnesium, high serum calcium increases urinary excretion of Magnesium, about 50 percent of the ingested magnesium is excreted.

Deficiency of Magnesium

Chromic alcoholism, cirrhosis of liver, sprue, severe vomiting, diabetic acidosis, therapy etc. cause Magnesium deficiency. Muscle tremor, nervous irritability, upset in muscle contraction and convulsions are the symptoms found in Magnesium deficiency. When increased absorption of Magnesium or reduced urinary excretion persists High blood magnesium levels occur. Extreme thirst, excessive warmth feeling, atrial fibrillation are the symptoms.

SODIUM

Salt has a unique position in human history. Salt was used as medium of exchange and so the word saltary is used even today. Body has about 92 grams of sodium or 235 grams of sodium chloride. Serium has about 142 mg/1 (1 gram= 43.5 mg/1) About 50 percent of body's sodium is present in extracellular fluid, 40 per cent in bone and 10 percent in intracellular fluid. In terms of concentration sodium content in plasma is about thirteen times that of intracellular fluid. Sodium content in gastrointestinal secretions is given in Table 7.5.

Table 7.5 : Sodium Content in Gastro Intestinal Secretions*

	Volume (ml) in 24 hours	*Sodium meg/1*
Saliva	1000	50
Gastric Juice	1000 – 2500	80
Pancreatic juice	500 – 1000	140
Bile juice	500 – 1000	100
Small bowel drainage	1000 – 3500	110
Distal ileumce-cum-drainage	1000 – 3000	80
Normal stool	100	50
Diarrhoea	500 – 15000	120

* Clibon U, Barriers SL. Enteric infections: Shigellosis and Salmonellasis J. Am. Pharmacent Assoc 1977; NS 117:80-87

The function of Sodium in our body are:

1. It maintains the normal osmotic pressure and water balance
2. It maintains the acid base balance of the body
3. It maintains the normal irritability of nerves and muscle contraction.

Recommended Daily Allowance

An average intake of sodium is 3–4 grams (7.5–10 grams of sodium chloride) a day can be easily supplied in a normal diet. In Tropical countries the requirement is more. When there is sweating, increased excretion of urine, vomiting, diarrhoea, etc., loss of water from the body takes place along with which sodium is also lost. So the exact requirement of sodium is not known. In Normal condition a normal man takes in about 5 to 20 grams of table salt which supplies about 70-350 meq of sodium. The sodium requirement is given in the form of sodim chloride requirement is given in Table: 7.6 because it is the only meneral which is taken in more or less pure form in addition to the naturally present amounts in food.

Table 7.6 : Sodium Chloride Requirement of Normal Persons

	Sodium chloride gms/day
Children	5
Adolescents	10–15
Adults	10–25

Dietary Sources of Sodium

The Principle source of sodium is sodium chloride. Natural sources of sodium are egg white, meant, fish, poultry, milk spinach, beet root, etc. Other vegetables, fruits and cereals are poor sources of sodium. The sodium content of various foods is given in Table 7.7.

Absorption

The absorption of sodium is almost complete and is very rapid. Kidneys regulate the sodium level in the body. When there is higher intake higher amounts are excreted and when there is lower intake lower amounts are excreted. When there is drastic restriction of sodium in the diet the urine has very very low or almsot nil excretion of sodium. The loss of sodium in sweat depends directly on the volume of sweat.

Hyponatremia

Depletion of serum sodium below 130 mg/litre is called Hyponatremia. Hyponatremia is caused due to (1) Prolonged vomiting and diarrhoea. (2) Poor re-absorption of sodium (3) Adreno cortical deficiency. (4) Diets poor in sodium (5) Starvation. The symptoms of sodium depletion are weakness, nausea, giddiness, lethargy, muscle cramps and circulatory failure if the depletion is severe. Usually Hyponatremia occurs along with dethydration. Because of dehydration volume of blood decreases and Red cell concentration increases. When the volume of blood decreases the blood vessels contract, Blood pressure decreases and pulse rate increases. Mental apathy, twitchings, convul-

Table 7.7 : Sodium Content of Some Foods

Food Stuff	*Sodium* mg/100g	*Food Stuff*	*Sodium* mg/100g
Cereals and Cereal Products :		Pink radish	63.5
Barley	16.1	Sweet Potato	9.0
Jowar	7.3	***Other Vegetables***	
Maize dry	15.9	Cauliflower	53.0
Rice flakes	10.9	Field beans	55.4
Raagi	11.0	Knol-khol	112.0
Wheat	17.1	Snake gourd	25.4
Pulses and Legumes :		**Fruits :**	
Bengal gram dal	73.2	Musk Melon	104.6
Black gram dal	39.8	Pine apple	34.7
Green gram dal	27.2	**Fish and other Sea Foods :**	
Red gram dal	28.5	Hilsa	52.0
Leafy Vegetables :		Katla	50.0
Amarnath	230.0	Prawn	66.0
Cabbage	14.1	Rohu	101.0
Coriander leaves	58.3	**Other Flesh Foods :**	
Fenugreek leaves	76.1	Goat liver	73.0
Spinach	58.5	Mutton	33.0
Roots and Tubers		**Milk and Milk Products :**	
Beet root	59.8	Buffalo's milk	19.0
Carrot	35.6	Cow's milk	76.0
Onion	4.0	Curds	32.0

sions and come are also seen. Oral feeds of 100–20ml fluid with salt should be given every two hours if the patient is able to drink and if he excretes about 1000 ml of urine a day. If the patient is unable to drink nasogastic feeds should be given. If both oral and nasogastic feeds are not feasible i.e. if the patient is vomiting a rectal drip can be given. In this method 1000ml of boiled drinking water with 5 grams of sodium chloride at room temperature can be given. The drip should be regulated at 15–20 drops a minute. Before starting rectal drip fecal matter should be evacuated from the bowel. The amount of saline should be in accordance with the amount of loss. In severe cases intravenous isotonic saline infusion should be given under medical supervision. Very vigorous treatment for low sodium is dangerous.

Hypernatremia

This is a condition where in sodium content of the body is more than normal i.e. serum sodium above 150 mg/litre. Causes for hypernatremia are (1) decreased water intake (2) increased sodium intake (3) deficient sodium excretion (4) Hyper activity of adrenal cortex as in cushings syndrome (5) Prolonged treatment with sex hormones, ACTH and Cortisone. The symptoms of hypernatremia are accumulation of water in the body is edema, increase in blood volume and increase in blood pressure.

CHLORIDE

Chloride exists as chloride in the body. About 100 gm is present in extracellular fluid. Chloride is very important in regulating osmotic pressure, water balance and acid base balance. The absorption and excretion of chloride is same as sodium. Chloride accompanies sodium and potassium. Chloride intake and deficiency parallels that of sodium.

POTASSIUM

Potassium is present in large amounts in all cells. It is present in smaller amount in extracellular fluid. It is about 250 grams as a whole in a adult man. Normally 20mg is present per every 100 ml of serum. Of the total 250 grams in the body 243 grams is present in the cells and 7 grams in the extracellular compartment. Potassium content in various gastro intestinal secretions are given in Table : 7.8.

Table 7.8 : Potassium Content in Gastrointestinal Secretions*

	Volume (ml) in 24 hours	*Potassium meg/l*
Saliva	100	20
Gastric Juice	1000 – 2500	15
Pancreatic juice	500 – 1000	5
Bile juice	500 – 1000	5
Small bowel drainage	1000 – 3500	5
Distal leumce-cum-drainage	1000 – 3000	8
Normal stool	100	25
Diarrhoea	500 – 15000	25

* Clibon U, Barrier SL, Enteri infections. Shigellosis and Salmonellosis J. AM. Pharmacent. Assoc 1977; NS 17: 80-87.

Functions of Potassium are:

1. It helps in maintaining acid base balance of the body
2. Potassium is very essential for synthesis of Glycogen
3. It is concerned with irritability of Nerves and all muscle
4. It is essential in growth and building of tissues.

Recommended Daily Allowance

Normal adults require about 2.5 to 4 grams of potassium. Infant need 0.5 – 1 gram and children need 0.6 to 4 grams of potassium daily depending on their age.

Dietary Sources of Potassium

Potassium is widely distributed in foods. Cereals, dried fruits, meats, fish and vegetables are good sources. Table 7.9 gives the Potassium content in different foods. The Potassium content in a cup of coconut water is 351 milli grams.

Absorption

Potassium is rapidly absorbed from the Gastro intestinal trac Though the digestive juice have a lot of potassium it is reabsorbed. The fecal loss of potassium is very low. When protein synthesis, glycogen formation and cellular hydration are in process potassium is rapidly removed from the circulation. When protein catabolism, dehydration or glycogenolysis are in progress potassium comes out of the cells. Excess of potassium ingested in excreted through urine. The kidney has a ability to conserve potassium in deficit is not as rigid as of sodium. Even when the intake of potassium is very low or zero kidney excretes about 20 mg per day.

Retention of Potassium

About 117 mg of potassium is retained with every 6.25 grams of muscle protein and for every one gram of glycogen stored in liver 14 mg of potassium is retained. When diabetic coma is treated with insulin and glucose, glycogen is rapidly formed in the liver. During this process potassium from the extracellular fluid is drawn and stored along with glycogen in the above mentioned ratio During this process severe hypokalimia occurs which may be fatal.

Hypokalimia

Deficiency of potassium in the body occurs due to (1) Deficient in

Table 7.9 : Potassium Content of Some Food Stuff

Food Stuff	*Potassium* mg/100g	*Food Stuff*	*Potassium* mg/100g
Cereals and Cereal Products :		*Other Vegetables*	
Bajra	307	Brinjal	200
Barley	253	Cauliflower	138
Italian millet	250	Drumstick	259
Maize dry	286	Papaya green	216
Ragi	408	Plantain	193
Rice	70	Sword beans	1800
Rice flakes	154	**Fruits :**	
Wheat flour	315	Amla	225
Pulses and Legumes :		Apricots	430
Bengal gram (Whole)	808	Cherries red	320
Black gram dal	800	Sweet lime	490
Cowpea	1131	Mango	205
Green gram dal	1150	Musk melon	341
Red gram dal	1104	Water melon	160
Leafy Vegetables :		Sapota	269
Amarnath	341	Seetaphal	340
Cabbage	114	**Fish and other Sea Foods :**	
Coriander	256	Hilsa	183
Spinach	206	Kotla	151
Roots and Tubers		Prawn	262
Carrot	108	Rohu	288
Colocasia l	550	Goat liver	160
Onion	127	Mutton	270
Potato	247	**Milk and Milk Products :**	
White radish	138	Buffalo's milk	90
Sweet Potato	393	Cow's milk	140
		Curds	130

take (2) Excessive loss from Gastrointestinal tract (3) diabetic acidosis (4) use of diureties (5) use of purgatives (6) Familial periodic paralysis (7) Over activity of adrenal cortex. (8) Use of steroids (9) Treatment of cardiac failure with digitalis (10) villous tumours of large intestine secrete mucus of high potassium concentration.

In Hypokalemic condition nausea, vomiting, hypotension, tachycardia, arrythmia, muscle weakness, electro cardiogram alternations paralytic ileus, etc., are seen. Heart may stop in diastole. A reliable serum potassium level cannot be measured by electrocardiogram. This situation can be corrected by administering fruit juices or commercial oral preparations orally or through nasogastic tube or intravenous depending on the patients condition. A concentrated solution of potassium stops the heart so it should not be given to the patient.

Hyperkalimia

High serum potassium level is called Hyperkalimia. It may result due to renal failure, rapid intravenous potassium transfusion and adrenal insufficiency. It is characterized by .brady cardia, peripheral vascular collapse, Anorexia, weakness of muscles, general apathy, paresthesias of scalp, face, tongue and extremities, poor respiration and cardiac failure may follow. Cardiac failure occur in systole. It can be treated by administering low potassium low protein, high carbohydrate diets. The high carbohydrate diet helps in formation of glycogen and movement of potassium into the cells. In acute cases glucose in administered intravenously along with insulin.

SULPHUR

Sulphur occupies 0.25 percent of body weight. It is present in all cells of the body. Connective tissue, nails, hair and skin are rich in sulphur. Thiamin, biotin, and aminoacids like cystine, cysteine and Methionine contain sulphur. A diet that fulfills body's need for sulphur containing aminoacids satisfies body's sulphur needs. Sulphur is absorbed completely from the intestinal tract. Sulphur is very essential in oxidation reduction reactions Table 7.10 gives the sulphur content in various foodstuffs.

IRON

Iron is a vital component of hemoglobin with transports oxygen to various tissues of the body. Life without iron is not possible for human beings. Except lactic acid bacteria all living organisms require iron for their life. Iron is present in Hemoglobin, Hyoglobin, cytochromes,

Table 7.10 : Sulphur Content of Some Food Stuff

Food Stuff	*Sulphur* mg/100g	*Food Stuff*	*Sulphur* mg/100g
Cereals and Cereal Products :		**Leafy Vegetables :**	
Bajra	147	Amarnath	61
Italian millet	171	Curry leaves	81
Ragi	160	Fenugreek leaves	167
Maize dry	114	Drumstick leaves	137
Rice	50	***Roots and Tubers***	
Rice flakes	105	Beetroot	14
Wehat whole	128	Carrot	27
Pulses and Legumes :		Potato	37
Bengal gram whole	179	Pink radish	31
Black gram dal	174	***Other Vegetables***	
Cowpea	165	Broad beans	53
Green gram dal	214	Cauliflower	231
Peas	189	Drumstick	137
Red gram dal	177	Knol Khol	143

catalase, peroxides, other enzyme systems, etc. Most of the iron in our body exists in complex forms bound to protein as porphyrin or heme or ferritin and transferrin. Hemoproteins and flavoprotein enzymes also possess Iron. The functions of Iron are :

(1) It is present in Hemoglobin which is essential for oxygen carriage.

(2) Cytochromes play a very important role in respiratory chain.

(3) Flavoproteins Zymes are essential for oxidation of several met.

(4) Catalase catalyses the decomposition of H_2O_2 formed in tissues to H_2O and O_2

(5) Myoglobin is a iron protei complex of the muscle which scores some oxygen for the immediate use by the cell.

The cor :entration of Iron fractions in Males and females with optimal body iron stores is given in Table 7.11.

Table 7.11 : Concentration of Iron Fractions in Normal Males and Females

Iron fraction	*Males*		*Females*	
	mg	Percent pool	mg	Percent pool
1. ***Functional Iron Compounds***				
a) Heme Compounds				
i) Hemoglobin	2766	66.00	2183	62.00
ii) Myoglobin	188	4.50	157	4.50
b) Heme enzymes	8	0.19	7	0.19
c) Non-Heme enzymes	420	10	360	10
d) Transport iron	7	0.17	5	0.14
2. ***Storage Iron Compounds***				
Ferritin	800	19	800	23
Total	4189	100	3513	100

Recommended Daily Allowance

Iron requirement depends on the availability of iron from the diet. Iron from vegetable origin is, not completely absorbed due to the presence of phytates and oxalates. Iron from Animal foods is easily absorbed. Iron requirement of various groups is given in Table 7.12.

Table 7.12 : Recommended Daily Allowance of Iron in Various Groups

Group	*Iron Requirement* mg
Man	28
Woman	32
Pregnancy	40
Lactation	32
Infants 0–12 months	1 mg/kg
Children 1–9 years	20–25
Boys 10–12 years	30–35
Girls 10–12 years	30–35
Boys 13–18 years	45
Girls 13–18 years	30

Dietary Sources of Iron

Cereals are the sources of iron in majority of population in India. Legumes, leafy vegetables, Jaggery are other sources. Animal foods like Meat, fish and eggs are good sources. Iron content of some foods is given in table 7.13. The Iron from vegetable origin may be poorly absorbed because of high phosphate content. Though Iron in spinach is high it is not absorbed completely. When foods are cooked in Iron vessels the iron content of the dish was observed to increase and thus the intakc is increased. Presence of vitamin c enhances the absorption rate.

Absorption

Iron is absorbed in ferrous state only. Normal 10 percent of the ingested iron is absorbed. But in patients with iron deficiency it may be absorbed upto 25 percent. Iron is absorbed from duodenum and Jejunum. Acidic medium helps in absorption of Iron white presence of phytetes trannins reduce the absorption. Presence of vitamin C amino acid cysteine, enhances the absorption of iron from the food. Heme present in Animal foods is absorbed to an extent of 60-70 percent. Its absorption is independent of the presence of Ascorbic acid. Non heme iron is the iron from vegetable origin and its absorption is enhanced in the presence of ascorbic acid. Absorption of iron is impaired in achlorhydria or Hypochlorohydria. Phytic acid and oxidic acid forms an unabsorbable complex with Iron and impair its absorption. Fecal iron is mostly unabsorbed dietary iron, sweat, desquamation, menstrual loss, etc., also account to the Iron loss from the body.

Iron Deficiency

Iron deficiency causes Anemia which is widely prevalent among adolescent girls, expectant and nursing mothers, women and children The oxygen carrying capacity is reduced due to low hemoglobin levels. Pallor, rapid exhaustion, weakness, anorexia, lassitude, difficulty in concentrating, headache, palpitations, loss of libido, craving for unnatural foods, decreased resistance to infection, dyspnoea on excertion, etc., are symptoms of iron deficiency Anemia.

Excess of Iron

Siderosis is the term used to describe excess of iron in the body. Hemosiderin stores the iron which is not available to the body. Excess intake of Iron or abnormally high absorption of iron from the intestine causes siderosis. It is chiefly deposited in liver, spleen, pancreas etc. which causes cirrhosis of liver, grey discolouration of skin, etc

Table 7.13 : Iron Content of Some Food Stuff

Food Stuff	*Iron* mg/100g	*Food Stuff*	*Iron* mg/100g
Cereals and Cereal Products :		***Other Vegetables***	
Bajra	8.0	Beans scarlet runner	2.6
Italian millet	2.9	Bitter gourd	2.0
Jowar	5.8	Cauliflower	1.2
Ragi	3.9	Cluster beans	1.2
Rice	3.1	Drumstick	0.9
Rice flakes	20.0	Onion Stalks	7.5
Puffed rice	6.6	Peas	1.5
Whole wheat flour	4.9	**Nuts and Oil Seeds :**	
Pulses and Legumes :		Almond	5.1
Bengal gram whole	4.6	Cashew	5.9
Black gram dal	3.8	Gingelly seeds	9.3
Green gram dal	3.9	Mustard seeds	7.9
Horse gram	6.8	**Fruits :**	
Red gram dal	2.8	Lemon	0.3
Soya bean	10.5	Water Melon	7.9
Leafy Vegetables :		Raisans	7.7
Amarnath spined	22.9	Sapota	2.3
Amarnath tender	3.5	Seetaphal	4.3
Cabbage	0.8	Strawberry	1.8
Cauliflower greens	40.0	**Fish and other Sea Foods :**	
Coriander leaves	18.5	Bacha	0.7
Curry leaves	20.0	Bombay duck (dry)	19.1
Fenugreek leaves	1.9	Crab (Muscle)	21.2
Gogu	2.3	Fishmeal	22.6
Mint	15.6	Herring	9.3
Spinach	1.14	Hilsa	2.1
Roots and Tubers		Mackerel	4.5
Beet root	1.2	Prawn	5.3
Carrot	1.0	**Other Flesh Foods :**	
Onion	0.7	Hens egg	2.1
Potato	0.5	Ducks egg	2.5
Sweet Potato	0.5	Liver (Sheep)	6.3
Tapioca	0.9	Mutton	2.5

8

Micro-Elements

Many elements occur in tissues and foods in small quantities. Hence these are called Micro Elements. These include Iodine, Copper, Zinc, Fluorine, Manganese, Cobalt Molybdenum, Selenium, Chromium, etc.

IODINE

Iodine is the essential constituent of the hormone thyroxine produced by Thyroid. Seaweeds were used in the treatment of goitre for centuries. In 1811 Courtois discovered iodine in the ash of seaweeds. Prout in 1855 introduced Potessiumhypo iodate in the treatment of Goitre. It was only in 1820 Coindet began using iodide in treatment of goitre. Chatim, in 1850, Bussin Gault in 1860, Baumenn in 1895, Kendell in 1914 and Fellenberg in 1923 helped in understanding iodine's role in curing goitre. Marine and Kimball in 1920 administered sodium iodide in school children diet and were able to cure Goitre. Charles Harrington in 1922 found the Chemical structure of thyroxine.

About 20 to 30 mg of iodine is present in thyroid gland in the form of Thyroglobulin. It is 2500 times greater than other tissues. Thyroid secretes about 100 micrograms of thyroid. Tyrosine an aminoacid incorporates four iodine atoms to form thyroxine. Serum protein binds 4 – 8 micrograms of iodine for every 100 milli liters.

Recommended Daily Allowance

It was Fellenberg who first gave the human requirement of iodine as 20 micrograms. This was suggested by comparing the iodine intake in both goitrogenous and non goitrogenous areas. Later in 1969 health and social security council recommended 150 micrograms. The mean recommended daily allowance is 75 - 150 micrograms. Puberty, menstruation, pregnancy, old age, cold weather increases iodine requirement.

Dietary Sources of Iodine

Foods of Marine origin are rich in iodine. Iodine is unevenly distributed through the soil and water. So the plants grown in the iodine bearing soil has iodine in it, the water in that region has iodine and the animals and human beings who consume the plants and water receives iodine. If iodine is not present in the water or foodstuffs it has to be supplied through iodised salt. Some foods have antithyroid effect also. The iodine content of various food is given in Table 8.1 The iodine content of plant foods depend upon on the iodine content of soil and in case of animal origin foods, it depends on iodine intake of the feed given to the animals.

Table 8.1 : Iodine Content of Foods

Food stuff	*Iodine Content Microgram/kg.*
Sea foods	300 – 3000
Fresh water fish	20 – 40
Fresh fruits	10 – 20
Fresh Vegetables (Except Spinach)	10 – 50
Spinach	200
Cereal grains	20 – 40
Meats	20 – 40
Milk	20 – 40
Eggs	90
Sea Salt	1 – 10
Iodized Table Salt	76000

Fletcher D. Dietary sources of iodine: an unlikely cause of allergic reactions. JAMA 1978, 239; 57

Absorption

Iodine ingested as organic iodine from foods is first reduced to in organic iodine. This iodine is transported by the circulation as free iodine and protein bound iodine. The circulating iodine is trapped by the thyroid gland. This iodine combines with tyrosine and forms mono ioditymsine. Two moniodityrasine molecules combine to form tetraiodine thyronine which is also called thyroxine. One mono iodothrosine combines with one diodotyrosine to form triiodothyronine which is more potent than thyroxine. Thiocyanates, perchlorates and other anions inhibit iodine absorption of thyroids. Absorption of iodine is dependent on activity of the gland. A small amount is excreted through feces and sweat.

Iodine Deficiency

Iodine deficiency produces endemic goitre. Goitre is a conditio where in the thyroid gland which usually measures 25 grams enlarges an weighs as much as 500 grams. If the treatment is started in early stage the change can be reversed. Iodine deficiency may be caused due t deficient intake or deficient trapping of iodine by the gland. It may als be due to insufficient thyrodine formation due to goitrogens an deficiency of specific enzymes needed for thyrodine synthesis. Which ca be hereditary. See sketch 8.1.

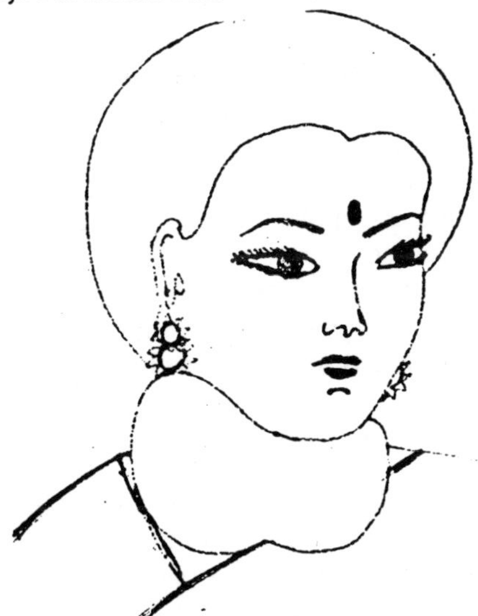

Sketch 8.1 : Goitre Patient

Because of Anti thyroid substances thyroxine secretion from thyroid is stopped which in turn leads to increase in thyrotropic hormone secretion. When thyrotropic hormone increases hypophysis occurs which leads to hypertrophy of thyroidgland. If this continues it leads to hyperplasticity of the gland and the cells of thyroid undergoes mitosis and thyroxine secretion is totally stopped.

Myxodema

Progressive destruction of epithetial tissue, over growth of non cellular components, formation of cysts and large colloidal space gradually reduces capacity of the gland to secrete thyroxin. This is apparent in people over 40 years age, more in females. Iodized salt, Iodized bread, Iodized Oil, etc., are used as preventive measure. The iodine supplied should meet the recommended daily allowances but shouldn't cause thyrotoxicosis.

Cretinism

Cretinism occurs in infants when pregnant woman has severe deficiency of iodine. Cretinism is characterized by muscular flabbiness, weakness, dry skin, low basal metabolism, severe mental retardation, enlarged tongue and thick lips. Administration of dessicated thyroid to the infant improves physical development and mental retardation.

Hyper Thyroidism

Excessive secretion of thyroxine and increased metabolic rate are seen in Hyperthyroidism. It is also known as exopthalmic goiter, thyrotoxicosis, Graves disease or Basedows disease. Thyroid gland with iodine deficiency becomes over active in a attempt to produce the hormone. When iodine is supplied excess of thyroid hormone is produced and thyrotoxicosis is produced. Large thyroid gland and prominent eyes are symptoms of exopthalmic goitre. Weight loss, nervousness, prominent types, enlarged thyroid gland increased appetite, weakness and signs of cardiac failure may be present.

COPPER

Hart and Elvejem of Wisconsin University in 1928 showed that copper is essential along with iron for curing iron deficiency Anemia. Human body has about 100-150 mg of copper. Serum coper is about 122 micrograms per 100ml. Traces of copper are present in all tissues but Liver, brain heart and kidney have higher concentrations. In blood 90% of Plasma copper is present as ceruloplasmin while 60% of erythrocyte copper is present as erthyrocuprein. Adult human liver has about 10 to 15mg copper, kidney has 10 mg and brain 10 mg.

Functions of Copper are:

1. It is essential in hemoglobin formation.
2. Copper is present in several enzymes like tyrosinase uricase, cytochrome oxidase, ferroxidase, etc.
3. Copper is essential for phospholipid synthesis, collagen synthesis and maintaining integrity of myelin sheath.

Recommended Daily Allowance

2 to 3 mg per day is considered to be safe and adequate for adults. In case of infants 1 mg and 1-3 mg for children is considered to be adequate.

Dietary Sources of Copper

Normal diets to supply 1 to 4mg of copper daily. The Copper content of the foods depend on the copper content of the soil where they grow. Cereals, pulses, meat and eggs are good sources of copper. Copper content of various food stuffs is given in Table 8.2. Milk is a poor source of copper.

Absorption

About 2 to 5 per cent of dietary copper is absorbed from the upper gastro intestinal tract and stomach. Molybdenum, Zinc and cadmium are antagonistic for copper. Absorbed copper is mainly excreted through bile and faces. About 48 micro grams of copper is excreted through urine in 24 hours.

Deficiency

Deficiency of copper is not common, Patients with nephritic syndrome. kwashior, sprue and occasionally Iron deficiency Anemia exhibits copper deficiency.

Excess of Copper

Excess intake of copper is toxic. Wilson's disease is a rare hereditary disorder. In this disease bio chemical abnormality is present at birth but clinical signs appear in adolescence. In this disease about 50 per cent of

Table 8.2 : Copper Content of Various Foods

Food Stuff	*Copper* mg/100g	*Food Stuff*	*Copper* mg/100g
Cereals and Cereal Products :		Potato	0.16
Bajra	1.06	Pink radish	0.08
Italian millet	1.40	***Other Vegetables***	
Jowar	0.46	Drumstick	0.01
Ragi	0.49	Mango	0.04
Rice	0.07	Peas	0.23
Rice flakes	0.37	Pumpkin	0.05
Wheat	0.69	Chillies	1.40
Pulses and Legumes :		**Fruits :**	
Bengal gram dal	1.34	Amla	0.18
Black gram dal	0.92	Banana	0.16
Cowpea	0.86	Gauva	0.14
Green gram dal	0.38	Jack fruit	0.13
Horse gram	1.82	Sweet lime	0.51
Peas	1.28	Orange	0.58
Red gram dal	1.20	Pineapple	0.13
Leafy Vegetables :		Seetaphal	0.42
Amaranath	0.08	Wood apple	0.21
Coriander	0.13	**Fish and other Sea Foods :**	
Drumstick leaves	0.07	Bacha	0.11
Tamarind leaves	0.02	Hilsa	0.14
Roots and Tubers		Katla	0.12
Beet root	0.29	Rohu	0.13

ingested copper is absorbed and deposited in brain, liver, kidney eye etc. Because of this cellular necrosis occurs and fibrosis follows. There are three types in this disease (i) Cerebral type (ii) Hepatic type and (iii) Both Cerebral and Hepatic type.

Cerebral Type

Neurological abnormalities arising from dysfunction of lenucular region of brain. Necrosis and sclerosis of the corpus structures lead to based ganglion syndromes. Cortical involvement leads to dementia.

Hepatic Type

Hepatic Cirrhosis occurs which leads to portal hypertension and hepatic failure. Hemolytic jaundice may also precede.

Both cerebral and hepatic type may be present in some cases.

ZINC

Zinc is primarily intracellular and thus it is proportionate to the lean body mass. Man has about 2 grams zinc in his body. It is distributed allover the body. Iris and retina of eye, liver, bone, hair, prostrate, spermatozoa, etc., have higher concentrations. 85 per cent of blood zinc is present in Red Blood cells. But each white blood cell has 25 times as much Zinc as that of Red cell. Bones has about 200 micro grams per gram, about 150-250 micro grams per gram of hair and 80-110 micro grams per 100 ml of plasma.

Functions of Zinc are

1. It is present in a number of enzymes as carbonic anhydrase, Alkaline phosphate, Alcoholdehydrogenase, Lactic dehydrogenase, etc.
2. It acts as co factor is synthesis of DNA and RNA
3. It enhances the action of FSH and LH
4. It helps in mobilization of vitamin A from Liver.

Recommended Daily Allowance

Zinc requirements for different age groups per day is as follows

Infants	-	3—5 mg
Children	-	10 mg
Adolescents	-	15 mg
Adults	-	15 mg
Pregnancy	-	20 mg
Lactation	-	25 mg

Dietary Sources for Zinc

Data of dietary sources of Zinc is sparse. Oysters, Liver meats, fish, cereals are good sources. Legumes nuts oil seeds, vegetables and fruits are fair sources. Zinc present income selected food are given in Table 8.3. Zinc present in animal foods is well absorbed than zinc present in plant foods because of phytates which interfere in zinc absorption.

Table 8.3 : Zinc Content of Selected Foods*

Food stuff	*Portion*	*Zinc (mg)*
Fish, light poultry meat, shell fish (Except crob and Oyster)	30 Z	2.0
Pork, veal, crab, dark turkey meat	30 Z	3.00 – 4.0
Beef, Beef liver	30 Z	4.0 – 5.0
Oyster	30 Z	5.0
Mature dried beans, lentils	½ cup	0.9 – 1.0
Cowpeas, black eyed peas	½ cup	1.5
Whole cow milk	1 cup	0.9
Cheddar cheese	3 slices	1.6
Cooked whole wheat cereal	1 cup	1.2
Corn flakes	10 Z	0.08
White wheat bread	1 slice	0.5
Cooked white rice	1 cup	0.8

* Murphy E W, Wills BW, Watt BH. Provisional tables on the zinc content of foods. JAM Diet Association 1975; 66: 345-55

Absorption

Phytates present in foods of plant origin bind Zinc and forms zinc calcium phytate which is insoluble. Zinc is mainly absorbed from duodenum and ileum. About 5 to 10 per cent of dietary zinc is absorbed. Of the absorbed 50 percent is retained and the rest excreted.

Zinc Deficiency

Hypogevsia which means lowered taste acuity, dysgensia means unpleasant perverted and obnoxious taste. Hyposmia which means lowered odour acuity and dysosmia which means disagreeable odor sensation are some of the consequences of zinc deficiency. These symptoms are severe in acute viral hepatitis, cirrhosis of liver malabsorption syndrome, hepatic coma and kurashiorkor. Growth Retardation and retarded genital development are seen in children with zinc deficiency. Permanent effect on developing brain, alopecia, skeletal abnormalities, lowered plasma insulin, etc., are found in experimental animals with zinc deficiency. In human beings wound healing following severe burns is delayed, activity of various enzymes like carbonic anhydrase, carboxy peptidase, etc., are decreased, formation of muscle tissue in children recovering from malnutrition was found difficult, Hypogevsia, dysgevsia, Hyposmia and dysosmia are found.

Zinc Toxicity

Zinc slats when administered 60 to 100 times the recommended daily allowance induces vomiting, diarrhoea and cramps with in 3 to 10 hours. These subside shortly. Consumption of foods stored in galvanized tins increases Zinc ingestion. Acidic foods or beverages increases zinc solubility and cause zinc toxicity.

SELENIUM

Selenium is present in all tissues. Liver, spleen, pancreas, testis and kidney has highest concentration. Blood has about 25 micro grams per 100 ml. Both selenium and Vitamin E act as anti oxidants. Selenium is integral component of glutathione peroxidase. It also functions in the oxidative phosphorylation of energy compounds. An estimated safe intake is about 0.06 to 0.2 mg selenium per day in adults and 0.01 to 0.1 mg in children, Sea foods are rich in selenium cereals, Meats, vegetables and fruits are rich in selenium cereals, Meats, vegetables and fruits are fair sources. The Concentration of selenium in plant foods depend upon the selenium concentration of the soil. Selenium deficiency in humans is not noticed. In animal excess of selenium produced alkalidisease which is characterized by stiffness, blindness, deformity of hooves, loss of fur and death in some cases. School children showed dental caries in seleniferous area.

FLUORINE

Flourine occurs in the body in association with Calcium salt in teeth & bones. Small amounts of Flourine reduces the chance of both decay by making the enamel more resistant to the action of acids produced in the mouth. Fluoride salts of Calcium are less readily lost from bone during immobilization or following menopause. The plasma level of fluorine is 0.04 to 0.20 ppm.

Normally drinking water provides the fluorine needed by the body in may regions. Water usually has 1-2 PPM (Parts per million) in drinking water. This does not harm the body. 2 to 4 mg per day is the safe adequate level of fluorine in adults. 0.1 to 1 mg for infants and 0.5 to 2-5 mg for children and adolescents is the recommended daily allowance. Fluorine occurs in all foods. Table 8.4 gives fluoride content of some foods. The amount of fluorine in plant foods depend on the concentration present in Soil and water.

Fluoride Deficiency

Fluoride deficiency in children causes dental caries. Fluorine forms Calcium Phosphate fluoride compound in teeth which resist the acids produced by the bacteria in the mouth and thus present dental caries.

Table 8.4 : Flouride Content of Foods*

Food Stuff	*Fluoride* mg/100g	*Food Stuff*	*Fluoride* mg/100g
Cereals and Cereal Products :		French beans	1.5
Whole wheat	2.9	Tomato	1.4
Wheat flour milled	5.4	Cluster beans	1.4
Rice	7.7	Brinjal	2.0
Bajra	1.9	Giant Chillies	1.7
Pulses and :		**Fruits :**	
Bengal gram flour	8.1	Banana	1.1
Bengal gram dal	3.8	Orange	1.7
Leafy Vegetables :		Mango	1.3
Amaranath	6.1	Apple	1.7
Cabbage	1.9	**Animal Foods :**	
Spinach	2.1	Hens egg	1.3
Roots and Tubers		Pomphret white	2.1
Potato	1.9	Bombay duck	3.8
Onion	2.1	Prawns	2.7
Carrot	3.4	**Beverages :**	
Other Vegetables		Tea	56.6
Cucumber	2.5		

* Lakadwala, Punekar B.D. Fluorid Content of water and commonly consumed foods in Bombay and Study of the fluoride intake, Indian . J. Med. Res 1973: 61; 1679-87

Fluorine is easily absorbed from the intestines. More than half the ingested fluoride is excreted through urine and rest is deposited in bones. Fluoride toxicity is called Fluorisis. Large excess of fluorine 20 to 80 mg daily for several years lead to fluorisis of bone & Dental fluorisis. Sclerosis and hypercalcification of bones of spine, Pelvis and limbs occur in skeletal fluorisis. The ligaments of spine becomes calcified and the back bone bends producing Pokersback. The joints become stiff and movement becomes painful. Slowly the patient becomes bed ridden. Thorax becomes stiff and respiration becomes difficult. In dental fluorisis teeth becomes mottled. The upper incisors are first involved. The enamel becomes dull and pitting occurs. Gradually dark brown stains occurs which are difficult to remove.

MANGANESE

Manganese exists as trace mineral in the body. About 15-30mg of Manganese is present in a adults body. Though it is distributed allover the body, kidney, liver, pancreas and pituitary have higher concentration. Human blood has about 2.5 microgram of manganese per every 100 ml. Manganese play an important role in brain function. An excess or deficiency effects the brain function. The recommended daily allowance of Manganese is roughly 4mg in adults and , 0.5 to 4mg in infants and children. Cereals, bran, coffee, tea and nuts are good source of Manganese. Normal diet supplies about 5 mg of Manganese daily which i absorbed from the gut. Manganses deficiency has not been observed in Man. Abnormalities of bone, ataxia and sterility are found in experimental animals. In Man excessive depositing is found in those who inhale manganese in mines and chemical factories. Excess of manganese shows changes in basalganglia and posterior pert of hypothalamus.

CHROMIUM

Chromium is a trace element in human and animal bodies. It is about 6 mh in adult human being. Blood has about 0.01 to 0.05 PPM of chromium. Chromium requirements range from 0.01 to 0.2 mg during the life time. Animal foods have high chromium content than plant foods. Absorption is about 0.5 percent. Deficiency of chromium exhibits impaired growth and disturbances in protein, Lipid and Glucose metabolisms. Corneal opacity developed in chromium deficiency. Oral administration of about 50 PPM of Chromium produced kidney and liver damage and growth depression.

COBALT

Cobalt was first discovered as dietary essential in 1935. In 1948 Vitamin B_{12} (Cyano Cobalamin) was found to possess cobalt. Cobalt occurs in small amounts in all tissues. Liver and kidney possess higher concentrations. The recommended daily allowances of cobalt are not determined as the deficiency is not observed. Normal diet meets the need of Cobalt. Excess of cobalt intake suppress iron absorption and caused Anemia and death in experimental animals. Animals other than ruminants developed Polycythemia, hyperplasia of bone marrow, reticulocytosis and increase in blood volume.

MOLYBDENUM

Molybdenum found in all tissues while liver and kidney has some what higher amounts. Pulses, cereal grains, leafy vegetables, liver and kidney are good sources while fruits are poor sources. Infants require about 0.05 mg, children 0.1 to 0.3 mg and Adults need 0.15 to 0.5 mg of Molybdenum every day. About 60 per cent of the ingested molybdenum is absorbed and 50 percent of it is excreted through urine. Excess of molybdenum produced loss of weight and anorexia in rats and severe diarrhoea in cattle. It can be cured by administering copper. Molybdenum reduces copper retention in cattle.

SILICON

Silicon plays a possible role in bone calcification. Silicon content is about 50-1000 PPM in human beings. Human blood has 2-5 kg per ml. silicon is absorbd as solid silica and mobosilicic acid. About one percent of the ingested is absorbed and a greater part of it is again excreted. Normall silicon is excreted in urin in soluble form. In certain circumstances it is precipitated as Calculi and obstruct passage of urine. Silicon content of skin and thymus decrease with age. Tissues of heart, muscle and kideny has no change. There is relationship between Calcium, silicon, magnesium and fluorine. Silicon helps in calcification of bone.

CADMIUM

Cadmium occurs in small quantities in human and animal tissues. Cadmium interacts with zinc and other trace elements. Adult human body has about 30 mg of cadmium of which 10 mg appears in kidney, 4mg in liver, blood has about 0.7 PPM. Cadmium deficiency usually does not occur in human beings. Excess of zinc and copper interferes with absorption of Cadmium and vice versa. Cadmium in excess reduced weight gain and increased the incidence of systolic hypertension in rats. Rabbits developed hyperplastic bone marrow and hypochromic microcytic anemia. Necrosis of ovaries, and injurious effects on tests were also observed in rats which received injection of excess of Cadmium.

·Function of Vanadium, Tin and Nickel and strontium have been shown to have a role in animal nutrition but their role in human beings, their requirements, deficiency and toxicity is not known.

Water and Electrolyte Balance

Water is the largest constituent of the body. Water comprises about 60–70 percent of body weight. Lean persons have higher percentage of body water than obese people. Water stands second only to air in nature in maintaining life. One can live without food for weeks but with water deprivation one can live only for few days. If the body looses 10 per cent of body water condition becomes serious and if it reaches 20 percent the person dies. Water content in soft tissues is 70–80 per cent while in bone it is 20 per cent. The functions of water in human body are

1) Water forms essential and major constituent of living cell protoplasm.
2) It helps in regulating body temperature.
3) It maintains the osmotic pressure in the cells.
4) Water serves as a medium of all body fluids.
5) All Physiological chemical reactions in the body occur in water medium.
6) Water forms a vehicle for dilution and transport of nutrients.
7) It also forms a vehicle for carrying waste products to excretory organs.
8) Water being good conductor of electricity is instrumental in deduction of nerve impulses.

9) Water is responsible for electrolyte balance in the body.

10) It acts as lubricant while talking, swallowing, etc.

11) It acts as mechanical buffer e.g. : amniotic fluid, fluids that both the joints, etc.

12) Water gives shape and size to body tissues.

Water Sources to the Body

Water is absorbed from small intestine rapidly than from stomach and large intestine. Water can be given through rectum in the form of enema.

Water is absorbed mostly, only 100 to 200 ml of water is excreted in feces. Large bowel has the capacity to absorb about 5 litres of fluid. Water needs of the body are fulfilled by

1. Intake of water and beverages
2. Water in food and
3. Water formed during the oxidation of food stuffs.

When 100 mg each of fat, carbohydrate and protein are oxidised 107, 56 and 41 ml of water are produced respectively. Some water loss from the body occurs independent of water intake are losses in feces, in respiration and in maintenance of Physicochemical equilibrium. The water balance in the body is given in Table 9.1. In normal person the water excreted approximates intake.

Table 9.1 : Water Balance in the Body

	Water in ml.
Water Intake :	
Drinking water and Beverages	2000–5000
In food	1000–2000
By oxidation of food stuffs	300
	3300–7300
Water loss :	
In urine	1000–1500
Perspiration	1800–5200
Respiration	400
Feces	100–200
	3300–7300

RENAL LOSS

About 170 litres of fluid pass through kidneys each day. Of it 168.5 litres is reabsorbed and only 1.5 litres form urine and is excreted. About 30 gms. of urea is formed in the body per day only 750 ml of urine is enough for its excretion. If urine formation is below 750 ml waste products are retained in the body.

SWEAT

Perspiration of sweat may be sensible or insensible. Insensible loss accounts to relatively constant amount which is proportional to surface area of the body. This water loss helps in maintenance of body temperature when there is lot of loss by perspiration urine gets concentrated by conserving body water.

RESPIRATION

Expired air has water. Any condition that increases rate of respiration increases loss of water.

Ex : Fever, Exercise, etc.

In a normal situation thirst is an accurate guide to supply the necessary amounts of water to the body and renal tubular reabsorption of water aids in maintaining water balance.

Regulation of Water Balance

The following factors regulate the water balance.

1. Endocrines : Antidiuretic hormone from posterior pituitary gland increases reabsorption of water from distal renal tubules and reduces the urine volume.
2. Hypothalamus : Dehydration causes osmoconcentration of Plasma, which stimulates thirst centre in hypothalamus and provokes the animal to drink the required amount of water.
3. Kidneys are important water regulating organs.
4. Autonomic vasomotor action of vaso constriction and vasodilation also helps in regulation of water balance.

Effect of excess of sodium chloride

When sodium chloride is taken in excess the plasma crystalloid osmotic pressure rises. Which inturn forces water to move from interstitial spaces to plasma. Sodium chloride diffuses into interstitial spaces which pulls water alongwith it. Thus the sodium chloride concentration increases uniformly in extracellular fluid. The rise inosmotic pressure of extracellular fluid leads to a flow of water from cells into extracellular fluid, which results in increase of volume in extracellular fluid and decrease in intracellular fluid volume.

Effect of Sodium Chloride Depletion

When sodium chloride depletion occurs in plasma the crystalloid osmotic pressure of extracellular fluid falls and water moves from interstitial fluid into the cells, which results in decrease in volume of extracellular fluid and increase in volume of intracellular fluid. The body weight, plasma volume and blood volume decreases which in turn decreases cardiac out put and may lead to circulatory failure.

Dehydration

When adequate amounts of water are not taken to make up the water loss from the body dehydration occurs. Severe diarrhoea and vomiting also causes dehydration. The Extracellular fluid (ECF) is reduced along with its electrolyte content, the osmotic pressure rises. So water is drawn from Intracellular Fluid (ICF) to ECF. The metabolism of the cells is disturbed which leads to breakdown of Protein and loss of Potassium. The Antidiuretic hormone (ADH) secretion increases and urine volume decreases. The excretion of electrolytes is increased. Due to the decrease in plasma volumes venous and capillary pressures fall while osmotic pressure of plasma proteins increases. Plasma electrolytes, urea and NPN increases and condition becomes serious. Water, electrolytes and glucose should be supplied intravenously.

WATER INTOXICATION

When excess of water is taken especially when there is (i) Renal Failure (2) Excessive Administration of Fluids (3) Hypersecretion of ADH. Symptoms of water intoxication are weakness, lethargy, confusion, vomiting, convulsions and coma. In severe cases hypertonic saline may have to be administered intravenously.

ELECTROLYTE BALANCE

An ion is an atom or group of atoms that carry electric charge. Cations carry positive charge. *Ex* : Na^+, K^+; Ca^{++}, etc., Anions carry negative charge: *Ex.* : Cl^-, HCO_3^-, HPO_4^- etc. Cations donate electrons and Anions accept electrons. In a solution total cations are equal to anions. Electrolyte is a substance which in solution dissociates into its component ions some of which transmit electric current.

Electrolytes like sodium, potassium, chloride, etc., are present in both extracellular and intracellular fluids. The concentration is effected by water balance and electrolyte intake the following mechanisms keep the electrolyte balance at constant level :

Constant Level

Electrolyte concentration of ECF : ECF includes Plasma, Interstitial fluid and lymph. These have higher proportion of sodium, chloride and bicarbonate when compared to potassium and phosphate.

Electrolyte concentration of ICF : Tissue cells and erythrocytes has higher concentration of Potassium, Phosphates and bicarbonates when compared to sodium and chloride.

Cell membranes are permeable to water, glucose, lactate, amino acids, acetoacetate and phosphate control of free movement. The active transport mechanism prevents the passage of sodium from ECF to ICF and Potassium from ICF to ECF for which chemical energy is used.

Wide variations like hypertonic, isotonic and Hypotonic changes occur in both ECF increase and decrease.

Increase in ECF Volume

1. Hypertonic expansion : When salt solution is ingested the ECF becomes hypertonic and fluid from tissue cells is drawn out causing dehydration of tissue. Here serum levels are high.
2. Hypotonic expansion : When excess of water is ingested the ECF becomes Hypotonic and fluid is drawn into the tissue cells. Here serum sodium levels are low.
3. Isotonic Expansion : This situation occurs when excess of normal saline is administered. ECF increases and water is retained in the body causing edema. Serum sodium levels are normal.

Decrease in ECF Volume

Hypertonic Contraction : When water intake is very low dehydration occurs or when large amount of urine is excreted ECF becomes hypertonic and fluid is drawn into ECF from the cells. Serum sodium levels are high and tissue dehydration results.

Hypotonic Contraction : Ingestion of water without electrolytes when a lot of sodium chloride is lost from the body leads to Hypotonic state of ECF. Chromic renal tubular dysfunction and addisons disease also present this situation. Water is drawn from ECF into the tissues. Thus ECF volume is reduced, circulatory and renal failure occurs. Serum sodium levels are low.

Isotonic contraction : In vomiting, diarrhoea and hemorrhage isotonic fluids are lost from the body, which decreases ECF volume. This leads to fall in blood pressure, circulatory and renal failure. The terms Hyponatremia, Hypernatremia, Hyperkalemia and Hypokalemia are discussed under the Chapter Minerals—Macro Elements.

10

Inter-Relationship Among Nutrients

Excess of deficiency of certain nutrients affect the requirement of some other nutrient. The inter-relationship between different nutrients can be divided under the following heads :

i) Protein Energy Inter-relationship

ii) Effect of Carbothydrates, Proteins, and Fats on Vitamin Needs

iii) Vitamin—Vitamin Inter-relationship

iv) Vitamin–Mineral Inter-relationship

v) Mineral–Mineral Inter-relationship.

PROTEIN ENERGY INTER-RELATIONSHIP

When sufficient amount of energy is not consumed tissue break-down occurs and negative nitrogen balance results. It the Energy restriction continues fat depots are depleted and catabolism of tissues continues finally it leads to the death of the animal. When the carbohydrate and fat intake does not meet the energy requirement dietary protein is used for energy purposes. If Nitrogen lost from the body is greater than

Nitrogen intake the body is said to be in Negative Nitrogen Balance. This condition is usually seen in persons suffering from under-nutrition, burns, surgery, fever, etc. When carbohydrate intakes are sufficient for the energy production, dietary or tissue proteins are not catabolised for energy production. This is called the "Protein sparing action".

EFFECT OF CARBOHYDRATE, PROTEINS AND FATS ON VITAMINS NEEDS VITAMIN A AND FAT

Absorption of Vitamin A requires fat. Vitamin A in any form as and carotene (Provitamin) need fat for its absorption. In absence of fat Vitamin A absorption is not possible. Rancid fats destroy the Vitamin A present in the diet. The Vitamin A stores of the body are mobilized by high protein diets. Low protein diets help in conserving the body Vitamin A stores.

THIAMINE AND CARBOHYDRATE

Thiamine pyrophosphate is a co-enzyme essential in the Oxidative decarboxylation of pyruvic acid which is the main end product of carbohydrate metabolism. High carboydrate diet needs high thiamine intake.

NICOTINIC ACID AND TRYPTOPHAN

Tryptophan present in protein gets converted to Niacin in the body. The Niacin needs of the body can be met by tryptophan of proteins to some extent.

PYRIDOXINE AND FAT

Pyridoxine needs in high protein diet always increases. Addition of essential fatty acids to the diets low in pyridoxine offers protection against the development of pyridoxine deficiency symptoms. So the pyridoxine requirements are influenced by both quality and quantity of fats and proteins.

CHOLINE AND METHIONINE

Methyl group from choline when transferred to homocystine forms methionine and vice versa. Vitamin B_{12} and folic acid are essential in this reaction.

VITAMIN–VITAMIN INTER-RELATIONSHIP

VITAMINS A, E, AND K

In rats when Vitamin A intake is increased and vitamin K intake is reduced they developed vitamin K deficiency symptoms. Vitamin E helps in storage of vitamin A in liver. In vitamin E deficiency liver stores of Vitamin A depletion increased.

VITAMINS OF B COMPLEX AND OTHER VITAMINS

Thiamine deficiency causes disturbance in Riboflavin metabolism and considerable loss of riboflavin occurs through urine. The blood riboflavin levels are increased in the deficiency of pantothenic acid due to increased mobilisation from liver. Thiamine, riboflavin and pantothenic acid give partial protection from Vitamin B_6 deficiency. Vitamin B_{12} levels in serum and liver are reduced when vitamin B_6 deficient diets are fed to rats. Vitamin B_6 enhances the absorption of Vitamin B_{12}. Biotin has a protective action on pantothenic acid deficiency.

VITAMIN MINERAL INTER-RELATIONSHIP

VITAMIN C AND IRON

Food iron is of two types heme iron and non-heme iron. Heme iron is derived from Animal foods and is not influenced by the composition of other nutrients in the diet. Non-heme iron absorption is dependent of the other nutrient composition of the diet ascorbic acid can reverse the inhibiting effect of tannins, phytates oxahates etc. Ascorbic acid forms a chelate with ferric iron at acid pH and remains soluble at alkaline pH of the duodenum and aids in absorption of iron.

RIBOFLAVIN AND IRON

Riboflavin deficiency decreases iron absorption of dietary iron and decrease the hepatic iron mobilisation.

VITAMIN D, CALCIUM AND PHOSPHORUS

Vitamin D enhances the absorption of Calcium and Phosphorus form the intestine.

VITAMIN C, LEAD, IRON AND MERCURY

Iron will increase lead toxicity but vitamin C is ineffective. Vitamin

C increases mercury toxicity but iron exhilarates it.

MINERAL-MINERAL RELATIONSHIP

Copper is very essential for incorporation of iron in hemoglobin. The presence of excessive amounts of phytates and phosphates in diet interferes the absorption of Iron and Magnesium. The presence of excess of Calcium adversly effects intestinal absorption of phosphorus and vice versa. Excess molybdenum in diet prevents copper absorption. Nickel supplementation increases copper deficiency symptoms than in Nickel deprivation.

11

Recommended Dietary Allowances

Professionals in nutrition field use the food composition tables and Recommended Dietary Allowances as their main tools. Using food composition tables one can formulate a nutritionally adequate diet which meets the need. The socio economic and cultural aspects are also taken into consideration. Adequate diet is the amount of food that keeps a person physically fit and to maintain good health. A good diet should provide adequate amounts of all nutrients. Many National and International Committees worked on this aspect and framed the recommended dietary allowances for various nutrients. (a) Nutrition expert group ICMR, India, (b) Food and Nutrition Board, National Research Council, USA (c) Panel on Recommended Allowances on Nutrients, Departments of Health and Social Services UK and (d) Recommendations of FAO/WHO expert group recommended nutrient allowances. Recommended dietary allowance are the levels of intake of essential nutrients to be adequate to meet the nutritional needs of practically healthy persons. Allowances are the amounts of nutrients to be consumed, loss during preparation and plate waste should be considered. Requirement is the individuals requirement which is dependent on physical, social, environmental, hereditary and other factors. It is not possible to determine every individuals need in the world. So different recommended allowances are formulated for different communities. The difference especially is found in energy allowances.

The disadvantages of these Recommended Allowance Tables are i) Data on trace elements is limited ii) recommended allowances are not suitable to the people who are ill, or who require an increase or decrease of particular nutrient or nutrients depending on pathology and medication. The RDA are translated into diets with a wide range of foods which are called food guides. The food guides are formulated separately for each region. Food guides of one region does not fit for people of other region because the food stuff availability, food habits cultural patterns and socio-economic status vary from East to West and from North to South.

CALORIES

While estimating the energy requrements Age, Sex, body composition, body size, climate, environment, physical activity and physiological state should be considered. The recommended energy levels are average requirements that maintain health and normal weight individual in adults and to support growth in children. The energy requirement vary from one individual to another.

PROTEINS

Proteins are necessary for growth and maintainance of the body. Physiological stress conditions increase the need of protein. The NPU of Indian diets is lower than western diets so the amount of protein in Indian diets should be more than western diets.

FATS

Fats are essential for the absorption of all fat soluble Vitamins. Fats serve an important role in maintaining the health of an individual. Fat supplies the essential fatty acids like linoleic, linolenic and arachidonic acids. In adequate supply of essential fatty acids leads to a deficiency disorder of the skin called phrynoderma. Excess fat in diet leads to Hypercholestremia and atherosclerosis.

CALCIUM

Calcium is essential for calcification of bone, clotting of blood, muscle contraction, transmission of nerve impulse, etc. calcium deficiency in children produces decreased growth rate, loss of calcium from bones, Hyperpure thyriodism, osteoporosis, fractures, etc. Hypercalcimia results in calcium deposition in soft tissues, vomiting, gastro-intestinal bleeding, anorexia, increase in blood pressure, etc. Optimal intake of calcium according to recommended allowances ensures strong bones and teeth.

PHOSPHORUS

Calcium and Phosphorus requirements are closely related phosphorus needs are 20 per cent more than calcium. Large amount of phytin is present in the cereals, pulses and nuts. This interferes with the utilisation of calcium and iron.

IRON

Iron is the most important elements in the body. Without iron life is not possible. Iron forms the hemoglobin which carries the oxygen to various tissues. On an average 10 per cent food iron is absorbed. The recommended allowance are framed based on this per cent absorption.

VITAMIN A

Vitamin A requirements are expressed in terms of Retional or - Carotene. In India many children have Vitamin A deficiency. Therapeutic doses of Vitamin A are available free of cost in PHC's. The cheap sources of vitamin A like papaya, leafy vegetables consumption should be encouraged.

THIAMIN

Thiamin requirements are directly proportional to the carbohydrate intake. Thiamin is essential in carbohydrate metabolism. Thiamin pyrophosphate is essential in oxidative decarboxylation of pyruvic acid an end product of carbohydrate metabolism.

RIBOFLAVIN

Riboflavin requirements are directly related to the caloric requirements. It plays an important role in metabolism of Carbohydrates proteins and fats. Riboflavin form Riboflavin Mononucleotide and Riboflavin adeninedinucleotide which are part of enzyme or act as coenzymes and act as hydrogen acceptors and play an important role in metabolism.

NICOTINIC ACID

Nicotinic acid requirements are also related to caloric requirements. NAD and NADP need Nicotinic acid for their formation. These are hydrogen receptors and are involved in many enzyme reaction.

PYRIDOXINE

Pyridoxine forms pyridoxal phosphate act in several enzyme systems like transaminase system, Amino acid decarboxylase system, conversion of Tryptophan to Niacin, etc.

FOLIC ACID

Folic acid conjugate by itself is not absorbed. Hence folic acid requirement is expressed in terms of free folic acid. Folacin is essential for DNA synthesis. Folacin inhibitors are used to inhibit tumor growth and cell proliferation.

VITAMIN B_{12}

Vitamin B_{12} occurs only in foods of animal origin. It needs an intrinsic factor for absorption. The recommended allowance for different age groups is given in Table 11.1.

ASCORBIC ACID

Ascorbic acid is also called vitamin C. It is rapidly absorbed from the intestines. It helps in absorption of Iron, biosynthesis of mucopoly saccharides, leucocyte function, etc. Adequate intake of Ascorbic acid is given in recommended dietary allowance table.

VITAMIN D

Vitamin D is essential for absorption of calcium and phosphorus. It aids in calcification process. Exposure to sunlight helps in meeting the Vitamin D needs of the body.

Table 11.1 : Recommended Dietary Intakes of Nutrients (as revised in 1981)

Group	Particulars	Net Calories (kcal)	Proteins (g)	Calcium (g)	Iron (mg)	Vitamin-A: Retional (μg) or	Vitamin-A: β-carotene (μg)	Thiamine (mg)
Man	Sedentary work	2400						1.2
	Moderate work	2800	55	0.4–0.5	24	750	3000	1.4
	Heavy work	3900						2.0
Woman	Sedentary work	1900						1.0
	Moderate work	2200	45	0.4–0.5	32	750	3000	1.1
	Heavy work	3000						1.5
	Pregnancy (second half of pregnancy)	+300	+14	1.0	40	750	3000	+0.2
	Lactation							
	0–6 months	+550	+25		32	1150	4600	+0.3
	6–12 months	+400						+0.2
Infants	0–6 months	118/kg	2.0/kg	0.05–0.6	1.0 mg/kg	400	..	59μg/kg
	6–12 months	108/kg	1.7/kg			.00	1200	54μg/kg
Children	1–3 years	1220	22.0			250	1000	0.6
	4–6 years	1720	29.4	0.4–0.5	20–25	300	1200	0.9
	7–9 years	2050	35.6			400	600	1.0
Boys	10–12 years	2420	42.5	0.4–0.5	30–25	600	2400	1.2
Girls	–do–	2260	42.1					1.1
Boys	13–15 years	2660	51.7	0.6–0.7	25	750	3000	1.3
Girls	–do–	2360	43.3		35			1.2
Boys	16–18 years	2820	53.1	0.5–0.6	25	750	3000	1.4
Girls	–do–	2200	44.0		5			1.1

(Contd.)

Table 11.1 : (Contd.)

Group	Particulars	Riboflavin (mg)	Nicotinic Acid (mg)	Vitamin B_6 (mg)	Ascorbic Acid (mg)	Folic Acid (μg)	Vitamin B_{12} (μg)	Vitamin D (I. U.)
Man	Sedentary work	1.4	16					
	Moderate work	1.7	19	2.0	40	100	1	
	Heavy work	2.3	26					
Woman	Sedentary work	1.1	13					
	Moderate work	1.3	15	2.0	40	100	1	
	Heavy work	1.8	20					
	Pregnancy (second half of pregnancy)	+0.2	+2	2.5	40	300		
	Lactation						1.5	
	0–6 months	+0.3	+4	2.5				
	6–12 months	+0.2	+3		80	150		
Infants	0–6 months	71mg/kg	780μg/kg	0.3	20	25	0.2	
	6–12 months	65mg/kg	710μg/kg	0.4				
Children	1–3 years	0.7	8	0.6				
	4–6 years	1.0	11	0.9				
	7–9 years	1.2	14	1.2				
Boys	10–12 years	1.5	16	1.6				200
Girls	–do–	1.4	15		40	100	0.2–1.0	
Boys	13–15 years	1.6	18	2.0				
Girls	–do–	1.4	15					
Boys	16–18 years	1.7	19	2.0				
Girls	–do–	1.3	15					

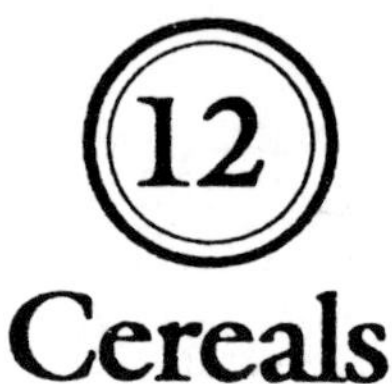

Cereals

Wheat and Rice forms the staple food in North and South India respectively. Apart from these Jowar, Maize, Barley, Bajra, Ragi, etc., are also used to some extent. Cereals are the sources of energy in poor population. Cereals have about $^{3}/_{4}$ carbohydrate and $^{1}/_{8}$ protein by weight. The Biological value of protein is less than Animal foods. Cereals have 0.5 to 4 per cent fat, 0.4 to 4 per cent Minerals and 0.1 to 2.7 mg per cent Thiamine Milling causes a great loss of vitamins and Minerals. The vitamin C content is low because the cereals are dried and stored. Germination helps in increasing the Vitamin C content.

GENERAL STRUCTURE

Cereals have kernel and ovary wall. Ovary wall gets attached to kernel and appears as one. The outer layer has cellulose minerals, thiamine etc. This layer gives protection to the kernel. Below this layer endosperm and embryo are present. Endosperm is present in the middle of the kernel. It has 75 per cent carbohydrate, and 4 to 13 per cent proteins. This provides the food for seedling until it synthesises its own food. Embryo forms the plant. Embryo has lipids, protein, minerals, thiamin and vitamin E. Kernel has about 13 per cent moisture. Because of this low moisture content we are able to store these grains for long time after drying. Milled cereals gets spoiled faster than unmilled. In the process of milling the outer bran layers are lost. The embryo is exposed to air and because of its Lipid content rancidity occurs. So, cereal grains should be stored without milling. The Nutritive values of different cereals and cereal product are given Table 12.1

RICE

South Indians use rice as their staple food. People of Bangladesh, Mainmar, China, Sri Lanka and Japan also use rice as their staple food. Rice can be easily milled when compared to other cereals. Rice can be grown in temperate climates where the temperature is not less than 25°C and rainfall more than 100 cm. Rice is grown well in delta areas. In India delta areas of Ganga, Krishna, Kaveri and Godavari yield good crop. Bengal, Bihar, Orissa, Andhra Pradesh and Tamil Nadu has good yield of rice. Kerala, Madhya Pradesh, Assam, Uttar Pradesh and Punjab gives medium yield.

STRUCTURE (See Sketch 12.1 on p. 168)

There are 5 parts in rice grain. They are :

1. **Husk** : It is loose coat which has no nutritive value. This coat is removed during milling.
2. **Bran** : It is the outermost coat of the grain. It has cellulose and some nutrients. It forms 5% of grain weight.
3. **Aleurone Layer** : This layer formed of polyhedral cells. It has proteins, phosphorus, thiamin and fat. It forms 8% of the grain weight.
4. **Embryo** : It is at the base of the grain. It is rich in lipids, Vitamin E and other nutrients.
5. **Endosperm** : It is rich in carbohydrate which is a source of energy. It forms 75 per cent of total grains weight.

Rice provides about 350 k cals of energy per every 100 grams of dry weight. It has about 7 per cent protein. Rice is deficient in an aminoacid lysine and methionine. Pulses and legumes are rich in lysine. So a combination of Rice and Pulse or Legume provides good quality protein or in other words increases the biological value of rice diet. Rice with milk or milk products also provides protein of improved biological value.

PROCESSING

The processing of rice includes removal of husk and bran. For this

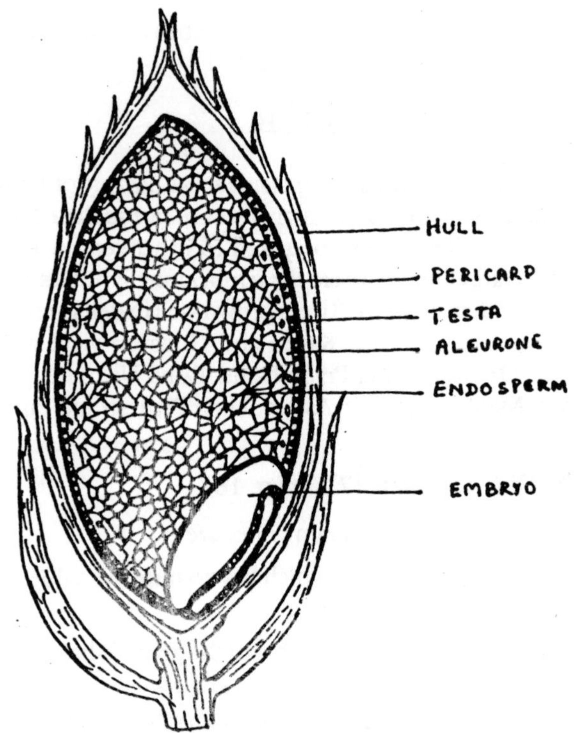

Sketch 12.1 : Cross Section of a Kernel of Paddy

removal three methods are employed.

1. Hand pounding
2. Machine milling
3. Parboiling followed by milling or hand pounding.

HAND POUNDING

This method is employed by the farmers. It is a laborious time taking process. A large mortar of 6 inch diameter, 8 inch depth and pestle of 6 feet length are used. The mortar is made of wood or iron or stone and pestle is of wood is iron. In this method the husk is separated and bran is preserved to some extent. Thus the vitamins and minerals are not lost.

MACHINE MILLING

In towns and cities rice is milled in machines. In this process bran, aleurone layer and embryo are lost. This is used as animal feed and is collectively called polishings. The advantages milling are : (1) It is quicker than hand pounding. (2) It is easily digested (3) Rice looks clean and attractive (4) lowered chances of contamination. The disadvantage is the Vitamins and Minerals present in bran and embryo are lost. The thiamine loss causes Beri Beri if rice is only food that supplies thiamine in the diet.

PARBOILING FOLLOWED BY HAND POUNDING OR MILLING

In South India parboiled rice is consumed. There are various methods of parboiling but the essential steps are :

1. Boiling paddy with water
2. Soaking paddy
3. Drying the paddy
4. Hand Pounding or Machine Milling the dried paddy

Previously paddy was soaked for 24 hours in water and is then boiled. During this process the B complex vitamins from the outer layer enters the grain. When the husk splits and opens, paddy is removed from water and is dried. The dried paddy is then dehusked by hand pounding or milling. Because of soaking for a long time paddy ferments and the rice has a unpleasant odour. C.F.T.R.I. developed a technique in which paddy is soaked in water at 65°C for 2 to 3 hours and then cooked. This short duration soaking does not develop any odours and thus increases its acceptability. The advantages of parboiling are :

1. Grain becomes harder
2. Polishing is easy
3. Parboiled rice when washed does not loose much nutrients as raw rice.
4. Parboiled rice can be preserved better.

The only disadvantage is, it involves additional process before polishing. But the advantages are more than disadvantages. Washing of raw rice before cooking looses 37 micro grams of thiamine where as parboiled rice loose about 21 micro grams. Methods of cooking also effect the nutrient loss. Cooking with just sufficient water is better than cooking with excess water which is later drained off. The different nutrient losses in different methods of cooking is given in figure 12.1. Cooking rice without much washing and with just enough water is recommended. Properly cooked rice leaves no residue so it is advised in a low residue diet. Rice diet helps in increased absorption of Iron. Fermented rice gives better nutrition. Rice in combination with black gram is fermented and cooked on vapour us idlis are good. These prevent fatty changes in liver. Fermentation doubles the vitamins Thiamine, Riboflavin and Nicotinic acid.

PRODUCTS OF RICE

Rice flakes and puffed rice are the products of rice apart from broken rice and rice flour. These need some processing to get transformed from rice to rice products.

Rice Flakes

Paddy is soaked in water at 65–70°C for 24 hours. Then water is drained off and the paddy is fried in a empty hot pan until the splitting of husk. Immediately paddy is hand pounded. The rice grain separates as a thin flake. Rice flakes are rich in iron content and these can be mixed directly to hot milk with or without sugar and consumed. This can be given to small children also.

Puffed Rice

Paddy is cooked, dried and dehusked. Then it is fried in hot sand quickly. Because of this quick frying the moisture in the grain forces out and the grain in puffed. The extent of puffing depends on moisture content of the grain. Immediately after frying puffed rice is separated by sieving. This puffed rice can also given to children.

WHEAT

Wheat is most widely used cereal in the world. It is grown next to rice in India. North Indians use wheat as their staple food. Wheat is grown in areas with cold climate and rainfall 50–100 cms. Wheat grows well in North Indian states.

STRUCTURE (See sketch 12.2 on p. 171)

1. **Bran** : It has cellulose and is 12 per cent weight of whole grain. It is a brown protective coat.

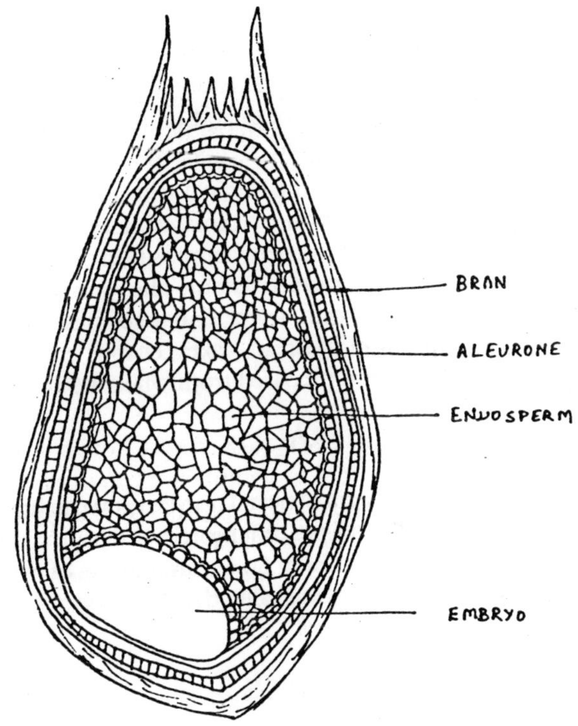

Sketch 12.2 : Cross Section of a Wheat Grain

2. **Aleurone Layer** : This layer is attached to bran and endosperm. It is a single layer cells and rich in protein usually it is removed alongwith bran.
3. **Endosperm** : It is about 85 per cent of whole grain. It is rich in carbohydrates and proteins.
4. **Embryo** : Embryo is situated at the base of the grain. It is rich in proteins, fat thiamine and vitamin E. It is also called germ.
5. **Scutellum** : It is a thin layer between germ and the main body of the grain. It is 1.5 per cent of total grain weight. It has 50–60 per cent of thiamine present in the whole grain.

Wheat provides about 350 k cals of energy per every 100 grams of dry weight. It has about 12 per cent protein. Wheat proteins are glutenin, and gliadin which are collectively called gluten. It is gliadin which causes celiac disease. Elimination of gluten from the diet results in remarkable improvement. Wheat is also limiting in amino acid lysine. When wheat is supplied with milk, pulses, soyabean and oil seeds and oil seeds the biological value of protein increased.

The flour remaining from the original wheat is called extraction percentage, with lowered extraction, percentage bran also decreases. But the energy value increases. The nutrient composition of high extraction flour is more than that of lower extracted flour. The wheat protein gluten absorbs water when mixed with water and becomes viscous. This property helps in preparation of bread, cakes, chaptis etc. Semolina is broken wheat and vermicelli is prepared from wheat flour.

RAGI

Ragi is cheaper than rice and wheat. It can be grown in hot climates. Where rainfall is low. Ragi 6 to 7 per cent protein and has the amino acid methionine which is limiting in Rice. So a combination of rice and ragi provides protein of better biological value than rice alone or ragi alone. Ragi is rich in calcium.

MAIZE

Maize grown in hot climates where rainfall is low. Maize provides about 11 per cent protein on dry weight basis. Zein is the protein present in Maize. Lysine is limiting amino acid in Maize. See sketch 12.3 on page 172 for structure of maize grain in cross section.

BAJRA

Bajra has very little bran so much loss does not occur during milling. Bajra provides 12 per cent protein. Hybrid varieties provide about 17 per cent. It has 5 to 6 per cent fat also. The limiting amino acids are lysine and threonine.

OATS

Oats were used as staple food in 17 and 18 centuries in Scotland. Oats take a very long time to get cooked. Now-a-days Oat flakes are made

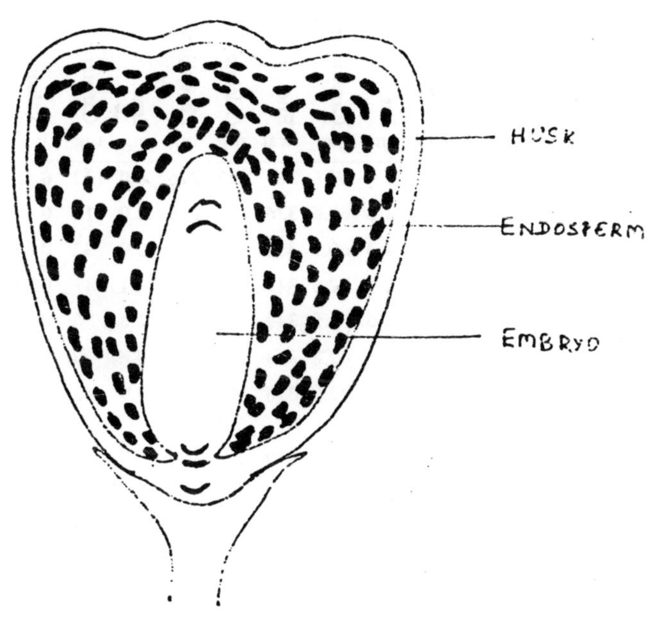

Sketch 12.3 : Cross Section of a Maize Grain

by passing the oat meal (debranned oats) is passed between hot rollers. These flakes are soaked in milk and consumed. Muffins, cookies, cakes, etc. are prepared with Oats.

BARLEY

Barley is also a hard grained cereal. In South India Barley water is given in convalescence, fever and in kidney diseases. Barley malt, beer and whisky are prepared from Barley. Apart from these cereals Italian Millet, Jowar, etc. are also used by a small number of population.

Table 12.1 : Nutritive Values of Different Cereals and Cereal Products

(Per 100 g)

	Protein gm	Fat gm	Carbohydrate gm	Energy kcal	Calcium mg	Phosphorus mg	Iron mg	Carotene mg	Thiamine mg	Riboflavin mg	Niacin mg	Vitamin C mg
Bajra	11.6	5.0	67.5	361	42	296	8.0	132	0.33	0.25	2.3	0
Barley	11.5	1.3	69.6	336	26	215	2.0	10	0.47	0.20	5.4	0
Italian millet	12.3	4.3	60.9	331	31	290	2.9	32	0.59	0.11	3.2	0
Jowar	10.4	1.9	72.6	349	25	222	4.1	47	0.37	0.13	3.1	0
Maize dry	11.1	3.6	66.5	342	10	348	2.3	90	0.42	0.10	1.8	0
Oat meal	13.6	7.6	62.8	374	50	380	3.8	0	0.98	0.16	1.1	0
Ragi	7.3	1.3	72.0	328	344	283	3.9	42	0.42	0.19	1.1	0
Rice (Parboiled milled)	6.4	0.4	79.0	346	9	143	1.0	--	0.21	0.05	3.8	0
Rice (parboiled hand pounded)	8.5	0.6	77.4	349	10	280	2.8	9	0.27	0.12	4.0	01
Rice (Raw hand pounded)	7.5	1.0	76.7	346	10	190	3.2	2	0.21	0.16	3.9	0
Rice (Raw milled)	6.8	0.5	78.2	345	10	160	0.7	0	0.06	0.06	1.9	0
Rice flakes	6.6	1.2	77.3	346	20	238	20.0	0	0.21	0.05	4.0	0
Rice puffed	7.5	0.1	73.6	325	23	150	6.6	0	0.21	0.01	4.1	0
Semolina	10.4	0.8	74.8	348	16	102	1.6	--	0.12	0.03	1.6	0
Vermicelli	8.7	0.4	78.3	352	22	92	2.0	0	0.19	0.05	1.8	0
Whole wheat	11.8	1.5	71.2	346	41	306	5.3	64	0.45	0.17	5.5	0
Wheat flour (Whole)	12.1	1.7	69.4	341	48	355	4.9	29	0.49	0.17	4.3	0
Wheat flour (Refined)	11.0	0.9	73.9	348	23	121	2.7	25	0.12	0.07	2.4	0

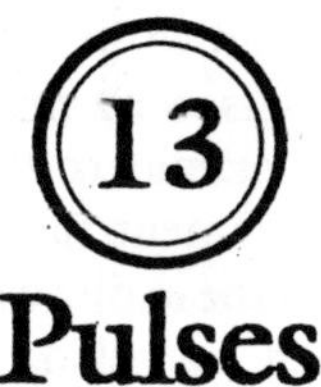

Pulses

Pulses belong to the family of leguminasae. Groundnut belongs to this family, because of its high oil content it is included under nuts and oil seeds for convenience. Pulses had a place in history since 5000 BC. Pulses are grown in South East Asia, middle east India.

Bengal gram, peas and green gram are consumed with or without splitting and removing the outer seed coat. Pulses are rich in proteins when compared to cereals. On an average pulses have 20 per cent protein on dry weight basis with an exception to Soyabean which has about 40 grams protein per 100 grams. Proteins have Methionine as limiting amino acid and abundant amount of lysine. A combination of pulses and cereals create a protein of high biological value because the limiting amino acid of one is abundant in other and vice versa. Pulses possess all B complex vitamins except Riboflavin which is present only in foods of animal origin. Milling does not effect the vitamin content in pulses. Soaking and fermenting increases the Vitamin content by 2 folds. During soaking the protease enzyme acts on the complex proteins and make it simple and available to the body. Fermentation decreases the phytate and trypsin inhibitors and enhances the ionisable iron content.

Bengal gram,. Black gram, Green gram, Red gram, etc., are growing in India. These are rich in carbohydrates, proteins phosphorus and Iron Germination increases the Vitamin C content. Vegetarians in India include 30 to 50 grams of these pulses in their daily menu. The unabsorbable part of the pulse in the large intestine produces a lot of gas when it gets fermented by intestinal bacteria resulting in flatulence. Nutritive values of pulses and Legumes are given in Table 13.1.

SOYABEAN

Soyabean is highly consumed in China and Japan. It is rich in proteins, carbohydrates and fats. Soya milk can be prepared which is similar to cow's milk in its vitamin content. Soya bean has trypsin inhibiting factor. This factor is neutralised by proper cooking. Iron absorption is decreased on Soyabean diet when compared to diet of egg or milk. But it was increased by baking Soyabean at 200°C or by supplementing 100 mg of Vitamin C. Soyabean when administered substitute of animal protein to patients with Type II hypercholesteremia, reduced plasma cholesterol by 23 per cent in males and 25 per cent in females.

GROUNDNUT

Brazilians first cultivated groundnuts. These are also called pea-nuts. It is grown in tropics and is cheaper where compared to other nuts and oil seeds. Groundnut provide 25.3g proteins, 40.1g fat, 567 k cals of energy per every 100 g. Groundnut protein is deficient in Methionine. Groundnut when supplied with milk forms an excellent source of protein. Ground nut is rich in Nicotinic acid. Which is deficient in Maize. So pellagra can be prevented by giving Groundnuts to the people whose staple food is Maize.

Fungus Aspergillus flavus grow on groundnuts in a moisture filled atmosphere. This fungus, produce toxins which are collectively called aflatoxins. These aflatoxins produced liver cirrhosis. If food contaminated with aflatoxins for long time produces Jaundice, Fever, Anorexia, Vomiting, Portal hypertension, Ascites and Swelling of Extremities. The nutrient content of Groundnuts is given in Table 13.1.

KHESARI DAL

This is called Lathyrussatives. It requires very little water so it is grown is para crop or in drought conditions. It provides about 28 grams protein, 345 k cals energy and little fat. It has a Toxin β (N) Oxalyl amino alamine which produce Lathyrism when the pulse is consumed as staple food for long time. This disease is discussed in detail in one of the next chapters.

Table 13.1 : Nutritive Values of Pulses and Legumes

(Per 100 g)

	Protein gm	Fat gm	Carbohydrate gm	Energy kcal	Calcium mg	Phosphorus mg	Iron mg	Carotene mg	Thiamine mg	Riboflavin mg	Niacin mg	Vitamin C mg
Bengal gram (whole)	17.1	5.3	60.9	360	202	312	4.6	189	0.30	0.15	2.9	3
Bengal gram dal	20.8	5.6	59.8	372	56	331	5.3	129	0.48	0.18	2.4	1
Bengal gram roasted	22.5	5.2	58.1	369	58	340	9.5	113	0.20	--	1.3	0
Black gram dal	24.0	1.4	59.6	347	154	385	3.8	38	0.42	0.20	2.0	0
Cow pea	24.1	1.0	54.5	323	77	414	8.6	12	0.51	0.20	1.3	0
Green gram whole	24.0	1.3	56.7	334	124	326	4.4	94	0.47	0.27	2.1	0
Green gram dal	24.5	1.2	59.9	348	75	405	3.9	49	0.47	0.21	2.4	0
Horse gram	22.0	0.5	57.2	321	287	311	6.8	71	0.42	0.20	1.5	1
Peas roasted	22.9	1.4	58.8	340	81	345	6.4	18	0.47	0.21	3.5	0
Rajmah	22.9	1.3	60.6	346	260	410	5.1	--	--	--	--	--
Soyabean	43.2	19.5	20.9	432	240	690	10.5	426	0.73	0.39	3.2	--

14

Nuts and Oil Seeds

Nuts and oil seeds are not much consumed. A nut is a fruit and the edible seed enclosed in a shell. These nuts and oil seeds are costlier than other food stuffs. The commonly consumed nuts are coconut, cashew nuts, groundnuts, almonds, pistachios, Brazil nuts, Spanish Chest Nuts etc. The nutrient density of nuts and oil seeds is more. Except groundnuts all others are not in reach of common man. Oil seeds have good amount of protein and fat. Because of its content it gives more calories but fat soluble vitamins lack. The nutritive value of different nuts and oil seeds is given in Table 14.1.

CASHEW NUTS

Cashew nuts were first cultivated in South America .40 per cent of the world's need are cultivated in India. Cashew nut provides about 21 grams protein, 46 grams fat and 600 k. cals energy per every 100 grams. Cashew nuts are enclosed in a hard shell. The shell has power of water proofing. It is used in preparing water proofing agents, warnish, ink, oil cloth paints, etc.

COCONUT

India occupies a prime position in coconut yield. 96 per cent of India's production is spread in South India. Coconut has a outer fibrous sheath, below which a hard shell is present which protects the white edible kernel and water. Fresh coconut provides 4.5 grams protein 41

Table 14.1 : Nutritive Values of Different Nuts and Oil Seeds

	Protein gm	Fat gm	Carbohydrate gm	Energy kcal	Calcium mg	Phosphorus mg	Iron mg	Carotene mg	Thiamine mg	Riboflavin mg	Niacin mg	Vitamin C mg
Almond	20.8	58.9	10.5	655	230	490	5.1	0	0.24	0.57	4.4	0
Cashewnut	21.2	46.9	22.3	596	50	450	5.8	60	0.63	0.19	1.2	0
Coconut dry	6.8	62.3	18.4	662	400	210	7.8	0	0.08	0.01	3.0	7
Coconut fresh	4.5	41.6	13.0	444	10	240	1.7	0	0.05	0.10	0.8	1
Gingelly seeds	18.3	43.3	25.0	563	1450	570	9.3	60	1.01	0.34	4.4	0
Ground nut	25.3	40.1	26.1	567	90	350	2.5	37	0.90	0.13	19.9	0
Ground nut roased	26.2	39.8	26.7	570	77	370	3.1	0	0.39	0.13	22.1	0
Linseed Seeds	20.3	37.1	28.9	530	170	370	2.7	30	0.23	0.07	1.0	0
Mustard Seeds	20.0	39.7	23.8	541	490	700	7.9	162	0.65	0.26	4.0	0
Pista chio nut	19.8	53.5	16.2	626	140	430	7.7	144	0.67	0.28	2.3	0
Piyal seeds	19.0	59.1	12.1	656	279	528	8.5	0	0.69	0.53	1.5	5
Safllower seeds	13.5	25.6	17.9	356	236	823	4.6	0	--	--	--	--
Sunflower seeds	19.8	52.1	17.9	620	280	670	5.0	0	0.86	0.20	4.5	1
Wal nut	15.6	64.5	11.0	687	100	380	2.6	6	0.45	0.40	1.0	0

grams fat and 444 k cals energy. Coconut water is used for intravenous therapy. Nutritive value of different coconut products is given in Table 14.2.

Details of groundnut are discussed in the Chapter 13. Oil is extracted from both groundnut and coconut. After extraction the meal is used in cooking. Other oil seeds such as Gingelly seeds, Linseed, Mustard seeds, Safflower seeds, Sunflower seeds also provide lot of oil, protein and energy. All these oil seeds are used for extracting oil and the meal of some are used as animal feed. Some seeds like Mustard and Gingelly are used in cooking. Sweet preparations with Gingelly seeds are also not uncommon. Especially children love the toffees made of Gingelly seeds.

Table 14.2 : Nutritive Values of Different Nuts and Oil Seeds

(Per 100 g)

	Protein gm	Fat gm	Carbohydrate gm	Energy kcal	Calcium mg	Phosphorus mg	Iron mg	Carotene mg	Thiamine mg	Riboflavin mg	Niacin mg	Vitamin C mg
Coconut fresh	4.5	41.6	13.0	444	10	240	1.7	0	0.05	0.10	0.8	1
Coconut dry	6.8	62.3	18.4	662	400	210	7.8	0	0.08	0.01	3.0	7
Coconut tender	0.9	1.4	6.3	41	10	30	0.9	0	0	0	0	2
Coconut milk	3.4	41.0	11.9	430	15	140	1.6	0	0.08	0.04	0.6	3
Coconut water	1.4	0.1	4.4	24	24	10	0.1	0	0.01	0	0.1	2
Coconut meal (deoiled)	23.8	2.8	47.9	312	112	646	69.4	.	0.13	0.57	6.0	5

15

Vegetables

Plants or parts of plants which are used for bringing colour, taste and flavour to the food we eat are called vegetables. Different parts of the plants are used as vegetables. Some parts are eaten raw and some cooked. Different parts have different composition. The protein, carbohydrate, vitamin and mineral content vary from plant to plant and from part to part of a same plant. Very few plants are eaten wholly. Vegetables according to nutrition are generally classified into three broad groups.

1. Green Leafy Vegetables
2. Other Vegetables and
3. Roots and Tubers

We can classify vegetables according to the different parts used in the plant. This classification is shown in Table 15.1.

Vegetables have pigments which give them a characteristic colour. These colours change while cooking different colours like green, yellow, red, orange, pink, white etc., are found in vegetables.

The green colour of the vegetables is due to chlorophyll in them. This chlorophyll is essential for manufacturing its food. Chlorophyll has 2.7 per cent magnesium and two ester groups. Chlorophyll is not soluble in water but it is, soluble in acetone, ether and benzene. Addition of sodium bicarbonate to green leafy vegetables enhances the green colour to dark green, cellulose softens but vitamins are lost. Where as if acid is added it changes to olive green. Addition of acid replaces magnesium

Table 15.1 : Classification of Vegetables (With Examples)

1. **Roots**	6. **Flowers**
Beet root	Brocoli
Carrot	Cauliflower
Radish	Banana flower
Sweet Potato	7. **Fruits, Immature**
Turnip	Brinjal
2. **Tubers**	Lady Fingers
Potato	Tomato
Yam	8. **Immature Legumes**
3. **Bulbs**	Bean
Onion	Chickpea
Garlic	Cowpea
4. **Shoots**	Peas
Asparagus	Soyabean
5. **Leaves and Stems**	9. **Fruits**
Cabbage	Tomato
Celery	10. **Fungus**
Kale	Mushrooms
Rhubarb	11. **Cucurbits**
Spinach	Cucumber
	Pumpkin

with hydrogen and so pheophytin is formed which is olive green coloured.

The yellow colour of the vegetables is due to carotenoids. These are soluble in fats but not water. Carotenoids give yellow, orange yellow and red pigmentation. Acid and alkaline mediums does not effect much. Anthocyanins are glucosides which give blue, violet and red shades. Anthocyanins gain red colour in acid medium and blue colour in alkaline medium.

Flavones and Flavanols give cream or light yellow colour to the vegetables. Both are glucosides and are not soluble in water, they are soluble in organic solvents. In alkaline medium the colour darkens but acid medium has no effect.

The strong flavour of the vegetables is due to the presence of sulphur. This sulphur is present as volatile compound or sulphate form. When vegetables are cooked at high temperature the protein and sulphur divide and give hydrogen sulphide. Vegetables grown on soil with high sulphur content gives a lot of hydrogen sulphide while cooking. Usually these volatile sulphur compounds are present in the form of glycosides. When these vegetables are cooked with acid, alkali or enzymes these glycosides form sugar, phenols, allysulphide and isothiocyanate. The smell of cabbage and turnip is due to the presence of plant acids and volatile sulphur compounds.

Vegetables are stored in 1. Cold storage, 2. Deep freeze, 3. Canning and Dehydration.

Cold storage is storing vegetables between 32° – 50° F temperature. Different vegetables need different temperatures. Vegetables can also be stored at low temperatures as 0°F. For longer time first the vegetables are cut into pieces and packed in suitable containers then frozen rapidly to 40°F and then stored at 0°F. Dehydration and canning of vegetables is similar to fruits but in place of sugar solution brine is used.

16

Fruits

Plants preserve their food in the form of fruit. These fruits bear seeds which help in the propagation of its species. The food stored in the seed supplier the essential nutrients to the germinating seedling. Fruits have moisture, acids, carbohydrates, pectin and fibre. Different fruits have different sizes. The fruit varies in size in different stages. The amount of moisture, carbohydrates, pectin and their characteristics also differ with the age of the fruit and its size. The acids in different fruits have different pH. Grapes and Tamarind fruit has tartaric acid, Lemons, Oranges and Mango has citric acid where as apple has malic acid. As the fruits ripen the organic acids change into sugars due to the action of enzytnes. The cellulose layers in the fruits have pectin which gives toughness to the fruit. As the fruit ripens changes occur in fruit and the pectins gets softened. The heat produced during ripening make the cellulose soft. During ripening the following changes occur in the fruit.

i) **Colour** : Usually the colour changes from green to the respective colour of the fruit. This is because of the pigments in it.

ii) **Texture** : Texture of a ripened fruit becomes soft. This is due to the changes in carbohydrates and pectin.

iii) **Taste** : Ripening imparts a sweet taste to the fruit.

iv) **Flavour** : Ripe fruits give a sweet flavour. Which is special and unique for every species.

The cereals, pulses and vegetables we use are also fruits of their respective plants but they do not have sweetness, juice lot of moisture or flesh. So, we do not consider them as fruits. Usually fruits we consider to consist seeds which are surrounded by juicy sweet flesh. The juiciness, moisture content and sweetness vary from fruit to fruit. Depending on the number of ovaries and its divisions fruits are classified into simple,. aggregate and multiple fruits. Simple fruit is again divided into 1. Berry, 2. Pepo, 3. Hesperidium, 4. Drupe and 5. Pome. The classification alongwith examples is given in Table 16.1.

CHEMICAL COMPOSITION OF FRUITS

Sugars

The sugars present in fruits are sucrose, fructose and glucose.. The total sugar content varies from 2 to 23 per cent. Table 16.2 gives the per cent sugar content of different fruits.

Ascorbic Acid

The ascorbic acid content of different fruits are not equal. Guava is richest source of Ascorbic Acid. Mango, Lemon, Oranges and Papaya are good sources, while Apple, Pears and Grapes are poor sources. Ascorbic acid content of different fruits is shown in Table 16.2.

Other Acids

Citric acid and malic acid occur in large amounts in fruits. Apples contain malic acid and grapes have tartaric and malic acids. Other organic

Table 16.1 : Classification of Fruits

Simple Fruits					Multiple	Aggregate
Berries	*Pepo*	*Hesperidium*	*Drupe*	*Pome*		
Blue berry	Cucumber	Orange	Apricot	Apple	Pine	Black berry
Gross berry	Dates	Lemon	Coconut		Custard apple	Straw berry
Grapes		Sweet lime			Pomogranate	
Banana						
Tomato						

Table 16.2 : Sugar, Ascorbic Acid and Total Acid Content of Some Fruits

Fruits	Sugar %	Ascorbic acid mg/100 g	Total Acid %
Apple	13.5	5	0.50
Banana	23.0	10	0.40
Black berries	12.0	--	0.90
Cashew fruit	11.6	60	0.50
Cherries	17.9	10	0.69
Figs	19.7	50	0.18
Grape fruit	10.1	40	2.22
Grapes	14.8	10	1.23
Gauva	12.5	300	0.81
Jack fruit	18.1	53	0.24
Lemons	2.2	45	5.10
Mango	14.5	62	0.32
Oranges	10.9	30	0.94
Papaya	9.5	45	0.25
Pears	15.8	4	0.30
Pineapple	13.8	24	0.72
Pome granate	17.7	16	1.00
Rasp berry	14.4	32	1.34
Straw berry	8.0	60	1.10
Water melon	6.8	6	0.03

acids are present in very small amounts. The total acid content of different fruits are given in Table 16.2.

Pigments

Various pigments present in fruits imparts them the attractive colours. Carotenoids, flavanols, anthocyanin etc., are some of them.

Polyphenols

These compounds impart the astringent taste to the fruits. Guava, Banana, Apple etc. contain polyphenols.

Enzymes

Several enzymes are present in fruits. These bring about enzymic browning of fruits. These are ascorbic acid oxidase, phenol oxidase, etc.

Fruits have very negligible amounts of fat and proteins. All fruits are not 100 per cent edible. 6 – 39 per cent on average forms the inedible parts of fruits such as skin, seeds, cellulose, etc. Water content in fruits vary from 7.5 to 83 per cent. In case of melon it is 95 per cent and papaya has about 90 per cent. The calcium present in plants products is in bound form which is not available for the body. Fruits are rich in Vitamin C. Yellow and orange fruits are rich in carotenoids. Drying, spoiling or damage causes loss of vitamin C. If the fruits are stored at 0°C immediately after plucking, this loss can be minimized. Cooking also makes the fruit loose a lot of Vitamin C. The energy content of fruits is very low. The nutritive value of different fruits is given in Table 1 of Appendix.

FLAVOUR OF THE FRUITS

Each fruit has its characteristic flavour. Aromatic compounds are responsible for this flavour. Usually these compounds are esters of methyl butyrate. Organic acids present in fruits are also to some extent responsible for this flavours. Whereas the taste is dependent on type and content of acid and the ratio of sugars present.

COLOURS OF THE FRUITS

Carotenoids impart yellow orange colour to the fruits. These carotenoids can be divided into carotenes and xanthophylls. When carotenes are oxidised xanthophylls are obtained and these can be easily oxidised. Anthocyanins are glucosides which give different shades of red and blue colours. Anthocyanins give blue colour at Alakaline pH and red at acidic pH. Apple, blue berries, Grapes and Plums contain these compounds.

Tannins are free phenolic acids or their glucosides. These have astringent flavour. These tannins can be divided into pyrogallol and catechol tannins. These are colloidal compounds. These in combination with Ferric acids from blackish violet colour and blackish green colours. The presence of tannins in coffee seeds give a special brown colour to them.

Pectic substances are complex colloidal carbohydrate derivatives which have anhydrogalacturonic acid. Protopectin is the water soluble pectic substance and yields upon restricted hydrolysis, pectin or pectinic acid. Pectinic acids are colloidal polygalacturonic acids which have more than a negligible proportion of methylester groups. These form gels with sugar and acid. Pectic acids are colloidal polygalacturonic acids and are free from methyl ester groups. All the above mentioned pectic substances are different form of pectin. Basically they possess 100 to 200 molecules of galacturonic acid. The first carbon atom which has the aldehyde of one molecule of galacturonic acid is linked to the fourth carbon of another galacturonic acid molecule by ether linkage. The molecular weights of pectins from different sources vary from about 20,000 to 4,00,000. The chemical structure of galacturonic acid and its methyl ester are shown in Figure 16.1 their linkage is shown in Fig. 16.2

Pectins are soluble in water forming colloidal solutions. The solutions are viscous which is related to molecular weight and degree of esterification of the pectin. Pectin concentration, molecular weight of pectin, sugar concentration and pH are the factors determining the gel formation of a fruit.

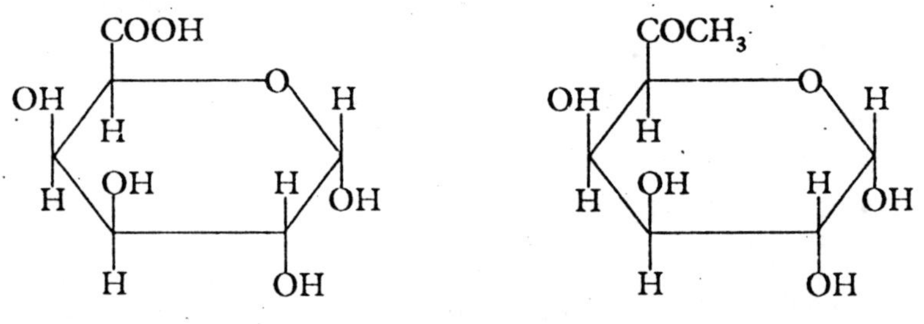

Fig. 16.1 : Galacturonic Acid and its Metyl Ester

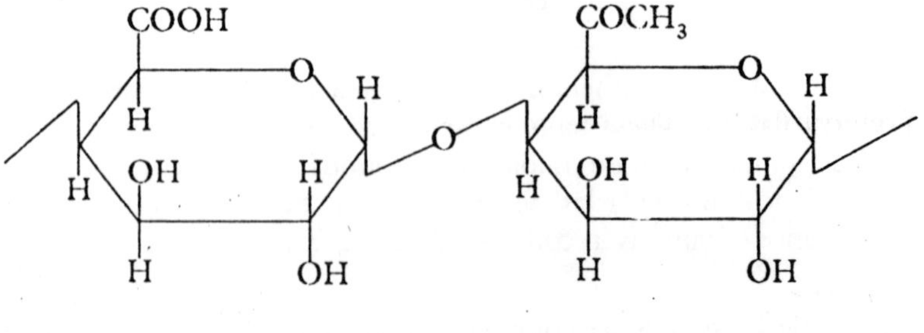

Fig. 16.2 : 1–4 Link between Galacturonic Acid and its Methyl Ester

Another substances called enzymes are present in fruits Oxidases and peroxidases are present in fruits which cause browning. Peroxidases are found in higher plant tissues. This decomposes H_2O_2 and form water and atomic oxygen. Oxidases can be divided into oxygenases, Tyrosinases and reductases. Oxygenases are aromatic substances. It has ortho dehydroxy group. Tyrosinase also takes part in many reactions and form brown black pigments called melanins. Reductase helps in reducing water to oxygen and hydrogen. Browning occurs in fruits. This may be due to enzyme participation also. Based on this the browning reactions are classified as 1. Enzymatic browning and 2. Non-enzymatic browning.

Enzymatic browning occurs in the presence of oxygen easily. If nitrogen compounds and sugars are present; organic acids and sugars are present or nitrogen compounds and organic acids are present browning occurs easily.

PREVENTION OF ENZYMATIC BROWNING

When fruits are cut browning can be prevented by

1. Changing the optimal condition
2. Addition of reducing agents
3. Removal of oxygen
4. Preventing oxygen to reach the fruit and
5. Inactivating the enzymes.

One can change the pH by dipping the fruit pieces in lemon juice or it can be stored at lower temperature. SO_2, salt and chlorides prevent browning for short time. CO_2 and nitrogen can be added to remove oxygen which reaches the fruit. The fruit pieces can also be dipped in boiled and cooled water or sugar solution which prevents oxygen contact with the fruit. Blanching inactivates enzymes and browning can be prevented.

Preservation and Processing of Fruits

Various products like canned fruits, Jams, Jellies, Marmalades, Juices, Squash, Cordials, Dried flakes, Dried fruits, etc. are made from fruits. The common methods used for preservation and processing of fruits are

1. Cold Storage
2. Freezing

3. Waxing
4. Canning
5. Fruit Juice Preparation
6. Jams, Jellies and Marmalades
7. Drying
8. Fruit Cereals Flakes
9. Fruit preserves
10. Candies, Glaced fruits, crystallised fruits, etc.

COLD STORAGE

Cold storage prevents action of micro organisms like bacteria, yeast and moulds. The enzyme action and loss of water from the fruit can be minimized. Fruits remain fresh for longer periods in cold storage.

FREEZING

Fruits are washed, peeled, sliced and are packed in bottles or cons in syrup and are stored at –50°C. Fruits are also stored in refrigerator containing higher amounts of carbondioxide which is called gas storage. This helps in preventing the gas loss from the fruit and helps the fruit to remain fresh.

WAXING

Wax emulsions with fungicides and bactericides are used to coat the fruits. This helps in destroying microorganisms on the fruit and also closes the pores of the fruit thus preventing loss of moisture. Fungicides like O-phenyl phenatol with sugar cane wax or microcry stalline petroleum wax are used, in which emulsifying agents like oleic acid or triethanolamine is used.

CANNING

Canning of fruits need the following steps. 1. Washing, 2. Peeling and Slicing, 3. Syruping, 4. Exhausting and sealing and 5. Heat processing and cooling. Washing removes dust, dirt and microflora from the surface of the fruits. Most fruits need peeling before canning. Peeling done by machines minimizes the chance of contamination. After peeling fruits are cut into slices and then transferred into cans filled with hot sugar syrup. Addition of sugar syrup aids in heat transfer and improving the taste of the fruits pieces. If the fruit has less citric acid, a small quantity of citric acid should be added to the syrup. Removal of air from the can before sealing helps in avoiding corrosion of the tin. The sealed cans are then sterilised by steam in a retort at atmospheric pressure for 35–45 minutes. After this the cans are cooled immediately under cold water.

FRUIT JUICES

Fruit juices are of different types. They can be divided into 1. Pure fruit juice, 2. Concentrated pure fruit juice, 3. Liquid fruits, 4. Squash, 5. Cordial 6. Fruit powder and 7. Carbonated fruit beverage.

JAMS, JELLIES AND MARMALADES

For preparation of Jams, Jellies and Marmalades the desired fruit should have adequate pectin. Jelly is a transparent and well set solid with original fruit flavour. It keeps its shape when removed from mould. Jam are cooked fruit pulp with sugar. Marmalade is fruit jelly with fruit pieces.

DRYING

Drying of fruits helps in storing them for a period of about 6 months. The commonly used dried fruits are raisins, dates, apricots, figs, pears and peaches. These fruits can be dried in sunlight or using artificial methods. First the fruits are cleaned, pickled, made into pieces and if needed dilute sodiumhydroxide or sodium carbonate are added, then passed through sulphurdioxide gas and finally dried. These treatments vary with the type of fruit. Mango pulp is strained and dried as thin layers and are stored as mango slabs. These slabs are treated with sulphurdioxide and stored in moisture proof packs.

FRUIT CEREAL FLAKES

Cereal flour is cooked with minimum amount of water, then it is blended with fruit pulp, sugar and citric acid. This mixture is dried on drum drier and flaked.

FRUIT PRESERVE

Under ripe nature fruits are selected for preparation of fruit preserve. Big fruits are cut into pieces and small ones are used as they are. These are cooked in sugar syrup until the pieces become transparent.

CANDIES, GLACED AND CRYSTALLISED FRUITS

Fruits impregnated with cane sugar, invert sugar and glucose and subsequently dried are called candies. Candied fruits covered with thin layer sugar which appears glassy is called glaced fruit. When candied fruit is covered with sugar crystals, it is called crystallised fruit.

17

Milk and Milk Products

Milk is a food item for all age groups. Milk has almost all nutrients so it is considered as a complete food. Vitamin C and Iron are limiting in milk. Children need approximately 1 litre of milk and adults 500 ml as minimum requirement. Milk is used to quench the thirst also. Many food items are prepared with milk.

Milk serum has lactose and many other mineral elements. Protcins are present dispersed in colloidal form. Fat is dispersed and forms an emulsion. Fat globules are of different sizes and can be observed in clusters. These globulês have a protein covering over them and when heated this covering becomes weak and breaks. Thus the globules coalesce. Milk has casein, fat globules and calcium phosphate in colloidal form. These reflect the light focussed on milk and so milk appears white in colour. But due to the presence of carotene and lactoflavin milk appears creamy white or light yellow in colour. Cow's milk has a lot of carotene so it appears to be light yellow in colour.

The presence of lactose gives the milk a special sweet taste. It is also dependent on the presence of other substances like chlorides and other gases dissolved in it. The dextrose forms acetyl methyl carbinol by the action of bacteria. This further gives diacetyl due to the presence of these two. Butter has a peculiar taste and flavour. Butyrin and caproin of the butter are also responsible for the flavour to some extent. Milk is slightly acidic in fresh condition. If there is large amount of cactic acid it shows fluctuation in its pH accordingly. The different nutrients present in the milk and composition of different milks is given in Table 17.1. Mean nutrient values of milk and some of its products are given in Table 17.2.

Table 17.1 : Composition of Different Milks

Nutrient	*Buffalo Milk*	*Cow Milk*	*Goat Milk*	*Human Milk*	*Assess Milk*
Protein (g)	4.3	3.2	3.3	1.1	2.1
Fat (G)	6.5	4.1	4.5	3.4	1.5
Carbohydrates (g)	5.0	4.4	4.6	7.4	6.5
Energy (k cals)	117	67	72	65	48
Calcium (mg)	210	120	170	28	80
Phosphorus (mg)	130	90	120	11	--
Iron (mg)	0.2	0.2	0.3	--	--
Carotene (mg)	--	6	--	--	--
Vitamin A (I. U.)	160	174	184	137	--
Thiamin (mg)	0.04	0.05	0.05	0.02	0.06
Riboflavin (mg)	0.10	0.19	0.04	0.02	0.03
Niacin (mg)	0.1	0.1	0.3	--	0.1
Free folic acid (mg)	3.3	5.6	0.7	1.3	--
Vitamin C (mg)	1	2	1	3	10
Sodium (mg)	19	73	11	--	--
Potassium (mg)	90	140	110	--	--

Table 17.2 : The Mean Nutrient Values per 100 ml of Milk and some of its Products

Nutrient	*Buffalo Milk*	*Cow Milk*	*Skimmed Milk*	*Skimmed Milk* powder	*Whole Milk* powder	*Curds*	*Cheese*
Protein (g)	4.3	3.2	2.5	4.1	3.5	3.1	24.1
Carbohydrates (g)	5.0	4.4	4.6	51.0	38.6	3.0	6.3
Fat (G)	6.5	4.1	0.1	0.1	26.7	4.0	25.1
Energy (k cals)	117	67	29	357	496	60	348
Carotene (mg)	160	174	--	Nil	1400	102	273
Thiamin (mg)	0.04	0.05	--	0.05	0.31	0.05	--
Riboflavin (mg)	0.10	0.19	--	1.64	1.36	0.16	--
Niacin (mg)	0.1	0.1	0.1	0.1	0.8	0.1	--
Folic acid (mg)	5.6	8.5	--	--	--	12.5	--
Vitamin C (mg)	1.0	2.0	1.0	5.0	4.0	1.0	--
Calcium (mg)	210	120	120	1370	950	149	790
Phosphorus (mg)	130	90	90	1000	730	93	520
Iron (mg)	0.2	0.2	0.2	1.4	0.6	0.2	2.1

The main protein in milk is casein and the rest is lactalbumin. Other proteins form a negligible portion. Casein forms casein calcium and phosphoprotein with calcium and phosphorus respectively. These proteins are easily digested and absorbed. These proteins have all essential amino acids. The main carbohydrate of milk is lactose which is important for growth of acid forming bacteria. In sour milk lactose is converted to cactic acid. The whey water after removing cheese is rich in lactose so cheese is a poor source of carbohydrates. The fat content is directly proportional to the protein content of the milk. If the protein content increases fat also increases but the water content decreases. The fat present in milk is in highly emulsified form. Homogenization of milk helps in even distribution of fat. This fat has Vitamin D also. Butyric and caproic acids are volatile fatty acids present in milk fat. All vitamins are present in milk. Vitamin C content is very little, which is lost when milk is heated. Milk is rich in calcium and phosphorus but it is a poor source of Iron.

Milk when processed becomes free from pathogenic micro organisms. Pasteurization, homogenization, sterilization, fortification, evapourization, concentration, freezing, fermentation, drying, etc., are the different processing carried on milk. Vitamin C is lost by these methods. Loss of thiamin and Vitamin B_{12} may also occur.

PASTEURIZATION

Pasteurization kills the pathogenic organisms present in the milk. Three methods are employed in this.

1. Milk is heated to between 62° and 65°C and kept for 30 minutes at this temperature,
2. Milk is heated to 72°C for 15 seconds and cooled rapidly. This is called high temperature short time method, and
3. Flash method in which milk is heated momentarily between 75°C and 77°C and cooled rapidly. Pasteurization does not alter the nutritive value of milk much only Vitamin C content is reduced by 20 per cent approximately.

HOMOGENIZATION

The fat present in unhomogenized milk is suspended in the form of different sized globules. These globules are split and made into 1/10th of their original size by applying pressure and forcing through fine appertures 40°C–65°C aids in this process. At 65°C a protein layer absorbs to the fat globules and does not combine with other globules.

Hence the fat globules in homogenized milk form a stable emulsion. But because of increased surface area rancidity occurs easily.

FORTIFICATION

Milk is rich in calcium and phosphorus. Vitamin D is essential for efficient utilization of these minerals in human body. So Vitamin D is added to the milk which is called fortification.

EVAPORISATION

In this method milk is heated in a vaccumpan to 60°C and 60% water is evaporated. In this method the milk gets concentrated and pasteurized. Vitamin C content is reduced. Vitamin D is usually added to evoprised milk. This milk can be diluted with water to make normal whole milk. The nutritive value does not differ much. This evaporised milk is filled in cans and heated to high temperature which facilitates in killing pathogenic organisms. Due to this heat treatment the colour, taste and flavour changes occur, which are pleasant. If sugar is added to the milk and then evaporised we can obtain sweetened condensed milk.

FREEZING

Pasteurized or homogenized milk is usually used for freezing. This milk should be stored below –10°F and should be immediately used after deforestation.

FERMENTATION

Bacteria ferment the lactose present in milk to lactic acid. Besides bacillus, moulds and yeast also ferment milk. Fermentation of lactose produces lactic acid and combines with calcium to form calcium lactate. Different bacteria produce different tastes and flavours. These fermented milk gives many product like curd and ghee. The vitamin content of milk is enhanced by fermentation. Fermented products of milk are comparatively better tolerated.

Milk is spray dried or roller dried and milk powder is obtained. Various concentration of milk can be obtained using this powder. Skimmed milk and whole milk can be used for this process. Milk powder can be stored for longer periods.

Milk is a good culture medium for growth of pathogens. Tuberculosis, undulant fever, scarlet fever, typhoid, paratyphoid, gastroenteritis, septic sour throat, amebic dysentery, bacillary dysentery, poliomyelitis, cholera brucellosis, anthrax, etc., are some of the diseases transmittable through milk. Cows and buffalos or any other milching animal should be tested for bovine tuberculosis and Brucella abortus. Apart from this milk should be stored and processed carefully.

18

Meat and Fish

Meat was the important food for pre-historic man. Many animal meats were used for this purpose. Animal flesh and organs like liver, kidney, pancreas and spleen contain protein of high biological value. Fish, prawns, crabs, snails, etc., are also consumed, but these foods are confined to areas with nearby water resources. Because of increased storage and transport facilities all foods are available all through the world irrespective of climate, season and sources.

STRUCTURE OF MEAT

Meat consists of muscle fibres bound together by a connective tissue matrix. Fibres are tubular structures with proteins, mineral salts, extractives and water. The connective tissue is composed mainly of collagen which yields gelatin on boiling. The amount of fat is dependent on cut of the meat and age and feed of the animal.

CUTS OF THE MEAT

Usually sheep, pig, cow or ox when cut have some soft parts and some bony parts. Usually bony parts are used for roasts. Meat from neck, belly and legs is tough and needs longer cooking time. In India mutton means meat derived form sheep. It is divided as (1) meat from thigh; (2) meat from ribs, (3) meat from back and (4) meat from neck regions. Meat from other parts is mixed up and sold for lower cost. Sketch 18.1 shows the division of various carcasses for obtaining meet.

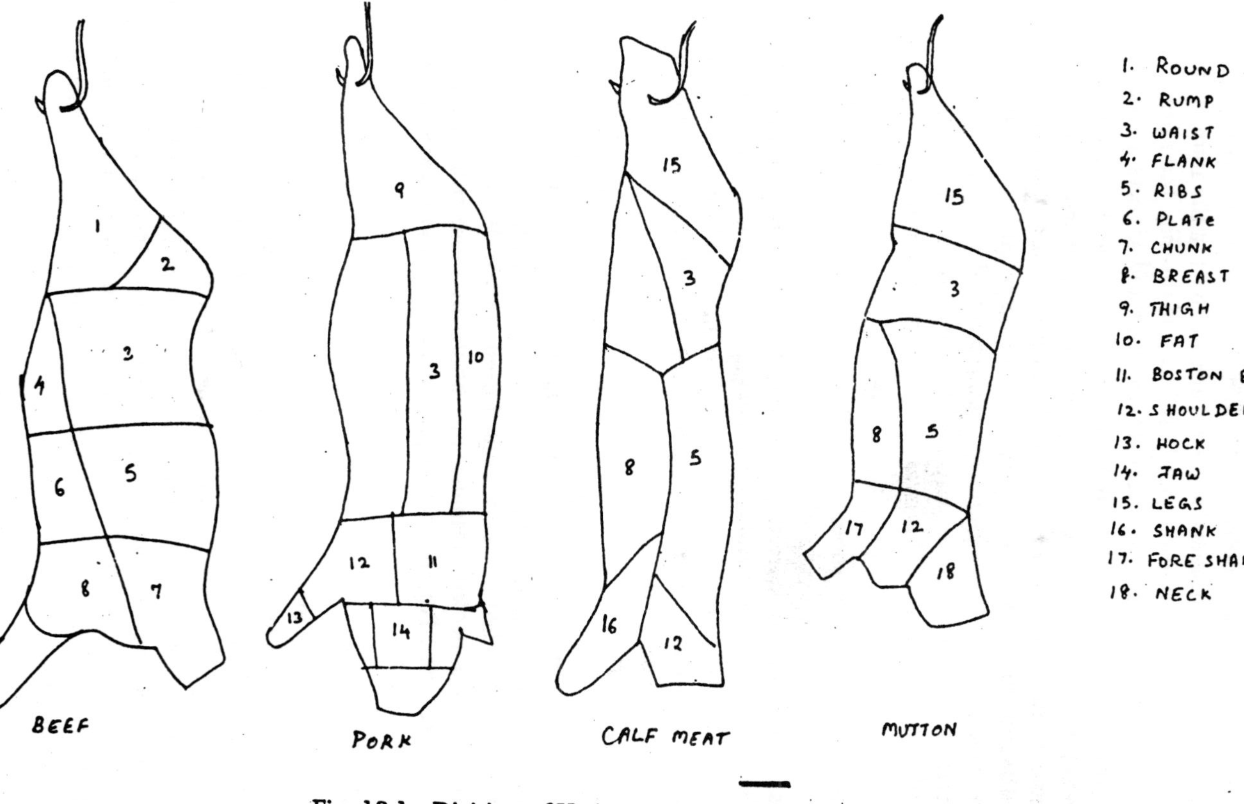

Fig. 18.1 : Division of Various Carcass for Obtaining Different Cuts

COMPOSITION

Meat contains highest amount of protein when compared to other animal foods. The carbohydrate content of meat is only one percent. Fat content varies from animal to animal age and feed of the animal. Meat is rich in Iron and phosphorus. Pork is rich in thiamin Meat from calf and chicken are rich in Niacin. Heart, liver and kidneys are rich in riboflavin, niacin and vitamin A. Vitamin C is very in meat and it is lost while cooking. In meat albumin, globulin, collagen and elastin are the protein substances. Albumin and globulin dissolve in dilute salt solution. Albumin dissolves in dilute acid and cold water. Albumin coagulates with moist heat where as globulin coagulates with dry heat. Collagen and elastin coagulates with dry heat. Collagen when heated with moist heat converts into gelatin. This is fastened in acidic medium.

Animal carcass stiffens immediately after sacrificing. This is called rigor mortis. Meat should never be used in this condition. After sometime meat looses stiffness and becomes soft. The carcass after sacrificing is stored at freezing point for 10 days to 6 weeks gets softened due to enzyme action and improves in taste. This meat is called ripened meat. This type of meat when cooked gives a golden brown colour and a very tasty gravy. Ripening more than 6 weeks produces rancidity due to the presence of fat.

POULTRY

The term poultry includes all birds which are reared at home. These birds are first beheaded, then the blood is allowed to drain and then feathers are pulled off. This is called dressed meat. Poultry with dark colour meat possess thiamine and riboflavin more than the light coloured ones. Poultry with fat gives good taste and juiciness to the recipe.

FISH

These live in water. These can be divided into fishes and crustaceans. Fish can further be divided into fresh water and sea water fishes. Fishes usually possess little fat (2%). Fishes like Halibut and Coal has about 5 per cent fat which is extracted from their liver. Protein efficiency ratio and biological value of fishes is more. Oysters are rich in iron, iodine, copper, calcium etc. Sea fish are rich in iodine Oysters are rich in riboflavin and thiamin whereas Salmon is rich in riboflavin and niacin. Fish lacks Vitamin C. Nutritive value of meat, fish and poultry are given in Table 18.1.

Table 18.1 : Nutritive Values of Meat, Fish and Poultry

	Protein g	*Fat* g	*Carbo-hydrate* g	*Energy* k cals	*Cal-cium* mg	*Phos-phorus* mg	*Iron* mg
Beef	22.6	2.6	--	114	10	190	0.8
Duck	21.6	4.8	0.1	130	4	235	--
Fowl	25.9	0.6	--	133	90	347	--
Goat meat	21.4	3.6	--	118	12	193	--
Liver goat	20.0	3.0	--	107	17	279	--
Liver sheep	19.3	7.5	1.3	150	10	380	6.3
Mutton	18.5	13.3	--	194	150	150	2.5
Pigeon	23.3	4.9	--	137	12	290	--
Pork	18.7	4.4	--	114	30	200	2.2
Snail	12.6	1.0	3.7	74	1321	147	--
Bacha	18.1	5.6	6.1	147	520	180	0.7
Bombay duck (dry)	61.7	15.1	2.5	293	1389	240	19.1
Catfish	21.4	--	--	86	10	230	--
Crab muscle	8.9	1.1	3.3	59	1370	150	21.2
Herring	20.3	3.2	2.2	119	429	305	9.3
Katla	19.5	2.4	2.9	111	530	235	0.9
Lobster	20.5	0.9	--	90	16	279	--
Mackrel	18.9	1.7	0.5	93	429	305	4.5
Mullet	19.1	7.8	2.1	155	357	175	4.4
Oil Sardine	19.6	2.0	0.1	97	357	349	6.1
Pomfrets (white)	17.0	1.3	1.8	87	200	290	0.9
Ribbon fish	18.1	3.2	0.6	104	214	218	13.9
Shark	21.6	0.4	0.8	93	357	262	1.4
Shrimp (dry)	68.1	8.5	--	349	4384	1160	--

The softness of the meat is dependent on aging, mechanical alteration, freezing at the time of rigor mortis, enzyme action, change in pH, use of acids, calcium and sugar etc. Aging brings softness in meat. This softness is different from meat to meat and this change in softness is sometimes fast and some times slow. Mechanical alteration i.e. grinding, beating, grating etc. also brings about softness in meat. If the meat is cut immediately after animal is sacrificed it acquires hardness which is relieved slowly. Usually a hard cut remains hard even after cooking. Use of enzymes like papain causes softness in meat. Proteolytic enzymes when spread all through the cut it softness easily but, it is a difficult task. Poultry immediately after sacrifice are given intravenous enzyme injection which causes softness of meat but this meat should be cooked immediately, else it want be advantageous in cooking. Enzyme can be brushed on the meat which causes softness on the top layers but in the middle it would remain hard. Addition of papain to the meat while cooking softens the meat and it would give good results when cooked between 55°C and 75°C. Freezing brings softness in beef. Aged animals meat does not get softness by this method. pH between 5.0 and 6.0 causes hardness of meat. It should be below 5.0 or above 6.0. This is because formation of gelatin from collagen is very little at pH 5–6. Intracellular proteins dissolve in salt. Salt increases the palatability of meat. The softness of meat after cooking is dependent on salt concentration. If the concentration of salt increases meat tends to be dry. Addition of 1.5 g of salt (per 100g of meat) increases taste, softness and weight of cooked meat. Addition of sugar alongwith salt gives softness to meat. It also increases the palatability.

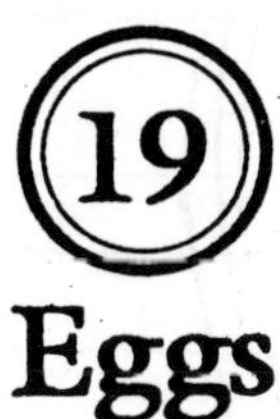

Eggs

Egg is a food stuff of high nutritive value. It has high biological value. Usually term egg refers to Hens egg. But nutritionally egg refers to all birds' eggs. It has balanced amounts of amino acids and is called reference protein.

STRUCTURE

Biologically egg has a living center surrounded by food material, protective membranes and shell. Above the shell there is a layer of mucin or bloom which protects the egg from bacterial invasions and water loss. The shell is made up of calcium carbonate mainly. Below the shell there is another membrane made of two layers, the inner and the outer. The outer layer sticks to the shell and is separated from the inner at large end by a air cell. Egg when laid has the temperature of hens body but later due to the temperature differences in the atmosphere air cell is formed. In a freshly laid egg the diameter of the air cell and the height are not more than 12mm and 3 mm respectively.

Different parts of egg are shown in the Sketch 19.1. The inner white yolk is surrounded by yolk which has a germ spot and is surrounded by a membrane called the vitelline membrane. The whole yolk is suspended in the middle of the egg by means of white thread like structures called chalazae. The germ spot is also called blastoderm and it has a latebra behind connecting the inner white yolk. The egg white or albumin surrounding the yolk is made of three layers of alternate thin and thick layers. Next is a double layered protective membrane. The

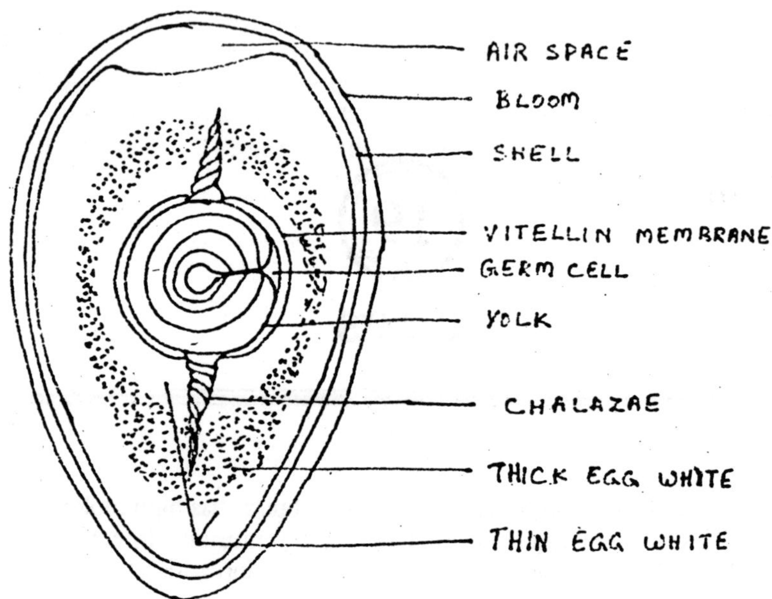

Sketch 19.1 : Different Parts of an Egg

inner membrane surrounds the egg white where as the outer membrane is attached to the shell. In between these two membranes the air cell is present. This is formed due to the temperature differences in the body of the layer bird and external temperature. Next is the shell, a brittle covering made of calcium carbonate mainly. The shell is surrounded by a thin film of mucin called bloom which is protective in function.

EGG YOLK

The colour of the yolk varies according to the feed and heredity. It ranges from pale yellow to orange. Egg yolk possess about 50 per cent water, 1/6 part of total protein, 1/3 part fats and 1.7 per cent minerals. It has different proteins. The following are important ones : 1. Phosphoproteins, 2. Lipoproteins, 3. Egg yolk has about 30 per cent lipids. It is a mixture of about 66 per cent triglycerides, 28 per cent phospholipids, 5 per cent of cholesterol and little of other lipids. Egg yolk has Iron, Phosphorus and Calcium. The sulphur content is lower when compared to egg white. Vitamin A, thiamin, riboflavin and vitamin D are also present in the yolk. Egg yolk has two lipoproteins at least, lipovitellein and lipovitellenin. Lipovitellin contains 17 to 18 per cent lipid, while lipovitellenin contains 36 to 46 per cent mainly lecithins. Lipoproteins by exhaustive extraction with 80% alcohol gives proteins vitelline and vitellenin. Vitelline contains 1% phosphorus and vitellenin contains 0.29 per cent approximately. Egg yolk has water soluble protein called livetin. The composition of egg yolk is 49% water, 32% fat, 16.7% protein, 1.8% ash and 50.5% total solids. Yolk is 31% of the total egg.

EGG WHITE

Egg white possess 88 per cent water, 10 per cent protein and traces of fat. Egg white contain several proteins of which ovalbumin measures to 55%. Table 19.1 gives the proteins and their percentage in Egg white.

Table 19.1 : Proteins in Egg White

Name of the protein	*Relative amount (%) in egg white*
Ovalbumin	55
Conalbumin	13
Ovomucoid	10
Lysozyme	3.4
Avidin	0.05
Ovo inhibitors	0.1
Other proteins	11.55

Ovalbumin is abundant in egg white proteins. It is a phosphoprotein with a small amounts of carbohydrate. It is readily precipitated by heat. Conalbumin binds the iron forming red coloured complex. Ovomucoid is a glycoprotein which has mannore and glucosamine. Lysozyme is a protein, basic in nature with high percentage of histidine, lysine and arginine. It is unstable with alkalies but is stable to heat, cold and other denaturing agents. Ovomucin precipitates on dilution with water at 6.4 pH. It is most difficult protein of the egg white proteins to handle as it is very insoluble and difficult to purify. Avidin is a protein which binds biotin. It is present in low concentration in egg white. Egg white has 88 per cent water, 0.05 per cent fat, 10 per cent protein, 0.82 per cent ash and 12.13 per cent total solids. Egg white is about 58% of the total egg. Egg white have sulphur, potassium, chlorine and sodium in appreciable amounts while phosphorus, calcium, magnesium and iron in smaller amounts.

EGG SHELL

Egg shell is brittle and acts as protective membrane to the contents inside. Shell is about 11% of the total egg. Shell is made up of calcium carbonate mainly. The composition of egg shell is as given in Table 19.2.

Table 19.2 : Composition of Egg Shell

$CaCo_3$	92.4
$MgCo_3$	1.29
P_2O_5	0.76
Organic matter	4.25
Water	1.4

COLOUR OF THE EGG

Shell

The colour of the shell is dependent of breed and inheritance. Some birds lay egg with white shells, some with brown shell, some with specks and some with other colours like blue.

White

Egg white has a opalescent appearance, as the pH raises the egg white becomes clear and transparent. Some times egg white appears with greenish colour which is due to its riboflavin content.

Yolk

The colour of egg yolk is dependent on the feed. The colour of the yolk varies from almost white through yellow and deep orange.

QUALITY OF AN EGG

The term quality of an egg denotes its value from nutritional, palatability and culinary stand points. Various methods like candling, yolk index, and observation of the shell quality are used to determine the quality of an egg.

Candling

This method is used to find the quality of egg without breaking it. A 40 watt bulb is illuminated in a narrow metallic container at one end and egg is rotated at the other end. The position and size of the yolk is seen as a shadow. The air space and meat spots if any can also be seen.

This is not a reliable method.

As the egg deteriorates, chalazae weaken and yolk tends to settle down rather remain suspended.

Yolk Index

The egg is broken and is poured into a flat plate. The height of the yolk and its width are measured in millimeters. The height divided width gives the yolk index. As the egg deteriorates the vitelline membrane breaks because yolk imbibes water from egg white, thus the yolk spreads off.

Shell

Shell should be devoid of any cracks and should not be washed. Washing the shell dissolves the protective layer bloom and renders free entry of micro-organisms into the egg. So egg if washed should be used immediately.

CHANGES DURING STORAGE

Physical Changes

1. Egg white becomes less viscous
2. Water is imbibed by the yolk from egg white thus increasing in size and resulting in breaking of vitelline membrane, and
3. Due to moisture loss, air cells increases in size.

Chemical Changes

The chemical changes are due to

1. Loss of water
2. Loss of carbondioxide
3. Change in pH
4. The breakdown of proteins
5. Increase in free ammonia
6. Deterioration in the flavour of eggs.

STORAGE

The purpose of storing the eggs is to prevent deterioration as long as possible. The alkalinity and bacterial count is kept lowest. The atmosphere in the storage is maintained to possess some Co_2 so that changes in pH can be minimized. At higher temperatures growth of the bacteria can be seen. So eggs are stored at cool temperatures. Moisture on the eggs helps the moulds to grow well. So moisture should be controlled. Temperature between 29°F and 31°F is optimal for storing eggs.

Dipping eggs in mineral oil at 10°F for a few seconds and then storing at 50°F to 60°F increases the storage life of eggs. Mineral oil should be at 10°F only. Any variations cause the egg to imbibe oil and spoil easily. The oil layer prevents the moulds entering the egg so that eggs can be stored for longer duration.

PROCESSING

Cold storage, freezing, drying and thermostabilization are the methods used in processing the eggs.

Cold Storage

Usually eggs are stored at a temperature slightly higher than freezing point (usually at 29°F – 31°F). Increase in temperature increases loss of carbondioxide from the egg and causes liquification of egg white. The humidity and air currents in the room should be regulated. Storing eggs at the above mentioned temperature in a atmosphere of carbondioxide or Ozone is preferable. In this method eggs can be stored for about six months.

Freezing

Freezing controls the growth of bacteria. In this method care should be taken upon the sterilization of equipment and avoidance of contamination of egg mass. In this method eggs should be freezed untill they are used. Eggs should be washed just before breaking and freezing should follow immediately. Usually winter pasteurization is done before freezing. Yolk is pasteurized at 61.6°C and white at 56.7°C for about two minutes. In this method 99 per cent of pathogens will be destroyed. Freezed egg white is better than freezed egg yolk. Freezed egg yolk become gummy, thick and viscous. This can be minimized if sugar is added to the yolk before freezing.

Drying

Previously eggs are dried using belt drying method. Now spray drying is used. The egg is broken and egg white or egg yolk or both are put into a automizer and is spray dried. Immediately the powder is stored without any moisture. Eggs can be preserved as whole eggs, or as separated yolks or whites. To retain their functional properties as well as colour, flavour egg white requires enzyme treatment for removal of last traces of glucose. If the drying temperature is at 40°F undesirable changes in taste and smell takes places. It is better to dry the eggs at 0°F.

Thermostabilisation

In this method eggs are heated for 16 minutes in oil or water at 130°F – 136°F. In this type of eggs white is more gummy and it is difficult to separate yolk and white. Foam volume of these eggs is lower than the untreated eggs so the cooked volume of these egg products is also low

20

Beverages

Beverage forms an undeletable item from our daily menu. Beverage not only refreshes a person but also helps in supplementing fluid. A day starts with a cup of strong coffee or tea for many. Serving a beverage to the guest is just as a hello. Beverage help to foster social contact as it is convenient to discuss over a cup of tea or coffee. The most commonly used beverages are tea, coffee, fruit juice and aerated waters. These are conveniently classified as

1) Coffee, tea and cocoa
2) Nonalcoholic beverages
3) Alcoholic beverages

COFFEE

Coffee can be called as a universal beverage. Coffee has alkaloid caffeine and tannins which give characteristic aroma and have a stimulating action, which remove the feeling of exhaustion. Coffee was born in Tropical Africa and spread throughout. It is cultivated throughout the tropical and subtropical areas. It needs 18.9°C to 25°C temperature, slight drizzling and sunlight. It is best grown at a height of 1500–2500 feet above sea level. Coffee fruits appear seven months after the appearance of flowers. It takes another three months for ripening. The ripe fruit has dark crimson colour. These fruits are collected from the tree and processed. The important varieties grown are : 1) Coffee arabica 2)

Coffee Robusta and 3) Coffee Liberica. Mostly Arabica and Robusta are cultivated in India.

PROCESSING

Two methods are followed one is plantation or parchment second is native or cherry. One is wet process and other is dry process.

Plantation or Parchment

In this method the mature fruit are sent into pulpers and the pulp is removed. Later it is fermented for 12 to 36 hours and washed. Then they are dried, the parchment membranes sticks to the seed. This membrane is removed in curing houses. This is called plantation or parchment coffee. Parts of a coffee fruit is shown in Sketch 20.1.

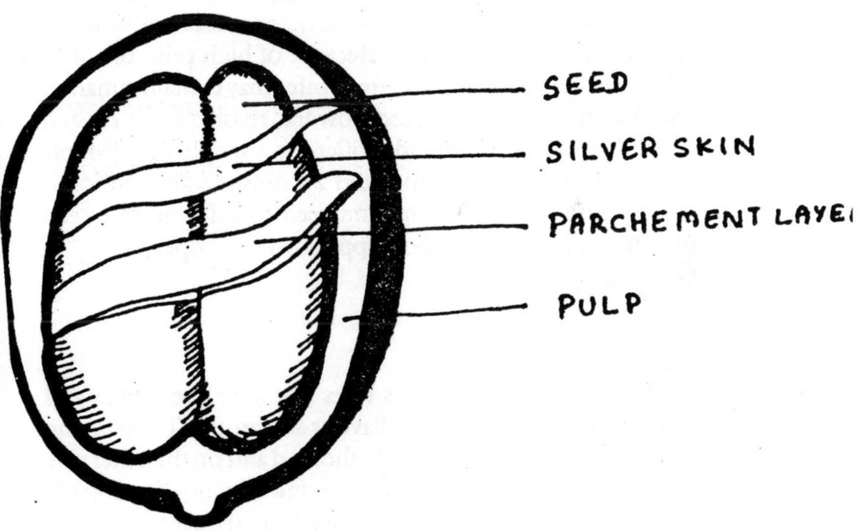

Sketch 20.1 : Parts of a Coffee Fruit

Native or Cherry

This is comparatively easy method. The fruits are dried until the parchment membrane become loose. Then the fruits are pounded in a mortar or sent into a huller and the husk is removed. This is called native or cherry coffee. The characteristics of different coffee's are given in table 20.1.

Table 20.1 : Characteristics of Different Coffees

Species	*Type of Process*	*Characteristics*
Arabica	Plantation	Long seeds, Greenish or greenish blue in colour
	Cherry	Dull coloured or brown
Robusta	Plantation	Smaller in size than Arabica and Greenish in Colur
	Cherry	Dull Coloured

Chicory a plant root imparts flavour to coffee. A blend of coffee and chicory is permitted by law provided it is declared on the label. Such coffee is called "French Coffee". Chicory is more soluble in water so french coffee gives a strong decoction. Because of high price of coffee adulteration became common. Adulterated coffee may contain tamarind seed powder, skin of tapioca, date seed powder, roasted peas, roasted husk, etc. This adulteration can be identified by a simple test. Sample coffee powder is taken on a filter paper and 2% caustic soda solution is dropped on it. If the coffee has tamarind seed powder or date seed powder as adulterant pink to red spots appear on the paper.

Roasted Coffee Powder

Roasting

Normally processed coffee seeds does not have the aroma and flavour. Roasting imparts the necessary flavour and aroma. The roasting should be carefully done the colour inside the seed and on the outer side should be same. Over-roasting and under roasting does not develop the flavour desired. Table 20.2 gives the roasting effect on quality of coffee.

Table 20.2 : Effect of Roasting on Quality of Coffee

Roasting	*Aroma*	*Extract Consistency*
Light Roast (Light brown colour)	Less Aroma	Light Extract
Medium Roast (Medium Brown Colour)	Good Aroma	Strong Extract
Over Roast (Dark brown colour)	Less Aroma	Strong extract with bitter taste

While roasting the Co_2 increases in the seed and the pressure due to which the seed becomes porous and increases in size. During this time seeds gives good aroma, become shing in appearance and makes splitting sound. Immediately the seeds are removed from the roaster. This roasting caramelises the sugar in the seed and imparts the colour to the brew to some extent. This caramelised sugar is soluble in water when medium roasting takes place. But when seeds are over roasted the seeds are charred and gives bitter taste to the brew.

The grinding of roasted seeds should be medium fine and if desired can be blended with chicory powder but it should not exceed 50 per cent. Instant coffee is made by extracting the coffee powder and spray drying the extract along with the recovery of volatile flavouring compounds.

TEA

Tea was known since 350 A.C. Tea was first cultivated in China. Tea is also grown in Tropical countries. Tea is cultivated extensively in India, China and Sri Lanka. Only the new green shoots are collected. As the size of the leaf increases the quality of the tea decreases. Tea has caffeine, Tannin which give characteristic flavour and aroma. Tea leaves are plucked in the beginning of spring and summer. Boston Tea Party of colonial period, Tea Ceremony of Japan tells us the importance of tea in history.

PROCESSING

Three types of tea are made depending on their processing methods. They are 1) Black tea 2) Green tea and 3) Oolong tea.

Black Tea

The tea leaves are collected and spread thinly on racks. After withering these leaves are passed between rollers due to which the cells walls rupture and releases of enzymes and juices takes place. These leaves are left at 70° to 80°C for fermentation during which the dark colour develops. The polyphenols like catechin and Grallo catechin are respon sible for this. These leaves are then dried at 100°C.

Green Tea

In this preparation the tea leaves are first steamed to destroy the enzymes and micro organisms. Then these leaves are passed under a roller to rupture the cells walls and then dried at about 100°C.

Oolong Tea

It is intermediate between black tea and green tea. The leaves are slightly withered and fermentation sets in. For this process the leaves are spread about 4 inches deep in baskets in shade. These leaves are derived after 4 hours at 200°C stirring continuously. This tea has the qualities of both the qualities of black tea and green tea. Formosa is famous for Oolong tea. The manufacture of instant tea is some what similar to instant coffee. The tannin content of the tea or coffee depends upon the type, method of preparation and the serving size.

COCOA

Cocoa and chocolate both goes hand in hands. Cocoa grows well at about 15 to 40°C and about 700 meters above sea level. Cocoa is not only stimulant is a health drink as it has good amount of protein, fat and vitamins. The nutrient value depends on the amount of milk the drinks has.

Processing

The Cocoa fruits which are fully mature and ripe should be selected. First the fruit is split into two and the following processing steps are followed : 1) Fermentation 2) Curing 3) Roasting 4) Grinding and defatting 5) Powdering.

Fermentation

The freshly harvested beans are split and heaped and allowed to ferment in wooden boxes which are perforated at the bottom to collect off the liquids Oozed during fermentation. The heat in the box should reach 40–60°C. Fermentation completes when the temperature begins to fall.

Curing

The fermented beans are dried in sun or hot air driers. During this process the shell becomes dark brown.

Roasting

Roasting improves colour and flavour of the bean. After roasting the bean is sent into decorticating machines to remove the seed coat after which it is called nib.

Grinding and Defatting

The nibs are ground. The heat of the grinder makes the cocoa melt because of its high fat content. The fat is pressed to obtain cocoa butter and the residue is pressed into cakes.

Powdering

The Cocoa is then treated with alkali to improve its colour and flavour. This is called Dutch process. In natural process cocoa is directly powdered.

Cocoa should be stored between 16 to 21°C and 50–65 per cent humidity in atmosphere. Heat and moisture spoils cocoa by forming grey surface called bloom. In chocolates and sugared cocoa bloom is calls sugar bloom which is gritty because sugar crystals. The flavour is lost in these conditions. So, cocoa should be stored carefully.

NON-ALCOHOLIC BEVERAGES

Non alcoholic carbonated beverages are consumed in large quantities now-a-days. These beverage preparation include three steps :

1) Preparation of acidified flavoured syrup
2) Addition of carbonated water
3) Bottling

The major ingredients used in manufacture of non-alcoholic carbonated beverages are sugar, flavouring agent, acid, water, colour and carbondioxide. Synthetic flavour, approved colour, phosphoric or citric acid, soft water and chemically pure carbondioxide should be used in the preparation. The 60–65% cane sugar syrup is prepared and sterilized. To which per cent phosphoric or citric acid is added with flavours desired. Edible permissible colours are added and filled in clean bottles. Carbondioxide is added to this water and then worked with metal caps or crowns.

FRUIT BEVERAGES

These are three types usually

1) Fruit juice
2) Squash
3) Cordial

Fruit Juice

This is fresh juice extracted from various fruits which contain sugar, small amounts of vitamins and minerals. The presence of organic acids gives an acid taste to it.

Squash

This is prepared by the addition of sugar, preservative and organic acids to freshly expressed fruit juice. This is diluted with water before consumption.

Cordial

This is different from squash that the suspended fruit pulp has been removed. This is also diluted before consumption.

COCONUT WATER

The water from tender coconut is used for quenching thirst. This water is very popular and it is sterile. In fresh state it can be used for intravenous therapy.

COCONUT MILK

Coconut milk is a emulsion expressed from fresh grated coconut. It is extracted by the addition of 6 times the amount of water.

NEERA

Freshly extracted sap of palm is preserved by the addition of calcium hydroxide. It is popular in India.

SUGAR CANE JUICE

Sugar cane is crushed and the juice extracted is mixed with little lemon juice. This is a very popular drink in summer.

SHARBAT

This is sugar syrup flavoured with artificial flavouring agents. These syrups need dilution before consumption.

ALCOHOLIC BEVERAGES

Alcoholic beverages are broadly divided into three classes.

1. Beer, Ale, Porter, Stout, Toddy, etc.
2. Wine and Cider

3. Distilled liquors as whisky, brandy, rum, grin, vodka and Arack.

All these are fermented products distilled or undistilled. They vary in their alcohol content and hop.

BEER

This is made by fermenting barley malt extract with yeast. The alcohol content varies from 2 to 5 per cent and are usually pasteurized and carbonated before botting.

ALE

It is made from regular beer ingredients but stronger in hop than beer and has a higher alcohol content i.e. 4 to 6 per cent.

PORTER

It is heavier ale with strongly roasted malt with less hops.

STOUT

It is heavier and sweeter than ale and porter. It is similar to protein other aspects.

TODDY

It is fermented sap of palms with yeast. It has 4–8 per cent alcohol.

WINE

This is preparation made by fermenting grapes with yeast. Table wines have less than 14 per cent alcohol but dessert wines have more than 14 and less than 20 per cent alcohol by volume.

Cider

It is apple wine. Apple juice is fermented with yeast and it has 8 to 14 per cent alcohol by volume.

WHISKY

Alcoholic distillate from fermented Rye or wheat or barley malt or corn. The alcohol content is between 30 to 35 per cent by weight.

BRANDY

This is an alcoholic distillate of fermented grapes, apples etc. The alcohol content is between 30 to 35 per cent by weight.

RUM

The alcoholic distillate of fermented molasses or sugar cane juice whose alcohol content varies between 30 to 35 per cent.

GIN

It is diluted and flavoured ethyl alcohol

VODKA

It is an alcoholic distillate of fermented rye or potato.

ARRACK

It is an alcoholic distillate of toddy whose alcohol content varies from 30 to 35 per cent.

The nutrient composition of some beverages is given in Table 20.3.

Table 20.3 : Nutritive Composition of Some Beverages

	Protein gm	Fat gm	Carbohydrate gm	Energy kcal	Calcium mg	Phosphorus mg	Iron mg	Carotene mg	Thiamine mg	Riboflavin mg	Niacin mg	Vitamin C mg
Orange Juice	0.2	0.1	1.9	9	5	9	0.7	15	0.06	0.02	0.4	64
Passion fruit juice	1.2	0.2	7.7	37	10	30	0.7	1968	0.01	0.02	0	13
Milk Buffalo's	4.3	6.6	5.0	117	210	130	0.2	160	0.04	0.10	0.1	1
Butter milk	0.8	1.1	0.5	15	30	30	0.1	--	--	--	--	--
Skimmed milk	2.5	0.1	4.6	29	120	90	0.2	--	0.45	1.64	1.0	5
Coconut milk	3.4	41.0	11.9	430	15	140	1.6	--	0.08	0.04	0.6	3
Coconut water	1.4	0.1	4.4	24	24	10	0.1	--	0.01	--	0.1	2
Neera	0.4	--	10.9	45	--	140	0.1	--	0.02	--	--	13
Sugar cane juice	0.1	0.2	9.1	39	10	10	0.1	6	--	0.04	--	--
Toddy sweet	0.1	0.3	14.3	59	150	10	0.3	--	--	0.04	--	--
Toddy fermented	0.1	0.3	1.8	38	--	--	--	--	0.01	0.01	0.2	--

21

Spices and Condiments

Spices are aromatic pungent substances. Condiments are processed spices. Spices and condiments are used in small amounts but they influence the flavour and aroma to a great extent. Recognition of this flavouring compounds lead to the preparation of artificial essence. Cinnamon aldehyde gives clove flavour, methanol gives mint flavour etc. These spices and condiments comes under intentional additives. These spices and condiments are responsible for laying foundation of foreign trade. With Europeans pepper, cardamom, coriander, cumin seeds, celery, nutmeg, cloves, etc., are being exported to a large extent.

These does not contribute much to the nutritive value of the food. It is because they are used in very small quantities in India per head 10 to 25 grams of spices and condiments are consumed every day. Nutritive value of different spices and condiments are shown in Table 21.1. Mint leaves, coriander leaves, curry leaves, etc., provide good amounts of vitamin C in fresh condition.

CARDAMOM

It is seed of the plant Elettaria cardamomum. 90% of world's cardamom crop comes from India. Cardamom grown well in cool mountain valleys; 750–1000 meters above sea level and 150–200 cm of rain fall. Cardamom has a sweet flavour which is appetizing. Essence is prepared from this cardamon. Tincture of cardamon has medicinal value. It has carminative action, cardamom is consumed along with betel leaves or as it is to get rid of bad smell of mouth or to mask some smells and it is also used in preparation of many dishes.

PEPPER

Black pepper is dried fruit of a plant piper nigrum. Pepper has an important place in condiments and spices. 93 per cent of India's crop comes from Kerala. It has an alkaloid piperine which is 5 to 8 per cent of weight and 1 to 4 per cent of volatile pepper oil. Pepper is used as medicine for cold and cough. The pungency of pepper is due to a resin, chavicine.

CLOVES

Cloves are dried flower buds of the plant engenie caryophyllate. East India Company introduced cloves in India. It is mostly grown in South India. Cloves are known to be used in history as stimulant, medicine and spice. Clove essence is used in sweet dishes. Synthetic vanilla is prepared from oil of cloves. It has a great medicinal value in dental science. It even produces skin anesthesia by spillage.

CINNAMON

Cinnamon is bark of a tree Cinnamomum Zeylanicum which is grown in South India. Cinnamon is used as stimulant. It is known to cure windiness. The oil of cinnamon has cinnamic aldehyde which is said to have anti-bacterial action and carminative action.

CHILLIES

Chillies entered in India in 17 century. 75 per cent of India's crop come from South India. Capsaicin (8 methyl-N-vanillyl-6-Nonenamide) is responsible for the hotness of chillies. Chillies in fresh condition have a lot of vitamin C. Capsicum is used as vegetable. There are the most spices used in Indian cookery.

GINGER

Ginger is the root of zingiber officinale. The pungency is due to oleoresin and gingerol. Ginger grows all over India. Crop from Kerala accounts to 53 per cent of total production in India. Ginger ale is prepared from this. Ginger is used as medicine also.

NUTMEG AND MACE

Nutmeg is dried kernel from seeds of the tree Myristica frangrance.

These entered India in eighteenth century. The crop is grown in South India. The thick covering of nutmeg is called Mace. Nutmeg when ripe sheds off this covering. This covering has a attractive colour, flavour and aroma. If it is removed before nutmeg is ripe, it does not have good colour and is very thick too. Nutmeg has a great medicinal and cosmetic value. The oil extract from its leaves have weedicidal and medicinal properties. Mace extract is used as a mordant too.

ONION

Onion is widely used in India. It is consumed raw by some people. It has allyl propyl disulphide which is responsible for its tearing action. Crop taken when the leaves are withering a strong tearing action.

GARLIC

Garlic is the bulb of the plant Allium Sativum. Garlic has medicinal value. It is used in the treatment of whooping cough, long diseases, stomach ailments, etc. It has sulphur containing organic elements which are responsible for its strong odour. It is used to reduce cholesterol in our body also.

CORIANDER

Coriander is the spherical dried fruit of the delicate plant coriandrum sativum. The leaves of this plant are also used. It is rich in Iron.

CUMIN SEEDS

The dry fruits of cuminum cyminum are used in cooking. They have thymol cumin seeds act as carminative.

MUSTARD SEEDS

Mustard is obtained from the plant Brassica nigra (Black mustard) Brassica alba (White mustard). Mustard is used extensively all over the world.

TURMERIC

It is the root of a plant curcuma domestica. It imparts yellow colour which is not permanent. It has carminative and anti bacterial action. It inhibits gastric secretion. It has a sacred place in Hindu culture.

TAMARIND

Tamarind is the fruit of the plant Tamarindus India. It is grown in

South India. It has tartaric acid and pectin. It is sour to taste. When ripe also imports sweetish taste.

ASAFOETIDA

This is a essential oil, gum and resin mixture obtained from the plant Ferula nathrex or Ferula fetide. Asafoetide has a strong odour. It has a carminative effect and helps in release of flatus.

Table 21.1 : Nutritive Composition of Some Spices and Condiments

	Protein	Fat	Carbohydrate	Energy	Calcium	Phosphorus	Iron	Carotene	Thiamine	Riboflavin	Niacin	Vitamin C
	gm	gm	gm	kcal	mg	mg	mg	mg	mg	mg	mg	mg
Asafotida	4.0	1.1	67.8	297	690	50	39.4	4	--	0.04	0.3	--
Cardamom	10.2	2.2	42.1	229	130	160	4.6	--	0.22	0.17	0.8	--
Chillies dry	15.9	6.2	31.6	246	160	370	2.3	345	0.93	0.43	9.5	50
Chillies fresh	2.9	0.6	3.0	29	30	80	4.4	175	0.19	0.39	0.9	111
Cloves dry	5.2	8.9	46.0	286	740	100	11.7	253	0.08	0.13	--	--
Cloves green	2.3	5.9	24.1	159	310	40	2.1	72	--	--	--	--
Coriander	14.1	16.1	21.6	288	630	393	7.1	942	0.22	0.35	1.1	--
Coriander leaves	3.3	0.6	6.3	44	184	71	18.5	6918	0.05	0.06	0.8	135
Curry Leaves	6.1	1.0	18.7	108	830	57	7.0	7560	0.08	0.21	2.3	4
Cumin seeds	18.7	15.0	36.6	356	1080	511	11.7	522	0.55	0.36	2.6	3
Fenugreek seeds	26.2	5.8	44.1	333	160	370	6.5	96	0.34	0.29	1.1	--
Garlic dry	6.3	0.1	29.8	145	30	310	1.2	--	0.06	0.23	0.4	13
Ginger fresh	2.3	0.9	12.3	67	20	60	3.5	40	0.06	0.03	0.6	6
Lime peel	1.8	0.5	29.4	129	710	60	2.7	--	--	--	--	--
Mace	6.5	24.4	47.8	437	180	100	12.3	3027	0.25	0.42	1.4	--
Mint	4.8	0.6	5.8	48	200	62	15.6	1620	0.05	0.26	1.0	27
Nutmeg	7.5	36.4	28.5	472	120	240	2.03	0	0.33	0.01	1.4	--
Nutmeg rind	1.0	0.4	11.2	52	40	10	2.0	4	--	--	--	--
Pepper dry	11.5	6.8	49.2	304	460	198	12.4	1080	0.09	0.14	1.4	--
Pepper fresh	4.8	2.7	13.7	98	270	70	2.4	540	0.05	0.04	0.2	1
Tamarind pulp	3.1	0.1	67.4	283	170	110	17.0	60	--	0.07	0.7	3
Turmeric	6.3	5.1	69.4	349	150	282	67.8	30	0.03	--	2.3	--

Nutritive Values of Indian Food Preparations

India is called a sub-continent. It has various climates and soils. Foods grown and consumed vary from place to place. Due to availability of market and transport facilities foods that are impossible to grow in our place are now available for us. This facilitates us to make wide variations in our daily menu. Though nutritive value tables are available for almost all the foods consumed, to get the nutritive value of a recipe one has to spend some time to calculate. CFTRI, Mysore published a booklet "Balanced diets and Nutuitive values of Common Indian Recipes". This booklet enables a common man to know the nutrient composition of Indian recipes.

Table 22.1 gives the nutritive values of common Indian cereal preparations. (Preserving and per 100 g).

Table 22.2 gives the nutritive values of common Indian pulse preparations (Preserving and per 100 g)

Table 22.3 gives the nutritive values of common Indian milk preparations (Preserving and per 100 g)

Table 22.4 gives the nutritive values of common Indian Egg, Fish and Meat preparations (Preserving and per 100 g)

Table 22.5 gives nutritive value of some ready to serve foods (per 100 g)

CEREAL RECIPES

The energy from cereal recipes vary from 84–487 k cals. The energy varies with the amount of pulses and fats added. The fat content is ranging from 0.15 – 33.8 per 100 grams of recipe. The protein content varies from 1 to 8.8 per cent depending on amount of other ingredients.

PULSE RECIPES

The energy from pulse recipes vary from 15 to 190 k cals. This is dependent on the amount of fat added. The protein and fat contents range 0.8 to 9.7 and 0.5 to 11 per cent respectively.

MILK RECIPES

The energy from milk recipes vary from 18 to 164 k cals depending on the fat and sugar added; protein content varies from 0.35 to 5.5 per cent depending on the amount of pulse added. Milk is rich in calcium and calcium content of the milk recipes range from 0.04 to 0.21 mg per cent.

EGG, FISH AND MEAT RECIPES

Protein content of non-veg recipes range from 9 to 21.8 per cent, energy content vary from 77 to 339 k cals depending on the amount of fat added.

READY TO SERVE PREPARATIONS

These constitute a wide range of cereals, pulses, nuts, oil seeds, milk and milk products and fruit and fruit products. So the energy, protein and fat content varies widely.

Table 22.1 : Nutritive Value of the Common Cereal Preparations (per serving and per 100 g)

Food Preparations	Quantity (per serving)	Wt. (per serving) (g)	Calories (Kcal)	Protein (g)	Fat (g)	Carbohydrate (g)	Calcium (g)	Phosphorus (g)	Iron (mg)	Vitamin A Value (I.U.)	Thiamin (mg)	Nicotin acid (mg)	Riboflavin (mg)	Vitamin C (mg)
Cereal and Millet Preparations														
Rice preparations														
Plain rice	1 plate	505	595	11.8	0.8	134.8	0.02	0.20	5.0	--	0.20	3.0	0.10	--
"	---	100	118	2.34	0.16	26.8	0.004	0.04	1.0	--	0.04	0.60	0.02	--
Sambar bath	1 plate	485	405	13.6	5.1	76.2	0.08	0.16	3.4	132	0.20	1.70	0.10	5.1
"	---	100	84	2.8	1.05	15.7	0.02	0.03	0.7	27	0.04	0.35	0.02	1.1
Curd bath	1 plate	255	220	6.0	7.0	33.4	0.20	0.10	1.0	242	0.08	0.10	0.20	2.3
"	---	100	87	2.4	2.8	13.2	0.08	0.04	0.4	96	0.03	0.04	0.08	0.9
Sweet rice	1 plate	175	430	3.6	12.0	77.4	0.01	0.06	0.6	265	0.04	0.50	0.04	--
	---	100	245	2.0	6.0	44.2	0.006	0.03	0.3	151	0.02	0.29	0.02	--
Idli	2 nos.	136	130	4.6	0.2	27.6	0.03	0.08	0.8	8	0.10	1.2	0.05	--
"	---	100	96	3.4	0.15	20.9	0.02	0.06	0.6	6	0.07	0.88	0.04	--
Plain dosai	2 nos.	100	216	4.1	9.7	28.2	0.03	0.07	1.5	239	0.10	1.3	0.06	--
Masala dosai	1 nos.	100	212	4.6	8.4	29.4	0.04	0.08	1.7	210	0.09	0.8	0.06	3.6
Pongal (hot)	1 plate	148	200	5.5	6.0	30.5	0.03	0.07	1.6	174	0.09	0.6	0.08	--
	---	100	135	3.7	4.1	20.6	0.02	0.05	1.1	118	0.06	0.4	0.05	--

(Contd.)

Table 22.1 : (Contd..)

Food Preparations	Quantity (per serving)	Wt. (per serving) (g)	Calories (Kcal)	Protein (g)	Fat (g)	Carbohydrate (g)	Calcium (g)	Phosphorus (g)	Iron (mg)	Vitamin A Value (I.U.)	Thiamin (mg)	Nicotin acid (mg)	Riboflavin (mg)	Vitamin C (mg)
Cereal and Millet Preparations														
Wheat preparations														
Wheat uppuma	1 plate	128	163	3.8	5.4	24.7	0.01	0.04	0.7	141	0.05	0.4	0.01	1.2
,,	---	100	118	2.8	3.9	17.9	0.007	0.03	0.5	102	0.04	0.3	0.007	0.9
Chappatis	2 nos.	57	193	5.0	5.5	30.8	0.02	0.13	3.0	128	0.20	2.0	0.05	..
,,	---	100	339	8.8	9.6	54.0	0.04	0.23	5.3	224	0.35	3.5	0.09	..
Puris	2 nos.	32	136	2.2	8.4	13.0	0.01	0.06	1.3	50	0.06	0.8	0.02	..
,,	---	100	425	6.9	26.3	40.6	0.03	0.18	4.1	15	0.18	2.5	0.06	..
Plain parathas	1 no.	66	304	4.5	19.6	27.3	0.01	0.12	2.7	466	0.08	1.7	0.04	..
,,	---	100	461	6.8	29.7	41.4	0.015	0.1	4.1	707	0.12	2.6	0.06	..
Ravai Idli	2 nos.	114	212	5.0	8.5	28.7	0.06	0.08	0.9	289	0.07	0.5	0.03	1.5
,,	---	100	186	4.4	7.5	25.2	0.05	0.07	0.8	253	0.06	0.44	0.026	1.3
Kesari bath	1 plate	90	282	2.0	14.6	35.3	0.04	0.02	0.40	350	0.03	0.3	0.01	..
,,	..	100	313	2.2	16.2	39.2	0.04	0.02	0.44	389	0.03	0.3	0.01	..
Millet preparations														
Ragi balls	1 no.	336	446	8.0	7.6	86.8	0.40	0.30	6.0	230	0.50	1.2	0.13	..
,,	---	100	133	2.4	2.3	25.8	0.10	0.09	1.8	68	0.15	0.36	0.04	..

(Contd.)

Table 22.1 : (Contd..)

Food Preparations	Quantity (per serving)	Wt. (per serving) (g)	Calories (Kcal)	Protein (g)	Fat (g)	Carbohydrate (g)	Calcium (g)	Phosphorus (g)	Iron (mg)	Vitamin A Value (I.U.)	Thiamin (mg)	Nicotin acid (mg)	Riboflavin (mg)	Vitamin C (mg)
Millet preparations (Contd.)														
Ragi roti	2 nos.	185	460	8.0	9.0	87.0	0.40	0.30	6.0	255	0.50	1.2	0.13	--
"	--	100	249	4.3	4.9	47.0	0.22	0.16	3.2	137	0.27	0.70	0.07	--
Maize roti	2 nos.	142	314	9.3	5.5	56.4	0.01	0.30	1.8	62	0.30	1.2	0.08	--
"	-	100	221	6.8	3.9	39.7	0.007	0.20	1.3	43	0.20	0.8	0.05	--
Jowar roti	2 nos.	150	252	7.5	1.3	52.5	0.02	0.20	4.5	90	0.24	1.3	0.08	--
"	--	100	168	5.0	0.87	35.0	0.01	0.13	3.0	60	0.16	0.87	0.05	--
Ragi pittu	1 plate	146	422	4.4	7.4	84.0	0.20	0.20	8.0	282	0.20	0.6	0.06	--
"	---	100	289	3.3	5.1	57.7	0.14	0.14	5.5	193	0.14	0.4	0.04	--

Table 22.2 : Nutritive Values of Common Indian Pulse Preparations (Per serving and Per 100 g)

Food Preparations	Quantity (per serving)	Wt. (per serving) (g)	Calories (Kcal)	Protein (g)	Fat (g)	Carbohydrate (g)	Calcium (g)	Phosphorus (g)	Iron (mg)	Vitamin A Value (I.U.)	Thiamin (mg)	Nicotin acid (mg)	Riboflavin (mg)	Vitamin C (mg)
Green gram dhal, cooked	1½ cup	142	171	7.0	7.7	18.4	0.08	0.09	2.7	33	0.14	2.4	0.11	1.6
,,	--	100	120	4.9	5.4	12.9	0.06	0.06	1.9	23	0.10	1.7	0.08	1.1
Red gram dhal, cooked	½ cup	96	110	6.4	2.0	16.4	0.05	0.07	2.6	64	0.13	0.7	0.7	--
,,	--	100	115	6.7	2.1	17.1	0.05	0.07	2.7	67	0.14	0.73	0.73	--
Dhal Rasam	1½ cup	196	29	1.5	0.9	3.8	0.03	0.03	0.9	72	0.03	0.2	0.2	1.5
,,	--	100	15	0.8	0.5	1.9	0.02	0.02	0.5	37	0.02	0.1	0.1	0.8
Amarnath Sambar	1½ cup	140	97	5.1	2.7	13.0	0.50	0.08	8.0	2009	0.07	0.07	0.03	53.0
,,	---	100	69	3.6	1.9	9.3	0.36	0.06	5.7	1435	0.05	0.05	0.02	37.9
Radish Sambar	1½ cup	196	101	4.1	3.6	13.1	0.04	0.07	2.2	73	0.07	0.5	0.03	3.0
,,	---	100	52	2.1	1.8	6.7	0.02	0.04	1.1	37	0.04	0.26	0.02	1.5
Green gram Sundal	1 plate	142	259	13.1	9.2	30.9	0.08	0.20	4.8	120	0.24	1.2	0.10	1.1
,,	---	100	182	9.2	6.5	21.8	0.06	0.14	3.4	85	0.17	0.9	0.07	0.8
Bengal gram Sundal	1 plate	142	272	9.7	11.1	33.2	0.11	0.15	5.5	198	0.16	1.4	0.08	1.1
,,	---	100	192	6.8	7.8	23.4	0.08	0.11	3.9	140	0.11	0.98	0.06	0.8
Cowpea Sundal	1 plate	142	255	13.5	8.8	20.2	0.05	0.20	2.5	71	0.30	0.9	0.15	1.1
,,	---	100	180	9.5	6.2	21.4	0.04	0.14	1.8	50	0.21	0.6	0.11	0.8

Table 22.3 : Nutritive Values of Common Indian Milk Preparations (Per serving and Per 100 g.)

Food Preparations	Quantity (per serving)	Wt. (per serving) (g)	Calories (Kcal)	Protein (g)	Fat (g)	Carbohydrate (g)	Calcium (g)	Phosphorus (g)	Iron (mg)	Vitamin A Value (I.U.)	Thiamin (mg)	Nicotin acid (mg)	Riboflavin (mg)	Vitamin C (mg)
Coffee	--	100	52	1.9	1.7	7.2	0.05	0.05	0.10	77	0.02	0.09	0.09	0.7
,,	1 cup	200	104	3.8	3.4	14.4	0.10	0.10	0.20	154	0.04	0.18	0.18	1.4
Tea	--	100	36	0.7	0.8	6.5	0.03	0.02	--	38	0.01	0.05	0.05	0.3
,,	1 cup	200	72	1.4	1.6	13.0	0.06	0.04	--	76	0.02	0.10	0.10	0.6
Cocoa	1 cup	200	174	7.5	7.0	20.2	0.20	0.15	0.30	306	0.08	0.2	0.34	2.7
,,	--	100	87	3.8	3.5	10.1	0.10	0.08	0.15	153	0.04	0.1	0.17	1.35
Wheat Payasam	1 cup	154	178	3.4	4.3	31.5	0.09	0.08	0.40	160	0.05	0.1	0.12	--
,,	---	100	116	2.2	2.8	20.5	0.06	0.05	0.26	104	0.03	0.06	0.08	--
Rice Payasam	1 cup	154	178	3.2	4.2	31.7	0.09	0.08	0.40	160	0.05	0.1	0.26	--
,,	---	100	116	2.1	2.7	20.6	0.06	0.05	0.26	104	0.03	0.06	0.17	--
Bengal gram dhal payasam	1 cup	140	221	7.7	5.1	35.9	0.07	0.14	4.7	197	0.05	0.2	0.40	--
,,	---	100	158	5.5	3.6	25.6	0.05	0.10	3.4	141	0.04	0.14	0.28	--

(Contd.)

Table 22.3 : (Contd.)

Food Preparations	Quantity (per serving)	Wt. (per serving) (g)	Calories (Kcal)	Protein (g)	Fat (g)	Carbohydrate (g)	Calcium (g)	Phosphorus (g)	Iron (mg)	Vitamin A Value (I.U.)	Thiamin (mg)	Nicotin acid (mg)	Riboflavin (mg)	Vitamin C (mg)
Sago porridge	1 cup	266	227	3.7	4.0	44.0	0.14	0.10	0.70	204	0.06	--	0.23	4.0
,,	---	100	85	1.4	1.5	16.5	0.05	0.04	0.26	77	0.02	--	0.09	1.5
Rice porridge	1 cup	280	263	7.6	6.2	44.3	0.30	0.20	0.7	306	0.10	0.3	0.34	6.0
,,	---	100	94	2.7	2.2	15.8	0.11	0.07	0.25	109	0.04	0.11	0.12	3.3
Wheat porridge	1 cuup	193	317	8.7	8.0	52.7	0.24	0.22	1.0	408	0.13	0.2	0.50	8.0
,,	---	100	164	4.5	4.1	27.3	0.12	0.11	0.52	211	0.07	0.1	0.26	4.1
Ragi porridge	1 cup	280	263	6.9	6.3	44.7	0.30	0.20	1.7	321	0.20	0.2	0.40	6.0
,,	---	100	94	2.5	2.2	16.0	0.11	0.07	0.61	115	0.07	0.07	0.14	3.3
Milk (Cow's)	1 cup	200	130	7.0	7.4	9.8	0.24	0.20	0.8	280	0.06	0.2	0.34	4.0
,,	---	100	65	3.5	3.7	4.9	0.12	0.10	0.4	140	0.03	0.1	0.17	2.0
Buffalo Milk	1 cup	200	216	8.4	16.0	9.3	0.42	0.30	0.8	368	0.06	0.2	0.42	3.4
,,	---	100	108	4.2	8.0	4.6	0.21	0.15	0.4	184	0.03	0.1	0.21	1.7

Table 22.4 : Nutritive Values of Egg, Fish and Meat Preparations (Per serving and Per 100 g)

Food Preparations	Quantity (per serving)	Wt. (per serving) (g)	Calories (Kcal)	Protein (g)	Fat (g)	Carbohydrate (g)	Calcium (g)	Phosphorus (g)	Iron (mg)	Vitamin A Value (I.U.)	Thiamin (mg)	Nicotin acid (mg)	Riboflavin (mg)	Vitamin C (mg)
Omelette	1	39	77	5.8	5.7	0.5	0.03	0.10	1.0	940	0.06	0.1	0.15	..
,,	..	100	197	14.9	14.6	1.3	0.08	0.26	2.6	2410	0.15	0.26	0.38	..
Minced Meat Curry	1 plate	128	220	11.6	18.0	2.7	0.10	0.01	2.1	277	0.10	0.9	0.20	2.4
,,	...	100	172	9.1	14.1	2.1	0.08	0.08	1.6	216	0.08	0.7	0.16	1.9
Meat Fry	1 plate	142	339	21.8	26.0	4.5	0.23	0.20	3.3	294	0.23	7.8	0.30	7.6
,,		100	239	15.4	18.3	3.2	0.16	0.14	2.3	207	0.16	5.5	0.21	5.4
Fish Fry	1 plate	100	220	17.5	16.2	1.4	0.05	0.45	1.2	216	0.11	1.3	0.02	1.0
Rice Mutton Pulav	2 plates	341	686	20.4	39.0	63.6	0.10	0.22	3.5	100	0.20	6.0	0.20	1.1
,,	...	100	201	6.0	11.4	18.7	0.03	0.06	1.03	29	0.06	1.8	0.06	0.32

Table 22.5 : Nutritive Values of Some Ready-to-serve Food Products (Value Per 100 g)

Food Preparations	Quantity (per serving)	Wt. (per serving) (g)	Calories (Kcal)	Protein (g)	Fat (g)	Carbohydrate (g)	Calcium (g)	Phosphorus (g)	Iron (mg)	Vitamin A Value (I.U.)	Thiamin (mg)	Nicotin acid (mg)	Riboflavin (mg)	Vitamin C (mg)
Cereal Products														
Biscuits	4	36	170	1.8	7.0	25.0	0.01	0.06	0.7	...	0.10	0.01	0.3	...
"	..	100	480	5.2	20.2	71.0	0.04	0.16	1.8	...	0.03	0.04	0.8	...
Bread, white	2 slices	50	135	4.4	1.6	25.2	0.03	0.05	1.2	...	0.02	0.02	0.3	...
"	...	100	269	8.7	3.2	50.4	0.05	0.09	2.4	...	0.04	0.04	0.6	...
Corn flakes	1 cup	25	96	2.0	0.1	21.3	0.01	0.03	0.5	...	0.01	0.01	0.1	...
"	..	100	386	8.0	0.4	85.2	0.02	0.12	1.8	...	0.04	0.04	0.4	...
Nuts														
Almond	15 nos.	30	196	6.2	18.0	3.1	0.07	0.15	1.1	...	0.07	0.04	0.8	...
"	...	100	654	20.8	60.0	10.4	0.23	0.49	3.5	...	0.24	0.12	2.6	...
Cashew nut, roasted	15 nuts	30	179	6.4	14.1	6.7	0.02	0.13	1.5	...	0.19	0.04	0.8	...
"	...	100	596	21.2	46.9	22.3	0.05	0.45	5.0	...	0.63	0.14	2.8	...
Pea nut, roasted	4 table spoons	40	219	10.7	16.0	8.1	0.02	0.16	0.6	...	0.36	0.07	5.7	...
"	...	100	549	26.7	40.1	20.3	0.05	0.39	1.6	...	0.90	0.18	14.2	...

(Contd.)

Table 22.5 : (Contd.)

Food Preparations	Quantity (per serving)	Wt. (per serving) (g)	Calories (Kcal)	Protein (g)	Fat (g)	Carbohydrate (g)	Calcium (g)	Phosphorus (g)	Iron (mg)	Vitamin A Value (I.U.)	Thiamin (mg)	Nicotin acid (mg)	Riboflavin (mg)	Vitamin C (mg)
Pulses														
Bengal gram (puffed)	5 table spoons	50	186	11.3	2.6	29.5	0.03	0.16	4.5	...	0.15	0.08	0.7	...
"	...	100	372	22.5	5.2	58.9	0.06	0.31	8.9	...	0.30	0.15	1.3	...
Peas (puffed)	5 table spoons	50	170	11.5	0.7	29.6	0.02	0.18	2.5	...	0.24	0.11	1.3	...
"	...	100	340	22.9	1.4	59.1	0.04	0.36	5.0	...	0.47	0.21	2.5	...
Dairy products														
Butter	1 table spoon	14	100	0.1	11.0	0.1	0.003	0.003	...	462	...	...	...	...
"	...	100	716	0.6	81.0	0.4	0.02	0.02	...	3300	...	...	...	...
Cream	1 cup	239	745	6.0	78.0	8.0	0.20	0.20	0.1	3200	0.06	0.29	0.1	...
"	1 table spoon	15	45	0.3	5.0	1.0	0.01	0.01	...	200	...	0.02	...	...
Milk Cow's whole	1 cup	200	130	7.0	7.4	9.8	0.24	0.20	0.2	280	0.06	0.34	0.2	4
"	...	100	65	3.5	3.7	4.9	0.12	0.10	0.1	140	0.03	0.17	0.1	2
Fruits														
Apple	1 medium	150	78	0.5	0.15	18.6	0.02	0.03	2.5	...	0.09	0.05	0.3	3
"	...	100	52	0.3	0.10	12.4	0.01	0.02	1.7	...	0.06	0.03	0.2	2

(Contd.)

Table 22.5 : (Contd.)

Food Preparations	Quantity (per serving)	Wt. (per serving) (g)	Calories (Kcal)	Protein (g)	Fat (g)	Carbohydrate (g)	Calcium (g)	Phosphorus (g)	Iron (mg)	Vitamin A Value (I.U.)	Thiamin (mg)	Nicotin acid (mg)	Riboflavin (mg)	Vitamin C (mg)
Banana	1 large	100	101	1.2	0.2	23.4	0.01	0.02	0.6	120	0.04	0.14	0.3	6
Guava	1 medium	100	66	1.5	0.2	14.5	0.01	0.04	1.0	...	0.03	0.03	0.2	212
Mango	1 medium	200	110	2.0	0.2	25.0	0.02	0.04	1.0	3720	0.16	0.18	1.8	90
"	...	100	55	1.0	0.1	12.5	0.01	0.02	0.5	1860	0.08	0.09	0.9	45
Orange	1 medium	150	74	1.4	0.5	15.9	0.08	0.03	1.5	475	0.18	0.09	0.45	10
"	...	100	49	0.9	0.3	10.6	0.05	0.02	1.0	350	0.12	0.06	0.3	68
Fruit Products														
Jam	3 tea spoons	20	56	..	...	14.0	...	...	0.2	...	0.01	0.02	0.1	...
"	...	100	280	0.1	0.1	70.0	0.02	0.01	1.0	...	0.04	0.08	0.4	...
Jelly	3 tea spoons	20	56	...	...	14.1	...	...	0.2	...	0.01	0.02	0.1	...
"	...	100	282	0.1	0.1	70.6	0.02	0.01	1.0	...	0.04	0.08	0.4	...
Orange juice	1 glass	200	96	1.4	0.2	22.6	0.02	0.04	2.0	400	0.18	0.08	0.8	122
"	...	100	48	0.7	0.1	11.3	0.01	0.02	1.0	200	0.09	0.04	0.4	61
Raisins (dried)	..	100	315	2.0	0.2	76.2	0.10	0.08	4.0	...	0.06	0.09	0.5	...
"	2 table spoons	25	79	0.05	0.5	19.0	0.03	0.02	1.0	...	0.015	0.02	0.1	...
Mango Juice	1 glass	200	120	0.8	0.2	29.2	0.02	0.04	2.0	3000	0.06	0.08	1.0	98
"	...	100	60	0.4	0.1	14.6	0.01	0.02	1.0	1500	0.03	0.04	0.5	49
Tomato juice	...	100	19	0.5	0.1	4.3	0.02	0.02	1.5	1050	0.03	0.03	0.4	16
"	1 glass	200	38	1.0	0.2	8.6	0.04	0.04	3.0	2100	0.06	0.06	0.8	32

23

Food Exchange Lists for India

Nutritive values of diets are calculated using Nutritive values given in food composition tables. This type of calculation is time taking and is not convenient for a common man. More over planning diets daily using these tables may cause boredom and the basic instinct of planning a diet would be lost due to this laborious work. In order to reduce this work food exchange lists are developed. The advantages of using a food exchange list are (1) Time saving, (2) Helps the patient to choose a wise variety of foods, (3) patients can formulate their own diets basing on the availability of foods, and (4) Monotony is well avoided.

The Indian diet varies a lot from the western type. Indian diet consists a generous amount of carbohydrate from cereals, fair amount of pulses and a little milk, meat, fish and eggs. Cereals form the energy giving source of the diet. As they form the major part of the menu they are the sources of Proteins, vitamins and minerals. Legumes and nuts have the supplementary role. Most consider milk as children food and meat, fish and eggs are used regularly and uniformly. Among nuts peanuts are consumed in appreciable amounts. The food exchange lists suitable for India are given in Table 23.1 to 23.10 and are briefly discussed below.

The different food exchange lists are :

Table 23.2	Cereal Exchanges	Carbohydrates with protein
Table 23.3	Roots and Tuber Exchanges	
Table 23.4	Sugar, Sago, Juice, Jam, honey etc. exchanges	Carbohydrates without protein
Table 23.5	Meat, Fish and Egg Exchanges	Protein Exchanges
Table 23.6	Milk Exchanges	
Table 23.7	Pulse Exchanges	
Table 23.8	Nuts and Oil Seeds Exchanges	
Table 23.9	Fat Exchanges	
Table 23.10	Vegetable Exchanges	

Definition of an exchange list

An exchange list is grouping of foods in which specified amounts of all foods listed are approximately equal in its carbohydrate, Protein and fat contents. An exchange list can also be defined as foods of similar composition in which they are comparable in their nutrient contents.

Table 23.1 : Food Exchange Lists

Food Exchange	*Carbo-hydrate* gm	*Protein* g	*Fat* g	*Energy* K cals
Carbohydrates with protein				
1. Cereal Exchange	15	1.2–2.9	0.5	71
2. Roots and tuber exchange	15	0.6–3.0		·64
Carbohydrates without Protein				
3. Sugar, Sago, etc., exchange	15	--	--	60
Protein Exchange				
4. Meat, Fish and Egg Exchange	--	7	0.1–7.2	28–92
5. Milk Exchange	12	6.5–10.4	0.3–47.5	76–661
6. Pulse Exchange	15	6	1	87
7. Nuts and oil seeds exchange	7	0.5–17	5	60
8. Fat exchange	---	---	5	45
9. Vegetable exchange	7	1–5	---	38

Table 23.2 : Cereal Exchange : Each Exchange Supplies 15 g Carbohydrate, 0.5 Fat, 2 g protein, and 71 K cals of Energy

Name of the Food Stuff	*Weight* gm	*Protein* g	*CHO* g	*Energy* K cals
Bajra	22	2.6	15	80
Barley	22	2.5	15	73
Jowar	21	2.2	15	72
Maize (tender)	61	2.9	15	76
Maize (dry)	23	2.5	15	78
Ragi	21	1.5	15	68
Rice parboiled and pounded	19	1.6	15	68
Rice parboiled milled	19	1.2	15	66
Rice raw milled	19	1.3	15	66
Rice flakes	19	1.3	15	67
Rice puffed	21	2.5	15	73
Wheat (Whole)	21	2.5	15	73
Wheat flour (Whole)	22	2.6	15	74
Wheat Semolina	20	2.1	15	70
Wheat vermicelli	19	1.7	15	68

Table 23.3 : Roots and Tuber Exchanges : Each Exchange supplies 15 g Carbohydrate, 0.6 to 3 g protein and 64 k cals of energy

Name of the Food Stuff	*Weight* gm	*Protein* g	*CHO* g	*Energy* K cals
Beet root	160	2.8	15	68
Carrot	150	1.2	15	72
Colocasia	66	2.0	15	64
Onion (Small)	111	2.0	15	65
Onion (big)	132	1.2	15	65
Potato	62	1.0	15	63
Radish (Pink)	206	1.2	15	66
Radish (White)	412	3.0	15	70
Sweet Potato	50	0.6	15	60
Tapioca	37	0.2	15	58
Turnip	226	1.2	15	65
Yam	54	0.7	15	60

Table 23.4 : Sugar, Sago, Juice etc., exchanges : Each exchange supplies 15 g Carbohydrate and 60 K cals of Energy

Name of the Food Stuff	*Protein* g	*CHO* g	*Energy* K cals
Honey	15	15	60
Jam	15	15	60
Orange Juice	240	15	60
Raisans (dry)	16	15	60
Sago	15	15	60
Sugar	15	15	60

Table 23.5 : Meat, Fish and Egg Exchanges : Each exchange supplies 7g of Protein, Energy varies from 28 to 92 K cals and Fat from 0.1 to 7.2 gm

Name of the Food Stuff	*Weight* gm	*Protein* gm	*Fat* gm	*Energy* K cals
Beef muscle	31	7	0.8	35
Duck	32	7	1.6	42
Duck's Egg	52	7	7.2	92
Hen's Egg	53	7	7.0	91
Fowl	27	7	0.2	30
Goat Meat	33	7	1.2	30
Liver (goat)	33	7	1.1	38
Liver (sheep)	35	7	2.7	53
Mutton Muscle	38	7	5.0	73
Pigeon	30	7	1.5	41
Pork	33	7	0.2	30
Cat fish	33	7	--	28
Crab Muscle	79	7	0.9	36
Crab	63	7	6.1	83
Herring	35	7	1.1	38
Katla	36	7	0.9	36
Lobster	34	7	0.3	31
Mackeral	37	7	0.6	34
Prawn	37	7	0.4	31
Sardine	33	7	0.6	34
Shark	32	7	0.1	29
Shrimp	10	7	0.9	36

Table 23.6 : Milk Exchange

Name of the Food Stuff	Weight gm	Protein gm	Fat gm	CHO gm	Energy K cals
Buffalo milk	240	10.3	21.1	12	289
Cows milk	280	9.0	9.5	12	188
Goats milk	260	8.6	11.7	12	190
Curds	400	12.4	16.0	12	240
Butter milk	2400	19.2	26.4	12	360
Skimmed Milk	260	6.5	0.3	12	76
Chana	150	20.4	35.0	12	444
Cheese	190	45.7	47.5	12	661
Skimmed buffalo milk Khoa	47	104.0	0.7	12	97
Whole Buffalo milk Khoa	54	85.0	18.3	12	246
Whole Cow's milk Khoa	48	96.0	12.4	12	198
Whole milk powder	32	8.4	8.5	12	158

Table 23.7 : Pulse Exchanges : Each Exchange supplies 15g Carbohydrate, 6gm protein and 87 K cals of energy, Soyabean is rich in Protein and Fat

Name of the Food Stuff	Weight gm	Protein gm	Fat gm	CHO gm	Energy K cals
Bengal gram (Whole)	25	4.2	1.2	15	88
Bengal gram dal	25	5.2	1.4	15	93
Bengal gram roasted	26	5.8	1.3	15	95
Cowpea	27	6.3	0.2	15	85
Green gram (Whole)	26	6.3	0.3	15	88
Green gram dal	25	6.1	0.3	15	87
Horse gram	26	5.7	0.1	15	84
Lentils	25	6.3	0.2	15	87
Peas (dry)	27	5.2	0.3	15	83
Peas (roasted)	25	5.8	0.3	15	86
Rajmah	25	5.6	0.3	15	84
Red gram dal	26	5.7	0.4	15	87
Black gram	25	6.0	0.3	15	87
Field bean	25	5.0	0.2	15	87
Soyabean	71	30.6	13.8	15	307

Table 23.8 :Nuts and Oil Seeds Exchanges : Each Exchange Supplies 5g fat and 60 K Cals energy.

Name of the Food Stuff	*Weight* gm	*Protein* gm	*Fat* gm	*Energy* K cals
Almonds	9	17.0	5	56
Cashewnut	11	2.7	5	64
Coconut (dry)	8	0.5	5	53
Coconut (fresh)	12	0.5	5	54
Gengelly seeds	12	2.1	5	65
Ground nuts	13	3.2	5	71
Ground nuts (roasted)	13	3.3	5	72
Pistachio	9	1.8	5	58
Piyal Seeds	9	1.6	5	56
Walnut	8	1.2	5	54

Table 23.9 : Fat Exchanges : Each Exchange supplies 5 g and 45 K cals energy

Name of the Food Stuff	*Weight* gm	*Fat* gm	*Energy* K cals
Butter	6.2	5	45.2
Ghee	5	5	45
Hydrogenated oil	5	5	45
Cooking oil	5	5	45

Table 23.10 : Vegetable Exchanges : Each Exchange Supplies 7 g Carbohydrate and 38 K cals of Energy Protein Content varies.

Name of the Food Stuff	*Weight* gm	*Protein* gm	*CHO* gm	*Energy* K cals
Beans Scarlet Runner	23	1.7	7	37
Broad beans	97	4.4	7	47
Bitter Guard	167	2.6	7	42
Brinjal	175	2.5	7	42
Cauliflower	175	4.5	7	53
Cluster Beans	65	2.1	7	10
Double Beans	57	4.7	7	48
Drum stick	189	4.7	7	40
French beans	156	2.7	7	40

(Contd...)

Table 23.10 : Contd..

Name of the Food Stuff	*Weight* gm	*Protein* gm	*CHO* gm	*Energy* K cals
Giant chillies	163	2.1	7	39
Green Peas	44	3.2	7	42
Jack fruit seeds	27	1.8	7	36.
Kovai	226	2 7	7	41
Ladies finger	109	2.1	7	38
Mango (green)	69	0.9	7	30
Onion Stalks	79	0.7	7	32
Papaya (Green)	123	0.9	7	32
Pink Beans	100	3.1	7	44
Plantain flower	137	2.3	7	47
Plantain (green)	50	0.7	7	32
Tomato (green)	194	3.7	7	45

24

Food Adulteration

Adulteration of foodstuffs is a common practice in India. Adulteration occurs if food contains any substance injurious to health, if it has any decomposed substance, if diseased animals or foods are used in preparation, if its preparation, handling and storage are done under insanitary conditions, if the container render the contents poisonous, if any substitutes have been used to conceal the inferiority, if its contains any flavour other than those permitted by law, if any valuable constituents are omitted and if it contains pesticide residues or any other harmful additives. In India first adulteration preventive measure was taken in 1860 but it was under Indian penal code and was in control of Municipality. First food adulteration bill was introduced in 1899 at Bombay. In 1937 Central Advisory Board of Health and Food Adulteration Committee were inaugurated. Central Committee for Food Standards started working from 1944. In 1947 Indian Standards Institute (ISI) was established. ISI Certification Marks Act came into being from 1952. Apart from ISI Agricultural Marketing Association or Agmark, Army Service Corps or ASC, Fair Average Quality Standards F.A.Q., Food Adulteration Committee FAC recommend the standards. Prevention of Food Adulteration Act came into beign from 1954. This act prohibits the manufacture, sale and distribution of not only adulterated food but also foods contaminated and misbranded foods. The Central Foods Laboratory at Calcutta and the Central Food Technological Research Institute at Mysore test the foods for adulteration. The State Governments has a food testing laboratory with public analyst and staff to test the suspected foods.

According to the Prevention of Food Adulteration Act, an article of food is said to be adulterated if

(a) The article sold by a vendor is not of the nature, substance or quality demanded by the purchaser and is to his prejudice, or is not of the nature, substance of quality which is purports or is represented to be;

(b) If the article contains any other substance which effects, or if the article is so processed as to affect, injuriously the nature, substance or quality thereof;

(c) If any inferior or cheaper substance has been substituted wholly or impart for the article, so as to affect injuriously the nature, substance or quality thereof;

(d) If any constituent of the article has been wholly or in part abstracted so as to affect injuriously the nature, substance or quality thereof;

(e) If the article had been prepared, packed or kept under insanitary conditions where by it has become contaminated of injurious to health;

(f) If the article consists wholly or in part of any filthy; putrid, disgusting, rotten, decomposed or diseased animal or vegetable substance or is insect infested or otherwise unfit for human consumption;

(g) If the article is obtained from a diseased animal;

(h) If the article contains any poisonous or other ingredient which renders it injurious to health;

(i) If the container of the article is composed, whether or in part, of any poisonous or deleterious substance which renders its contents injurious to health;

(j) If any colouring matter other than that prescribed in respect thereof and in amounts not within the prescribed limits of variability is present in the article;

(k) If the article contains any prohibited preservative or permitted preservative in excess of the prescribed limits;

(1) If the quality of purity of the article falls below the prescribed standard or its constituents are present in quantities which are in excess of prescribed limits of variability.

Intentional addition, substitution or abstraction of substances which adversely affect the quality of foods, incidental contamination of foods with deleterious constituent such as toxin, insecticides, pathogenic bacteria and fungi, etc., due to ignorance, load of proper storage facilities or negligence and contamination during production, storage and handling are considered as adulteration.

All the substances added to the food during preparation, preservation, packing etc. are called food additives. These are classified into intentional additives and accidental additives. Intentional additives are those which are used to enhance the quality of the food without any toxic side affects. The use of these intentional additives are :

1. To Improve the nutritional value of the food

   Ex. : a) Addition of vitamin D to milk

   b) Addition of Iodine to salt

   c) Addition of vitamin A to Margarine

2. To improve the preservation quality

   Ex. : a) Addition of Antioxidants to fats

   b) Addition of anti-microbial agents to meats.

3. To make the food attractive

   Ex. : a) Addition of condiments

   b) Addition of bleaching agents

4. Use of leavening agents, stabilizers, sequestrates, etc.

Fertilizers and pesticides used on plants, antibiotics, tranquilizers, enzymes, hormones, toxic substances or chemical residues from the packing material etc., are called accidental or incidental additives.

Some common food adulterants are shown in Table 24.1.

Table 24.1 : Common Food Adulterants

Food Stuff	*Common Adulterants*
Cereals and Cereal Products:	
Wheat and Rice	Stones
Wheat flour	Tapioca flour
Semolina	Tapioca Semolina
Pulses and Pulse Products	
Bengal gram dal	Kesari Dal
Bengal gram Flour	Flour coloured with yellow dye
Red gram dal	Coloured with yellow or coal tar dye
All dals	Stones
Milk and Milk Products :	
Milk	Addition of water, removal of butter, Addition of hydrogenated fats, milk made from skim milk powder, addition of starch or dextrins
Milk powder	Starch and dextrins
Butter	Other fats
Ghee	Vanaspati
Ice cream	Artificial sweetness, non-permitted colours and jelling agents.
Oils and Fats	
Vegetable oils	Cheap non-edible oils, Argemone oil, mineral oil etc.
Hydrogenated fats	Animal fats.
Beverages	
Tea	Exhausted tea leaves other leaves coloured.
Coffee	Exhausted coffee powder, Roasted Tamarind seed or date seed powder, roasted husks
Soft drinks	Non permitted colours, Artificial sweetness like sac charin.

(Contd.)

Table 24.1 : Contd.

Food Stuff	Common Adulterants
Spices and Condiments	
Turmeric Powder	Starch coloured yellow by coal tar dye, yellow earth, talc coloured yellow.
Black pepper	Dired papaya seeds
Asafoetide	Resins and other plant gums
Chilly powder	Starch or talc coloured red
Mustard seeds	Argemone seeds
Miscellaneous	
Supari	Other nuts broken and coloured
Honey	Cane sugar syrup
Cinnamon	Bark or other trees

25

Food Poisoning and Food Borne Infection

Food hygiene aims at studying the methods of production, preparation and presentation of safe food. Handling of foodstuffs, utensils, method of preparation, treatment gives service, consumption and supply are all included in this subject. The care of the food poisoning bacteria originating from the host supplying food is also very important. Food should be free from all noxious material. It should be nourishing and should be served attractively. Chemicals may enter the food accidentally during cultivation, preparation, storage etc. These chemicals though present in small quantities cause a great damage. Micro organisms may enter the food directly by contamination or may be present in the host itself. Moulds and bacteria which grow in the foods may release poisonous substances and cause food poisoning. The knowledge of food poisoning helps in knowing the nature of these dangers and measures to prevent them.

Food poisoning is characterised usually by vomiting and/or diarrhoea and various other abdominal disorders. Centuries ago detailed information on foods to be eaten and food to be avoided, alongwith methods of preparation, storage etc. are given in medical books. Swine, Mice, rats, lizards etc., are then itself prohibited foods. It is recently identified that all these excrete and harbour salmonellae. Scavengers like eagle, vulture, seagull, etc. are prohibited. Among the water borne animals only fish with fins and scales are adviced. Shell fish, cru staceans, mammals of sea, etc. are prohibited.

Almost all the food poisoning cases we come across are due to the contamination of food by germs which grow actively in the food. All these growing organisms alongwith other harmful and harmless micro organisms are studied in the subject micro biology. Microbiology covers bacteriology, virology, mycology and parasitology.

Bacteriology	–	Greem word Bactron means a rod. The first appearance of the germs seen through micro scope is like rods.
Virology	–	Study of Viruses (smallest micro organisms)
Mycology	–	Study of fungi and moulds
Parasitology	–	Study of parasites.

The study of all the above was initiated by Van Leuwan Hock in 1675. He is a Linen draper in Delft of Wolland. His hobby is to make lenses and magnifying apparatus and observe nature through them. One day while observing a drop of pond water he saw tiny rods which moved very actively whithin the field. He took scrapings from his own teeth and found same type of organisms in it also and noted all in the form of drawings. After 200 years Louis Pasteur, a French Chemist and Bacteriologist proved Van Leuwan Hock's observations. Pasteur developed methods for culturing bacteria. Pasteur was able to show clearly that the theory of spontaneous generation, life arising from the in animate was false. When a food is sterilized by heat, living bacteria would not be appear excepting contamination from air, hands or from some other infected material. Some of the historical developments in food microbiology are given in Table 25.1.

One cannot prevent microbial contamination during primary processing. But one can try to minimize contamination and subsequent growth of micro organisms. The equipments used during processing also are good source of contamination. The quality of air and water used may also caused contamination. So let us first know the primary sources of micro organisms founds in foods.

Soil and water micro organisms are ofter one and the same. The bacteria in soil and water that are expected in foods Acinetobacter, Alcaligenes, Bacillus, Citrobacter, Clostridium, Corynebacterium,

Table 25.1 : Historical Developments in Food Microbiology

(a) Food Preservation	
1782	Introduction of canned vinegar
1810	Preservation of food by canning
1813	Use of SO_2 as meat preservative
1813	Post processing incubation of canned foods
1825	Patent for preserving food in tin cans was granted in U.S.
1835	Patent for making condensed milk granted in England.
1839	Use of brine bath to raise the boiling temperature of water
1840	Introduction of fish and fruit canning
1842	Patent for freezing foods by immersion in ice and salt brine was issued to H. Bejamin in England
1843	Sterilization by steam was attempted
1845	Canning was introduced in Australia
1853	Patent for sterilization of food by autoclaving was granted to R. Chevallier-Appert.
1854	Investigations of fermented urine by Pasteur
1855	Powder milk was produced in England
1856	Patent for the manufacture of unsweetened condensed milk was granted in United States.
1861	Introduction of brine baths to the United States.
1865	Freezing of fish on commercial scale began in United States.
1874	Steam pressure cookers were introduced
1880	Pasteurization of milk was started in Germany
1882	Destructive effect of Ozone on spoilage bacteria identified.
1886	Mechanical process of drying fruits and vegetables was carried out.
1887	Malted milk was introduced.
1889	Freezing of eggs was introduced.
1890	Commercial pasteurization of milk was begun
1890	Refrigeration of fruits was started

1907 Isolation of Lactobacillus bulgaricus from yogurt

1908 Sodium benzoate was given permitted preservative status in some foods.

1917 Quick freezing of foods was achieved

1917 Preserving fruits and vegetables under CO_2 was give patent.

1928 Commercial use of controlled atmosphere storage of apples was introduced in Europe.

1929 Use of high energy radiation for the processing of foods was given patent in France.

1943 Ionizing radiation to preserve hamburger meat was employed in United States.

1955 Sorbic Acid approved as food preservative.

(b) Food Poisoning

1857 Milk was idenitified as transmitter of typhoid fever

1870 Theory of Ptomaine poisoning was advanced by Frances Co Selmi

1888 Salmonella enteritidis isolated from meat which caused food poisoning.

1894 Staphylococci found to be associated food poisoning

1896 Clostridium botulinum was discovered by Van Ermengen

1926 Streptococci was identified to be associated with food poisoning.

1938 Campylobacter enteritis were traced to milk in Illinoss.

1939 Gastroenteritis caused by yersinia enterocolitica was first recognised.

1945 Etiology status of clostridium perfringens was proved.

1951 Vibrio parahemolyticus was shown to be an agent of food poisoning.

1960 Aflatoxin production by Aspergillus flavus was first reported.

1969 Enterotoxin of clostridium perfringens demonstrated.

1969 Clostridium botulinum type A was first isolated

1975 Salmonella enterotoxin was demonstrated.

1978	Food borne gastroenteritis caused by Norwalk virus recorded in Australia.
1983	Campylnbacter jejuni enterotoxin described.
	(c) Food Spoilage
1659	Occurance of Bacteria in milk identified
1680	Leuwan Hoek observed yeast cells
1780	Lactic acid identified as the principal acid in sour milk.
1839	Kircher found that organisms that produce slimyness in beet juice and sucrose solution to be identical.
1857	Pasteur demonstrated that the souring of milk was due to growth of organisms in it.
1873	Microbial deterioration of eggs was first reported
1873	Streptococcus lact is isolated in a pure culture
1887	Forster demonstrated the ability of pure bacteria cultures to grow at 0°C.
1888	First study on thermophilic bacteria was done by Miquel.
1895	Spoilage of canned corn due to improper heat processing was traced.
1902	Micro-organisms that can grow at 0°C were called psychrophile.
1912	Yeast that grow well at high osmotic pressure were called Osmophilic.
1915	Bacillus Coagulans was isolated from coagulated milk.

Enterobacter, Micrococcus, Protens, Pseudomonar, Serratia, Streptomyces etc. Molds participate in degradation of both plant and animal matter. Aspergillus, Rhizopus, Penicillium, Trichothecium, Botrytis, Fusarium etc. are found in soil. Bacteria that are associated with plants in addition to the above are Acetobacter, Erwinia, Flavobacterium, Kurthia, Lactobacillus, Lenconostoc, Listeria, Pediococcus and Streptococcus. The genus saccharomyces, Rhodotorula and torula are molds associated in many plant products. Bacteria found in intestinal tract are Bacteroides, Esherichia, Lactobacillus, Protens, Salmonella, Shigella, Staphy Lococcus, Streptococcus, Clostridum, Citrobacter, Enterobacter and Pseudomonas.

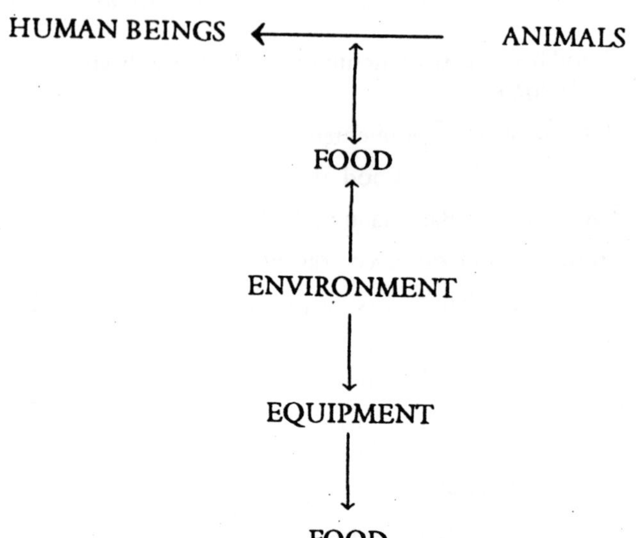

Fig. 25.1 : Pathways of Infection

COMMON FOOD BORNE BACTERIA

Aceto Bacter

These are gram-negative, rod shaped cells and are aerobes. These are found in grain mash, beer, wines, souring fruits and vegetables.

Acromonas

These are gram-negative, rod shaped cells and facultatively anerobic which display fermentative metabolism. These are normal inhabitants of fish intestines.

Alcaligenes

These are gram negative rods. At times they stain gram positive. They are widely distributed in nature in all decomposing matter of all types, in poultry products, milk etc.

Alteromonas

These are gram negative straight or curved rods and are aerobes. These require sodium growth and they are non-fermentative. These are common on marine fish.

Bacillus

These are gram positive, aerobic organisms that can produce endospores. Most of them are mesophiles with some psychrotropic and a few thermicphilic whose spores are heat resistant.

Brochothrix

Brochothrix thermasphacta is the recognised species in this genus. It is found mostly on processed meats stored in gas impermeable packages. Exponential phase cells are rods while stationary phase cells are cocoids.

Campylobacter

These are slender, spirally curved rods and posses flagella at one or both ends. They are found in oralcavity and intestinal canal. Some are pathogens.

Citrobacter

These are gram negative rods, slow lactose fermenting organisms. They can use citrate as sole carbon source. These are found in commonly infecal matter, water and some foods.

Clostridium

These are gram positive, spore forming rods. These are of great importance in canning industry because of their extreme heat resistance of their endospores. These are widely distributed in soil, water, man animals etc. High protein content, neutral pH and low oxygen availability promote the exotoxin productioin of these organisms especially C. botulinum.

Corynebacterium

These are gram positive rods often show granules, club snaped swellings and aerobic organisms. Most of them are mesophiles and a few are psychrotrophs. These organisms are present in some plants like wheat, beans and tomatoes, in intestinal tract of human beings and spoiled foods.

Enterobacter

These are gram negative short organisms. They are distributed widely in nature on plants, water, intestinal tract etc.

Erwinia

These are gram negative rods which grow within the psychrotrophic range. They cause galls, wilts, soft rots etc. in plants.

Escherichia

These are gram negative short rods. They are present in intestinal tract of man. Presence of E. aerogenes in foods is indication of fecal contamination.

Flavobacterium

These are gram negative rods, many are psychrophilic while most are mesophiles. They are found in soils water fish and plants. They can be isolated from decaying plant materials.

Lactobacillus

These are long, gram positive, non-sporing rods. Mostly these are found in plants and dairy products. These are used in producing fermented milk and cheese. These are used in microbiological assay of amino acids and B vitamins due to their exact growth requirements.

Leuconostoc

They are gram positive, spherical to oval shaped organisms found among plants. They are found in milk and dairy products.

Micrococcus

These are gram positive cocci. Most of them are mesophiles while some can survive and grow at psychrophilic range. They can tolerate high sodium content. These are distributed on skin of man, dust, soil, water and foods.

Moraxella

These are very short, plump, gram negative rods and are sensitive to pencillin.

Pediococcus

These are wide spread in nature especially on plants. Most of them are used as starters in some fermented foods.

Protens

These are gram negative rods which are aerobic. These are found on decaying materials, intestinal tract of man and animal etc.

Pseudomonas

These are gram egative, short, aerobic rods with a signle polar flagellum. Both Meso philes and psychrotrophic species ocist in this genus. They are distributed in soil, water, plants and intestinal tract of man and animals.

Salmonella

These are gram negative aerobic and short rods. They ferment glucose but not Lactose usually. They are found in intestinal tract of many species. Both pathogenic and non-pathogenic varieties exist.

Serratia

They are gram negative, protealytic, mesophilic and aerobic rods. They are found in water, soil, decaying plant and animal matter.

Shigella

They are short, non-motile, aerobic, mesophilic and gram negative rods. These are found in polluted water, intestines and feces.

Staphylococcus

These are gram positive cocci. Their presence in foods is undesirable. The toxin produce is a heat stable enterotoxin.

Streptococcus

They are gram positive, spherical to avoid in shape and micro aerophilic in nature. These are widespread on plants, plant parts and dair starter cultures. The presence of some species in foods indicate fecal contamination.

Vibrio

They are straight or curved rods which are facultative anerobes capable to fermentative metabolism and all utilize glucose. They require sodium.

Yersinia

These are gram negative rods. This genus includes the agent causing plague Y. enterocolitica causes gastroenteritis in man.

COMMON FOOD BORNE YEASTS

Brettanomyces

These are acid producing asporogenous yeasts that produce oval, elongate, spherical or olive shaped cells. These are found in European ales, spoiled pickles and beer.

Candida

These are asporogenous yeast which produce pseudomycelium. They reproduce by fragmentation of mycelium or by budding. They are found in fresh and cured meats. One species cause rancidity of margarine.

Debaryomyces

These are ascorporogenous yeast. These reproduce sexually and also by multipolar budding. These are found on surface of spoiling foods such as meats, pickle brine, wines and sausages.

Hansenula

These are ascosporogenous yeast that produce spherical, elongate or oval cells with a pseudomycelium. They reproduce by multipolar budding and sexually too. They are common on citrus fruits, olive brine, fruit juice concentrates, grapes and grape products.

Mycoderma

These are asporogenous yeast found on surface of beers, pickle brine, vinegar, fruit juice etc.

Rhodotofula

These are asporogenous yeasts. They reproduce by multipolar budding. They are found in air dust.

Saccharomyces

This group is very important in brewing, backing and distilling industries. These are a sporogenous yeast which produce oviod, spherical or elongate cell. These are found on fruits and vegetables where fermentation of sugar leading to CO_2 and ethanol formarion.

Schizosa Ccharomyces

These are ascas porogenous yeast that reproduce by fission or arthrospores or sekual means. They are found in sugar and other related products.

Torula

These are asporogenous yeast which produce spherical or oval cells. These reproduce by multipolar budding and psendomycelium. They are found on refrigerated foods.

COMMON FOOD BORNE MOLDS

Aspergillus

This mold produce straight upright conidiophores that terminate in a globore. The milds appear yellow to green to black in large number. Some produce a flatoxins and ochra toxins. This species is found on fruits, vegetables meats, cakes, etc.

Botrytis

This mold produce long slender conidiophores. It appears gray in mass on plants and plant foods.

Cladosporium

Dark conidiophores variously branched at apex of middle portion and septate mycelium is the special character. C. herbarum produces black spots on beef.

Fusarium

Thes molds have extensive mycelium and conidia are canoe shaped. They cause spoilage of many fruits and vegetables. Toxins like T_2, Vomitoxin and Zearalenone are produced by these molds.

Helminthosporium

This genus has plant pathogens and saprophytes. The conidiophores are short or long, septate simple or branched.

Mucor

These molds possess non-septate mycelia with conidiophores that bear columella and sporangium at the apex. They are found on foods.

Pencillium

These produce septate mycelia with conidiophores. In foods the colour ranges from blue to blue green. They are found in soil, air, dust bread, cakes, fruits etc. Some cause soft rot of fruits.

Rhizopus

This have non-septate mycelia with stolons and rhizoids. Sporangiophores arise at nodes bearing columella and sporangia. Spores are black in colour. These are found on fruits, bread, cakes, etc.

Sporotrichum

This molds have septate mycelia these can grow below 0°C and produce white spot on refrigerated beef.

Bacteria multiply by simple division into two every 20 to 30 minutes. Thus one cell becomes 2 million in 7 hours after continuous growth. The growth continues if there is a suitable environment and sufficient amount of nutrient. The life span of the cell depends on its type and the environment it is growth. Some produce spores which survive in dormant condition in unfavourable condition and develop as soon as the favourable conditions like moisture, food and temperature return they germinate into actively growing bacteria again. In laboratory meat broth base set into a firm gel by means of agar is used. Agar is extract from seaweed which melts at high temperature and sets into a gel at low temperature. Addition of blood, serum, milk or any other protein enriches the medium. Bacteria are innoculated on the media and left over night at 37°C which is suitable for their growth. The cells divide and heaps of bacteria is formed which has millions of cells, called colonies. Thus bacteria grow actively in foods during summer causing food poisoning.

Harmful organisms grow at body temperature. Majority grow between 15°C and 45°C. C. perfringens grows well even at 47°–50°C. Non sporing organisms die when heated to above 60°C but the duration of heating varies. Spores require boiling for above 5 hours. Using stead with pressure kills spores faster. Toxin produce by staphylococci needs boiling for about 30 minutes to be destroyed. Toxin produced by C. botulinum is destroyed more easily. cold temperature does not allow the bacteria to multiply but cannot kill. So, refrigeration only delays the spoilage of foods.

Human beings and animals host the disease causing orgaisms which may be passed to the food stuff and grow as soon as suitable conditions prevail.

Bacterial food poisoning causes disturbance of the gastro intestinal tract such as abdominal pain, diarrhoea and vomiting. Onset of symptoms occur within one to forty eight hours. Details of incubation period and duration of illness are shown in Table 25.2.

Table 25.2 : Bacterial Food Poisoning, Incubation Period and Duration of Illness

Cause of Food Poisoning	*Incubation period (hours)*	*Duration*
Salmonella	60–36	1–7 days
Stophy cococcus aureses	2–6	6–24 hours
Clostridium perfringens	8–22	24–48 hours
Clostridium botulinum	12–96	Death in 24 hours or Slow recovery over 6–8 months
Vibrio para hemolyticus	2–48	2–5 days
Bacillus Cereus	1–16	12–24 hours
Escherichia coli	12–72	1–7 days
Strepto coccus	3–22	24–48 hours

Salmonella reach food from excrete at the time of slaughter, from the hands in kitchess, from utensils, by using polluted water, etc. If the number of bacilli are few it may not be harmful. But, if the food is left for longer time in warm temperature sufficient number of bacteria will develop which are sufficient for causing food poisoning. Fever, aching of the limbs, headache, diarrhoea and vomiting are the symptoms of poisoning.

Staphylococcus are usually found in skin and in nose. This bacteria usually causes poisoning in food which are eaten cold Staphylococcus is readily destroyed by pasteurization. The onset of poisoning symptoms appear rapidly. The symptoms are vomiting, diarrhoea, abdominal pain, cramps and collapse.

Clostridium perfringens is found usually in excreta, meat products and on plants grown on night soil sewage. This bacteria produces spores which are heat resistant. Abdominal pain, nausea and diarrhoea are the symptoms of C.perfringens poisoning.

Clostridium botulinum is anerobic spore forming bacillus which produces a toxin that effects nervous system. The spores are heat resistant and survive boiling. Fatigue, headache, dizziness are the primary signs of C. botulinum poisoning. Diarrhoea is preceded by constipation. Disturbance in vision, speech difficulty, paralysis of throat muscles and paralysis of respiratory centres cause death.

Bacillus cereus are aerobic spore bearing organisms. These spores survive cooking and produce toxin when favourable condition like warm temperature is provided. Acute vomiting and diarrhoea are the symptoms of Bacillus cereus poisoning.

A thorough knowledge of food poisoning, food borne infection their causes, symptoms and prevention helps in preparing and consuming foods free from a chance of infection. The following are the measures to control bacterial growth.

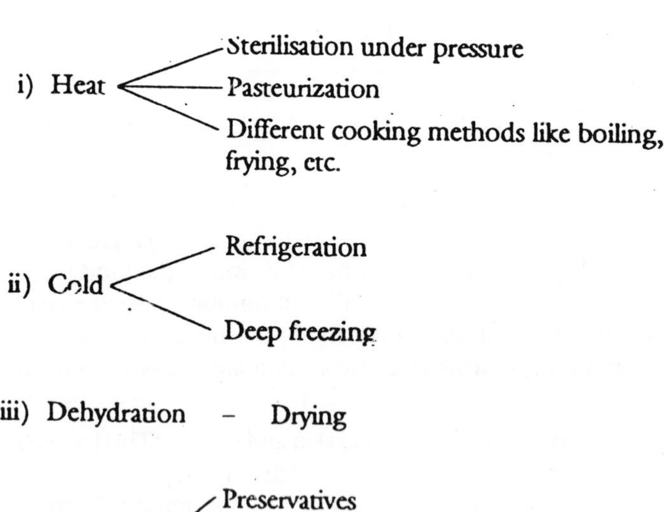

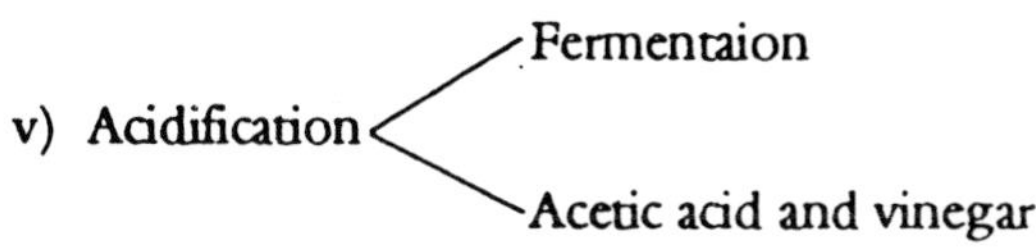

vi) Antibiotics

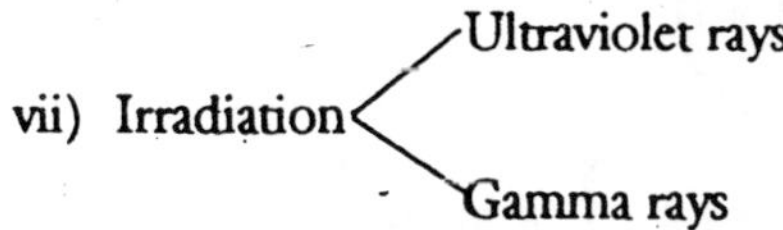

The food handler should not touch any of the body parts while preparing or serving the food. Hands should be washed before and after handling foods. Use of disposable paper towels than ordinary linen should be preferred. Persons with lesions should not handle the food. Smoking, tasting, coughing sneezing, etc., should not be done while handling the food. Nails should be short and clean. Bactericidal soaps should be used. Hair should be covered with net or cap and apron should be worn while handling the food control of flies, rat, mice, cock roaches and other insects is a must. The kitchen should be clean, well ventilated and the illumination should be bright. With all these precantions the chances of food poisoning can be minimised.

26

Toxicants in Foods

Some foods consumed by man contain some toxicants occuring naturally in them. Man with his experience started avoiding them. But some people because of illiteracy, traditions, superstitions and taboos consume these foods and are affected. Some toxicants affect immediately and some on habitual consumption show the ill effects. Some of them are discussed below.

ACKEE FRUIT POISONING

Ackee fruit is extremely popular in Jamaice and Nigeria. Usually unripe fruit causes poisoning. The poisonous properties are due to an unusual amino acid, hypoglycin-A and its glutamyl derivative, hypoglycin-B. Both has strong hypo glycemic action. Vomitings, drowsiness, stupor, turitching, convulsions and coma are the symptoms. This is because of severe depletion of liver glycogen and rapid fall in blood sugar resulting in coma and death. To save life treatment is intravenous glucose therapy as early as possible. Untreated cases die.

FAVISM

Ingestion of fresh or uncooked broad or faba beans cause favism. These beans have some glycosides containing pyramidine bases divicine and isouramil cause reduction of glutathione and glucose-6-phosphate dehydrogenase activity in RBC and cause hemolytic anemia.

HEMAGGLUTININS

Hemagglu tinins are present in legumes. These are proteins which have the ability to agglutinate the red blood cells. The most familiar agglutinin is Ricin found in castor seeds. Thorough heat treatment makes the castormeal detoxified.

LATHYROGENS

Lathyrism is a crippling disease characterised by paralysis of leg muscles after consuming the seeds Lathyrus satives over long period. These seeds have a toxin called β-(N) Oxalyl Amino Alamine (BODA). These seeds are commonly called Khesari dal. This crop can give good yield in drought conditions also. Naturally people take these seeds as their staple food. This crippling mostly is experienced by young male adults. Knee joints and ankle joint paralysis is experienced during midnight. Weakness is felt in the limbs. In the second stage patient cannot place the foot completely on the floor. He walks on toes with the help of sticks. In the thrid stage patient has severe pain in back and back bends. In the fourth and last stage patient cannot stand even with support he moves in sitting position. Finally patient becomes be ridden and awaits death.

Decortication, cooking, germination, fermentation etc. cannot detoxify this dal. This disease occurs only when the dal is consumed as staple food. So, the amount of consumption of this dal should be reduced. Giving up this dal immediately after noticing the first stage symptoms helps in aggravation of the disease. This dal can be detoxified by soaking it in water about 4 times the dal for 1 hour. 90 to 95% toxin is dissolved in water. The water removed should not be used. Then the dal is dried in sunlight. This dal can be used along with any cereal. Though some vitamins like thiamine and riboflavin are lost in this process final dal is 90 to 95 per cent free of the toxin.

TOXICANTS IN SPICES

The toxicants in spices usually give irritating sensation of mucous membranes. If consumed habitually over long periods or in excessive amounts toxic effects may be observed. Brown mustard seed when crushed with moisture gives allyliso thiolyanote which is a potent irritant. Capscium has capsaicin which is highly irritating and acts as a vesicant. Nutmeg and mace has myristicin which produces headache, cremps and nausea when consumed in excessive amounts. Other spices like giner, cloves, pepper etc. cause irritation to mucus membrane when consumed excessively.

GOITROGENS

Foods from Brassicae family possess goitrogens. The different goitrogens present are indolyl acetonitrite, thiocyanate, isothiocyanote, phenolic glycosides and Thio oxazolidone derivates. Cabbages and turnips have thio-oxazolidone derivative called 1–5 vinyl 2 thio oxazolidone. Mustard seeds rape seeds etc. contain thioglycosides which form isothiocyanate. Thicyanogen in some foods form cyanoglycosides. Phesolic glycosides present in the red skin of ground nut has goitrogenic property. In dolylacetonitrile present in brassicae family acts as goitrogen.

ATRIPLICISM

The young shoots of atriplex littralis caused toxic symptoms whose onset sudden. It ching and tingling of hands, edema of hands and face are the symptoms which later lead to gangreme.

AMERICAN WATER HEMLOCK

Consumption of this plant causes convulstions and unconsciousness leading to death.

BUSH TEA

Herbal infusion are very popular in tropics. Usually they are taken as tonics or medicines. The species senecio and crotolaria used in this infusion causes veno occlusive liver leading to cirrhosis.

CAMAS

Zigadenus venenoses resembles the edible camos and are frequently mistakingly consumed. This produces hypotension and cama.

DJENKOL BEANS

These are seeds of leguminous plant pitheco lobium lobatum benth. These beans have Djenkolic acid. Alkaline urine does not precipitate any problem. But if the urine is acidic this acid forms crystals and cause necrosis of ureter. The urine may possess Red Blood Cells, white blood cells and crystals of djenkolic acid.

LEU CAENA GLAUCA

This plant has an amino acid mimosive which is present in leaves and seeds chemically minosive is α-N-β-hydroxy pyriodine-4) amino propionic acid. This toxin causes loss of hair (baldness) and depression in growth.

SOLANINE

Potato has a toxic glycoside alkaloid in its peels called solanine. Sprouting potato and injured potato has higher concentration of solanine. Vomiting, abdominal pain and diarrhoea occurs within 10 hours after consumption of potatoes with more than 50 mg solanine per 100 grams. White snake root, Eupatorum urticae folium and aplo pappus laterophyllus are the plants which possess trimetol an unsaturated alcohol which on ingestion produces anorexie, vomiting, constipation ketosis and coma.

LIMA BEANS AND CASSAVA

Cyanogenetic glucosides yield hydrocyanic acid on hydrolysis which is highly poisonous. Consumption of lima bean (phaseolus lunatus) and cassava (manihot utissima) containing the toxin causes acute poisoning. The fodder of these plants also possess hydrocyanic acid is poisonous for cattle too.

SEA FOODS

Morayeel poisoning causes death due to paralysis of diaphragm, ciguatera poisoning causes death due to respiratory paralysis, puffer fish. Poisoning, results in intensive muscular paralysis and convulsions, cyclostoma, elasmobranch, turtle, oyster etc. also cause poisoning.

FATS AND OILS

Grossypol a phenolic compound of cotton seed oil, sanguinarine a alkaloid in Argemone oil are toxic to man and causes epidemic dropsy. Hydro carbon solvents used in extraction of oils are carcinogenic and may some times become fatal. Fumigation or insecticidal spray of oil seeds may leave residues in the seeds and may prove toxic.

MINERALS

Foods and water may possess excess of minerals,due to various reasons toxicity due to the presence of excess minerals is discussed in the chapters macro-minerals and micro-minerals.

FUNGAL TOXINS

Aspergillus Species : Four toxic products of aspergillus species are identified. They are aflatoxin B-1, B-2, G-1 and G-3 aspergillus poisoning was observed in animals. Consuming peanut meal. This aspergillus grows on ground nuts or ground nut meal in humid atmosphere to produce aflatoxins. This food stuff when consumed for sometime causes fatty liver and liver cirrhosis.

CLAVICEPS PURPUREA

Rye when infected with claviceps purpurea produces toxic compounds which are alkaloidal in nature. The disease caused it called ergotism. The alkoloid causing the disease is ergotamine may be responsible for the numbness, cyanosis, itching and peripheral gangrene.

MUSHROOM POISONING

Large size fungi of the class Basidiomyceties are called mushrooms. Aminita muscaria and aminita phalloides contain toxic. Aminita muscaria has an alkaloid–Muscaria which is highly toxic. Aminita phalloides has hepato toxic factros which produces severe necrosis of liver leading to death.

PENCILLIUM SPECIES

This is a common fungi. The toxin produces causes hepato renal damage and carcinoma.

BACTERIAL TOXINS

Staphylococeal poisoning is due to the enterotoxin produced by the staphylococci. Salivation, nausea, vomiting, diarrhoea, abdominal cramps and sweating are symptoms. Botulism is caused due to clostridium botulinum. They develop a neuro toxin due to which headache, nausea, dizziness, double vision, difficulty in swallowing, vomiting, paralysis and death may occur. Bacillus cereus occuring in cereals, milk and vegetables produce a toxin which on consumption causes symptoms of acute vomiting and diarrhoea. Salmonella poisoning is another important bacterial poisoning. The sources of food are infected poultry, eggs, meat and fish. The symptoms of salmonella poisoning are headache, vomiting, nausea, abdominal pain, diarrhoca, chills and faintness sometimes. Streptococci cause sore throat and scarlet fever. The synptoms of streptoccal poisoning are vomiting diarrhoca and abdominal pain. Shigella cause loose motions with nucus and blood usually accompanied by abdominal pain. Flies are the common carriers of this bacteria.

27

Food Allergy

The term allergy was first used by a Viennese doctor, Bara Clemens Von Pirquet in the year 1906 to mean altered activity. He use this term to describe some reactions in his patients. He was a paediatriciar He explained these reactions as marked reactions to certain foods, poller insect stings, development of immunity to infection, etc. Von Pirque was principally concerned with reactions involving the immune systerr the set of cells that protect our bodies from infection. Allergy to him i any altered response to the environment. Environment includes a external things that can affect the body, whether in food or water, in th air we breathe or things that come into contact without skin. Allerger is the substance that bring about the changed reactions. Both the word allergy and allergen are coined by Von Pirquet.

The commonly used terms to describe an adverse reaction to food include food allergy, food intolerance, hypersensitivity, sensitivity and false food allergy. All these terms are not synonymous. Food allergy and hypersensitivity are the adverse immunological responses to specific substance with characteristic symptoms and occurs whenever that food is ingested. Food intolerance does not involve the immunologic mech-anism and it may be due to an enzyme deficiency or other factors. The difference between food allergy and food intolerance are the symptoms occur within few minutes or hours following ingestion of food and it occurs whenever the food is consumed in first case and the symptoms occur in hours or days after ingestion of food and the condition tends to improve spontaneously or following a period of elimation of the food from the diet.

Food sensitivity is a umbrella terms for food allergy, food intolerance and other adverse reactions to food except where these are purely psychological in origin. False food allergy is a special type of non-immunological reaction, seen with particular foods, in which substance in the food triggers the mast cells directly. The reaction is not really an allergy at all, the immune system is not at fault and the body does not over produce IGE. But because the most cells releasing their chemical messengers the symptoms are exactly like those food allergy.

Allergy can be classified as shown below :

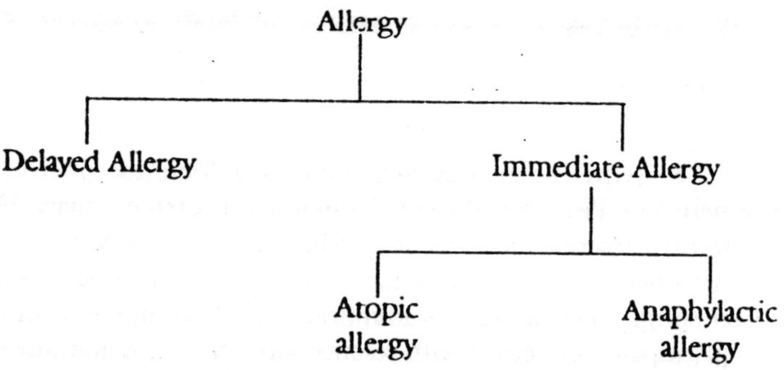

Delayed allergy is due to modified white blood corpuscles. The cells after the contact with allergen gets activated and are called sensitized cells.

In immediate allergy specific antibodies are formed by the plasma cells and react with allergen. These reactions leads to cellular damage and liberation of histamine; 5 hydroxy tryptamine, acetyl choline, etc. Atopic allergy is of hereditary nature. Undetectable antibodies are present in the individuals which manifest as rhinitis, asthma hayfever, etc. Classical allergic disorders such as hay fever, perrinial rhinitis, asthma and utricaria tend to run in family. Children of parents who has allergic disorders are more likely to be atopies. Children may have eczeme in baby food, lose the symptoms by 2–3 years old but develop asthma. This is called atopy. It is also possible for parents with no obvious atopic symptoms to produce atopic child. Both are probably carrying genes that contribute to atopy. Anaphylactic allergy is a condition where normal immunoglobulins are at work. This reaction is immediate and can be observed as soon as allergen reaches the circulation of a sensitized person.

The discovery of immunoglobulin E in 1960's helped in widening the rift between orthodox and unorthodox food allergists. Orthodox allergists described allergic reactions to be associated with classical reacuons such as rapid symptoms like swelling of lips, mouth and tongue, utricaria, vomiting and collapse. Unorthodox food allergists believed in delayed symptoms too.

In a allergy the immunoglobulin antibodies are produced in response to an innocuous antigen such as food molecule. These antibodies are usually found on surface of special immune cells known as mast cells that are present thoughout the body. If the antibodies on surface of the mast cell bind to their specific antigen, they stimulate the mast cell to release several chemical messengers. The normal purpose of these chemicals is to organize a more effective immune response, but in sufficient quantities they produce symptoms of allergy.

Allergens do not necessarily cause the symptoms where they first enter the body. They can enter the body by any route and show the symptoms elsewhere. The different symptoms of allergy are shown in Sketch 27.1.

In 1921 two German scientists Carl Prausnitz and Heinz Kustner demonstrated that blood is also involved in allergic reaction and produces violent reactions. Kustner was allergic to fish and developes utricaria. He injected a small amount of his blood serum to prausnitzs arm and next day fish extract was injected into the skin at the same place which produced a red itchy bump. They gave the name reagin to the factor present in blood which caused the reaction. This test is known as Prausnitz-Kuster test or passive transfer test. It is in 1960's that reagin was discovered to be an antibody by Japanese couple Kimishige and Teruko Ishizaka. This antibody is now called IgE.

These antibodies are special molecules produced by the body to fight off infections. These bind firmly to the bacteria or virus that causes an infection and stops it. Antibodies are 'Y' shaped molecules at whsoe tip of each arm is a specific antigen binding site. The antibodies are of 5 different types called as isotypes. They are IgG, IgA, IgM, IgD and IgE. Ig stands for immunoglobulin and suffix for antibody.

IgE molecules have their origin from B cells similar to other antibodies. Once they are produced IgE milecules behave differently

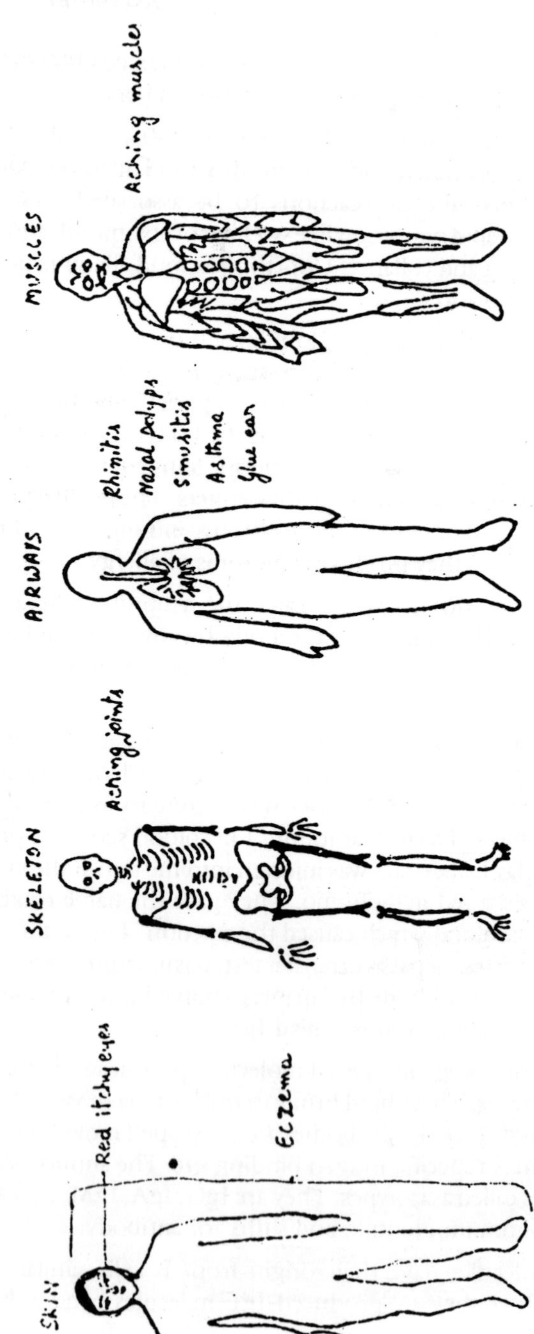
SKIN
Red itchy eyes
Eczema
SKELETON
Aching joints
AIRWAYS
Rhinitis
Nasal polyps
Sinusitis
Asthma
Glue ear
MUSCLES
Aching muscles

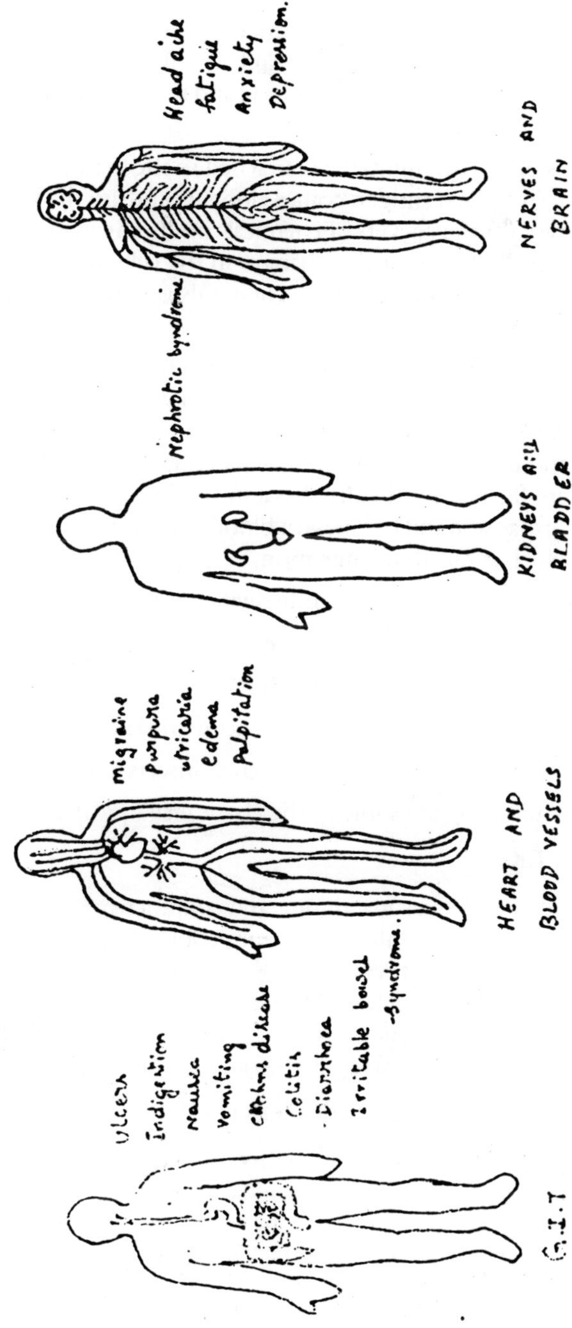

Sketch 27.1 : Symptoms of Allergy

from other antibodies in that they attach themselves to mast cells and basophils. Though both cells book slightly different under microscope basophils are found floating in the blood and mast cells embedded in the solid tissue of the body.

The stem of IgE molecule is attached to the mast cell the binding site are still free when antigen comes along it binds to the binding sites which trigger off the packets of chemicals inside the mast cell.They act as messengers and cause major changes in the cells and tissues around them. The process of releasing the chemicals is called degranulation.

The chemicals released by the mast cells are mediators. These mediators have effect on the body in different ways. Some make the blood vessels dialate some make them leaky so that blood escapes through the wall, some make the smooth muscles of lungs, stomach, intestine and bladder to contract. The parasites in the gut are loose the grip and are flushed out by diarrhoea in cases. For the parasites in the blood the expansion and leakiness of blood vessels produces redness and swelling which is called inflammation.

Allergens can be conveniently divided into 4 groups.

1. those we eat—food allergens or ingestants
2. those we breath in—inhalants
3. those which come into contact with skin—contactant and
4. those which are injected such as insects—injectants

The following are some of the classical allergic diseases in brief.

HAY FEVER

It is also called seasonal rhinitis and conjunctivitis by some. Pollen carried on the wind cause allergy to some people which is called hay fever. Mast cells in the nose and eyes respond to the proteins of the pollen grain. The mediators that are released cause inflammation of delicate membranes in nose and eyes and cause red, itchy, watery eyes and a runny or a congested nose. Some may suffer from itchy mouth and ears also.

PERENNIAL RHINITIS OR CONGESTED NOSE

Patients of hay fever suffer only in summer but patients of perennial rhinitis suffer all round the year. Moulds, dust, etc., cause this problem. Nose is connected with middle near by eustachian tube. So, perennial of rhinitis may cause a problem to ears. This tube becomes blocked with mucus from nose and air cannot reach middle ear and the secretions from ear cannot pass easily. This makes the mucus stick to the delicate bones of the ear and causes deafness. This condition is called chronic secretory otitis media (C SOM). Rhinits cause allergic sinusitis and nosal polyps also. Sinusitis is inflammation of membranes which may result from infection. Polyps are harmless but may obstruct the nasal passage and make breathing difficult. Another problem is past nasal drip where the mucus from nose trickles back of the throat into the trachea which has to be coughed off.

ASTHMA

In halnts which cause rhinitis also cause asthma. The target changes from nost to trachea dings and bronchi. The inflammation of membranes lining these tubes thicken and produce mucus which restricts passage of air causing asthma.

NETTLE RASH AND ODEMA

The mast cells in the lower layers of the skin releases mediatory which have a powerful effect on capillaries around. These capillaries become leaky and serum seeps out into the skin causing swelling and itching. Where there is a great deal of seepage from the blood vessels the tissues below skin become filled with serum casing localised Odema called Angiodema.

ATOPIC ECZEMA

Red itchy rash which tends to flake and then weep as it progresses. This becomes infections it scratched if bacteria attacks.

ASSESSMENT OF FOOD ALLERGY

Detection of food allergy requires caution, patience, skill and exeperience.

History

Though this is painstaking and time taking procedure it helps in accurate diagnosis of the allergen. Patient himself can predict the approximate allergen by this method. In case of infants and yound children mother should maintain a record and watch the reactions.

Diet Diaries

Patient should record each and every detail of the food ingested and the reactions found from time to time. Usually these are maintained on doctors advice.

Elimination Diet

This is a common procedure adopted for the detection of food allergy. Patient omits one of the suspected food each day and maintain records of diet and symptoms.

Immunological Test

Skin Prick Test, Radio Allergo Sorbent Test (RAST), Passive Transfer Test, etc. are used in this method. These tests are quite reliable but violent reactions and death may follow in some cases. So, these tests should be used cautiously. Another disadvantage is some extracts fail to give positive reactions though they are the culprits.

Leukopenic Index

This test involves the drop in the number of white blood cells after the ingestion of suspected food. The test is not reliable and does not give consistent results.

Trial Elimination Diets

The suspected food is eliminated from the diet for about 2 to 4 weeks. Then a trial dose of suspected food is given in a dose of 8–10 mg and results are observed.

Provocative Diet

The suspected food is introduced in disguised form without the knowledge of the patient to provoke allergic symptoms. If it gives positive result the offender is isolated.

Treatment

Corticosteroids (different from ones used by atheletes) have a general suppressive effect on inflammation, Antihistamines (which counter act the effect of mediator histamine) and bronchodilators used in asthma. Other options are as follows :

1. Avoid foods causing allergy
2. Know the contents of the food
3. Even if some food stopped giving allergy do not try to eat large amounts because allergy reoccurs.

4. Carry a syringe with adrenalin for allergy caused due to consumption of small amounts of allergin.
5. Apply food to fact except to mouth if this produces a rasn. leave the food.
6. Food additives also cause allergy so read the labels carefully.

Nutrition of Normal Infants

Genetically acquired characteristics, parental quality of nutrition and adequacy of post natal diet determines the growth and development of an infant. Mammals produce milk to feed their offspring during their early life. Milk is a specifically and specially designed nutriton for infant mammals. Milk of a particular mammal is ideal food for its infants. But, due to various other reasons infants may not be in a position to obtain milk from their mother. In such cases milk from other mamals is utilized making some modification like dilution, addition of sugar, etc. Usually cow's milk is used as substitute for human milk.

Growth and development are two distinctive terms that go hand in hand in case of normal children. Growth is an increase in size of the body or any parts of the body. Where as, development is maturation of body tissues organs and systems so that all functions can be carried out. After birth growth occurs very rapidly in the first year of life. In the first 5 to 6 months infants gain about 150 to 250 gms, a week and doubles the birth weight. In the next 6 months they gain 100 to 150 gms a week thereby triplling the birth weight by the time of first birthday. Normally birth length varies between 50 to 55 cm and reaches 75 to 80 cm at the end of first year.

At birth an infants possess 75 per cent water, 12 to 15 per cent fat and poorly developed muscle. By first birth day body fat increases to about 20 to 25 per cent ad water content decreases to 60 per cent. Bones contain more of water and cartilage at birth. The total calcium content of the skeleton at birth is 25 to 30 gms. which is trippled by the end of first year.

Growth and development of brain is rapid in fetal life and first 6 months of infancy from 6 months of age brain does not grow but it develops uptil the age of 5 years. 80 to 90 per cent of adult size is achieved by fourth birthday. The digestive system is not fully developed in infants. They will be unable to digest proteins, fats and simple carbohydrates. From 3rd month gastric secretion starts increasing. Salivation starts by 2nd or 3rd months. As we all know small sized animals have rapid heart beat when compared to large sized ones. This rule applies to infants also. At birth an infants heart beats 120 to 140 times per minute. The respiratory rate is also higher i.e. 20 times per minute. These rates gradually comes to normal as the infants grow. Even the kidneys cannot function normally and completely until the first birth day. Muscular co-ordination is also very poor in infants. At birth a baby has only rooting reflex. That is sucking, swallowing and breathing are the only functions carried out with muscular co-ordination. For about 3 months baby can only suckle. Later tongue movements are co-ordinated and solid food when kept on the tongue can be taken into the mouth and is swallowed. This is called extrusion reflex. By the age of 6 months an infant has better muscular co-ordination.

NUTRITIONAL REQUIREMENTS

The primary basis for the nutritional requirements of an infant is the amount of milk from mother ingested by a healthy infant. This data would be sufficient for calculating the nutritional needs of a infant upto first 6 months. The requirements for the next 6 months is based on the consumption of a formula and mixture of solid foods. The requirements of the different nutrients are briefly discussed below :

Protein

A healthy infant adds about 3 to 4 grams of protein daily to her body. Normal breast fed infant receives 1.5 to 2 grams of protein per kilogram per day. Which furnishes about 2 to 2.5 grams of protein per kilogram per day during the first few days of birth. Later it goes down to 1.5 grams by six months. Protein from cow milk is less efficiently utilized than protein from human milk. The protein requirement per kilogram body weight can be met with 1.6 gram of human milk protein or 2 gram of cow milk protein.

Energy

Infants have a high skin surface. Infants body spend a lot of energy to regulate their body temperature and metabolic activities. They energy needs of infants for the first 6 months range from 95 to 140 kcals per kilogram and 80 to 130 k cals per kilogram in the next 6 months. Half of this energy is used for maintaining the needs of basal metabolism. Babies who cry a lot and who are active need much more energy

Carbohydrate

Lactose is the main carbohydrate in an infant diet which accounts to about 40 per cent of calories from human milk. Lactose helps in the absorption of calcium and phosphorus and in maintaining a normal intestinal microflora. Other carbohydrates which are added to cow's milk in preparation of formulas or commercial fees are sucrose, cane syrup and dextrimaltose. Sucrose is easily available and cheap and has an advantage over lactose that it is easily digested and absorbed more rapidly but less than glucose and maltose. So, it is usually added to infant feeding formulas.

Fat

About 40 to 50 per cent of calories in human milk and in most formulas are supplies by fat. Fat provides essential fatty acids essential for infants. About 5 per cent of the calories are derived from linoleic acid in breast fed infants. In case of infants fed on other animal milk derive only 1.5 to 2 per cent. So, addition of vegetable fats rich in linoleic acid is desirable to other animal milk formulas when given to infants. Cholesterol is also essential for synthesis of bile salts and for the development of central nervous system. But the desirable level of cholesterol in an infant diet is not known.

Minerals

The infant needs may minerals for proper growth. These minerals are to be suplied in the milk. Human milk and Cow's milk fulfill all the mineral needs except for iron. So, infant foods based on animal milk should be fortified with iron. Infant foods based on soyabean and peanut should be fortified with iodide because these food stuffs possess goitrogenic properties.

Vitamins

Infants fed on unfortified cow's milk need vitamin A, D, E, C and niacin in additional amounts. Cow's milk is low in above vitamins so infants fed on animal milks need a supplement.

NUTRITIONAL REQUIREMENTS OF A INFANT

The nutritional requirements of infant are given in Table 28.1.

Table 28.1 Nutritional Requirements of a Infant

Nutrients	*Age*	
	0 – 6 months	6 –12 months
Energy (K cals)	118/kg	108/kg
Proteins (g)	2.0/kg	1.7/kg
Calcium (g)	0.5–0.6	0.5–0.6
Iron (mg)	1	1
Retional (mg) or	400	300
-Carotene (mg)	----	1200
Thiamine (mg)	59/mg/kg	54mg/kg
Riboflavin (mg)	71 mg/kg	65 mg/kg
Niacin (mg)	780 mg/kg	710 mg/kg
Vitamin B_6 (mg)	0.3	0.4
Folic acid (mg)	25	25
Vitamin B_{12} (mg)	0.2	0.2
Vitamin D (I.U.)	200	200
Vitamin C (mg)	20	20

Superiority of Human Milk Over Cow's Milk

Human milk is superior to other animal milks in many ways. It helps the normal get bacteria to develop and suppress the invasion of pathogenic bacteria. Other animal milks or formulas have the danger of geeting contaminated while storing, transferring and bottling.

Immunoglobulins

Breast milk has immunoglobulins that fight against micro organisms. IgA, IgG and IgM are the immunoglobulins that are present in human milk. These show antibody activity against E.coli, Poliovirus, Pneumococci and Streptococci.

Lymphoid Cells

Breast milk has lymphoid cells which produce IgA and mediate cell immunity as well as macrophages with phagocytic activity. Human milk also has 1000 to 4000 leucocytes per millimeter square during the first fortnight after delivery which prevent infection in gastrointestinal tract of the infant and the mamary glands of the mother.

Lactoferrin

Breast milk possess lactoferrin an iron binding protein which has bacteriostatic effect on E.coli—the important bacterial pathogen in new born. Human milk also possess 2 mg/ml of lysozyme which has antibacterial activity cow's milk has very little amounts of lysozyme and lactoferrin.

Lactobacillus Bifidus Factor

Breast milk possess a specific growth factor for promoting the growth of Lactobacillus bifidus a specific species of lactobacillus. The intestinal flora of infants fed on cow's milk formula is a mixed variety whereas infants fed on breast milk have only lactobacillus bifidus. This is evident by the acid reaction of the stools of infant. Breast milk when compared to cow's milk, has higher contents of vitamin C, iron, polyunsaturated fatty acids, and cystine in proteins. Adding to this it has low curd tenstion, high albumin content, low buffering capacity and less load on kidney. A comparison of human milk with other animal milk can be seen Table 17.1 of chapter 17 i.e. Milk and Milk Products.

Milk supplies a greater part of the required nutrients to the infants. Other foods like fruit juices, egg yolk strained vegetables, fruits, meat and pre-cooked cereals provide the nutrients that are lacking in milk. Fruit juices given to infants are orange and tomato. These provide vitamin C and the organic acids which help to lower the curd tension of milk and aid in absorption of calcium. Egg yolk is fair source of iron which is lacking in human milk. Yolk can be added to infants diet from 5th month. Strained fruits, vegetables and meat can be given from 5th to 6 months onwards. Pre-cooked and iron fortified cereals are also given to infants and these form the first solid foods of the body.

29

Nutrition of Pre-School Children

The growth and development of a pre-school child is entirely dependent on their diet. Infections and infestations attack immediately when the diet is poor in quality. During the second year the child increases in height by 7 to 8 cm and gains 3–5 kg. During 3, 4 and 5 years the weight gain is 2 kg per year approximately. and height gain is 9 cm, 7 cm 6 cm approximately. The water content of the body decreases gradually with addition of adipose tissue and mineralisation of the bone. The body protein increases to 18 per cent of body weight by four years of age from 14 per cent at the frist birth day. At this stage a deficit of as little as 10 K cals per kilogram body weight leads to growth failure and reduced nitrogen retention even when the protein intake is adequate. A well nourished child would be alert, vigorous, quickly recovering from fatigue, sleeps well at night, normal in height and weight has clear bright eyes, straight well formed teetch, pink unbleeding gums, lustrous healthy hair, firm muscles, good appetite and regular bowel movement.

NUTRITIONAL REQUIREMENT OF PRE-SCHOOL CHILD

The nutritional requirements of a pre-school child are given in Table 29.1.

Table 29.1 : Nutritional Requirements of Pre-school Child

Nutrient	Amount
Energy (K cals)	1220
Proteins (g)	22
Calcium (g)	0.4 – 0.5
Iron (mg)	20 – 25
Retinal (μg) or	250
-Carotene (μg)	1000
Thiamine (mg)	0.6
Riboflavin (mg)	0.7
Niacin (mg)	8
Vitamin B_6 (mg)	0.6
Folic Acid (μg)	100
Vitamin B_{12}(μg)	0.2 – 1.0
Vitamin D (I. U.)	200
Vitamin C (mg)	40

Young children have a very keen taste of sensitivity. Mild flavoured foods are preferred by pre-school children. The temperature of the food also should not be hot or cold. The foods given should not be sticky or gummy. Foods that can be picked up with fingers are relished by the children. Plain fruit juices, milk, milk beverages, chesse, cookies etc. can be given to pre-school children. Children enjoy colourful meal than a monotonous colours. They also enjoy eating by their own than fed. They have a very little span of attention i.e. they are readily diverted so the food should be attractive and tasty according to the child's like. A child should be fed when hungry. Energy foods, vitamins and minerals should not be dumped with over enthusiasm as it may cause other health problems.

Protein calorie malnutrition and other deficiency diseases may occur easily with faulty food habits. Children are great imitators and they imitate their elders and parents. So it is the parents duty to cultivate good food habits in the family. Non-availability of foods, ignorance, superstitions and poverty are the factors responsible for nutritional disorders in children.

For children milk is the important food which is good source of all nutrients except iron, which is easily accepted by children. Eggs, meat and fish are rich sources of protein and B-complex group of vitamins. But the cost of these foods is far off reach for common man. So, a common man can use legumes which are easily available and are almost equal to animal foods. Nuts and oil seeds provide good amount of protiens and fats.

Ignorance and illiteracy of mothers are responsible for malnutrition and faulty food habits of children. So, education of mothers is very essential to improve the nutritional status of the family. Table 29.2 gives a balanced diet formula for children between 1–3 years.

Table 29.2 : Balanced Diet for Pre-school Children (1–3 years)

Food Item	*Vegetarian* gm	*Non-vegetarian* gm
Cereals	150	150
Pulses	50	40
Green leafy vegetables	50	50
Other vegetables, Roots and Tubers	30	30
Fruits	50	50
Milk	300	200
Fats and Oils	20	20
Meat & Fish and Eggs	--	30
Sugar and Jaggery	30	30

30

Nutrition of Children and Adolescents

The nutrition of a school going child is easy when compared to a pre-schooler or on adolescent. A pre-schooler should change from a milk based diet to solid foods and a adolescent has a variety of changing tastes. So in both cases planning menu of the child's choice is difficult. But in case of a school going child group acceptance plays a major role. The child learns to accept foods from different cultural patterns and different family habits from peer group. Another advantage is child tries new foods in a group easily than trying alone at home.

The growth pattern of the school going children and adolescents varies from males to females. Boys gain 4 to 8 cm height and 3 to 7 kg weight per year between 5 and 14 years. Girls gain 5 to 7cm height and 2 to 5 kg weight per year between 5 and 13 years. Rate of growth in both height and weight tends to decline from 14th year in boys and 13th year in girls. Table 30.1 gives the recommended dietary allowances for shcool children and adolescents.

Adolescents are greatly influenced by their peer group. They strive for approval by their peers. In this thought the children who have good food habits also tend to make new habits with unbalance diets. In this crucial time they would be away from home for studies, sports and other activities. Meanwhile they develop, some wrong notions on foods and leave some nutritious foods. Especially girls have a notion that they are over weight, they are not satisfied by their structure and starts slimming down programmes by omitting meals which leads to nutritional disorders. On the other hand boys want to weight more and they think gain in weight is gain in muscle and indication of strength. The competition in all fields of life and emotional difficulties of teens, make the adolescents restless. They listen more to their friends than parents. So giving nutrition education to a child is very important before he/she enter eleventh or twelvth year of life. Choosing foods rich in all nutrients should be taught to every child. Table 30.2 gives balanced diets for children and Table 30.3 gives balanced diets for adolescents.

Table 30.1 : Recommended Dietary Allowances for School Children and Adolescents (I.C.M.R., 1981)

Nutrient	Both Sexes		Boys			Girls		
	4–6 years	7–9 years	10–12 years	13–15 years	16–18 years	10–12 years	13–15 years	16–18 years
Calories (Kcal)	1720	2050	2420	2660	2820	2260	2360	2200
Proteins (g)	29	36	43	52	53	42	43	44
Calcium (g)	0.4 to 0.5	0.4 to 0.5	0.4 to 0.5	0.6 to 0.7	0.5 to 0.6	0.4 to 0.5	0.6 to 0.7	0.5 to 0.6
Iron (mg)	20 to 25	20 to 25	20 to 25	20 to 25	20 to 25	20 to 25	35	35
Retinol (μg) or β-Carotene (μg)	300 1200	400 1600	600 2400	600 2400	750 3000	600 2400	600 2400	750 3000
Thiamine (mg)	0.9	1.0	1.2	1.3	1.4	1.1	1.2	1.1
Riboflavine (mg)	1.0	1.2	1.5	1.6	1.7	1.6	1.4	1.3
Nicotininc acid (mg)	11	14	16	18	19	15	15	15
Vitamin B_6 (mg)	0.9	1.2	1.6	2.0	2.0	1.6	2.0	2.0
Ascorbic acid (mg)	40	40	40	40	40	40	40	40
Folic acid (μg)	100	100	100	100	100	100	100	100
Vitamin B_{12} (μg)	1.0	1.0	1.0	1.0	1.0	1.0	1.0	1.0
Vitamin D (I.U.)	200	200	200	200	200	200	200	200

Table 30.2 : Balanced Diet for Children

Food Item	4–6 years		7–9 years		10–12 years	
	Vegetarian (gm.)	Non-Vegetarian (gm.)	Vegetarian (gm.)	Non-Vegetarian (gm.)	Vegetarian (gm.)	Non-Vegetarian (gm.)
Cereals	200	200	250	250	320	320
Pulses	60	50	70	60	70	60
Green leafy vegetables	75	75	75	75	100	100
Other vegetables						
Roots and tubers	50	50	50	50	75	75
Fruits	50	50	50	50	50	50
Milk	250	200	250	200	250	200
Fats and Oils	25	25	30	30	35	35
Meat and fish eggs	--	30	--	30	--	30
Sugar and Jaggery	40	40	50	50	50	50

Table 30.3 : Balanced Diets for Adolescent Boys and Girls

	Boys				Girls	
	13–15 years		16–18 years		13–18 years	
	Vegetarian (gm)	Non-Vegetarian (gm)	Vegetarian (gm)	Non-Vegetarian (gm)	Vegetarian (gm)	Non-Vegetarian (gm)
Cereals	430	430	450	450	350	350
Pulses	70	50	70	50	70	50
Green leafy vegetables	100	100	100	100	150	150
Other vegetables	75	75	75	75	75	75
Roots and tubers	75	75	100	100	75	75
Fruits	30	30	30	30	30	30
Milk	250	150	250	150	250	150
Fats and Oils	35	40	45	50	35	40
Meat and fish	--	30	--	30	--	30
Eggs	--	30	--	30	--	30
Sugar and Jaggery	30	30	40	40	30	30
Groundnuts	--	--	50*	50*	--	--

* An additional 30 gm. of fats and oils can be included in the diet in place of groundnuts.

31

Nutrition in Old Age

Old people are valuable source of experience, talents and skills. With aging there is a progressive decline in water content, lean body mass and adipose tissue. With increasing age skin looses its flexibility, collagen in the body increase and bones become fragile. old people become frail; physically disabled and lonely. Many may be suffering with diseases with one kind or the other. The medication they take may interfere the absorption and utilisation of some nutrients in the body.

Changes that take place in old age are as follows :

Cellular Changes

The number of functional parenchymal cells decrease. This is evident in the tissues with no regeneration capacity like brain, heart, kidney, etc. The reduction in number of taste buds reduces taste activity and modifies acceptance of food.

Function of Gastrointestinal Tract

Secretion of saliva decreases which causes difficulty in swallowing. Some people may loose the teeth and some may have ill fitting dentures which causes difficulty in swallowing. The acidity of the stomach decreases which interferes the absorption of calcium, iron, zinc and vitamin B_{12}.

Cardiovascular System

Progression accumulation of athermatous plaques reduce the lomen and elasticity of blood vessels which inturn reduces the cardiac output and increased resistance to flow of blood. The functioning capacity of the heart decreases with the change in character of the heart muscle.

Nervous System

The reaction time decreases especially when higher centres are involved, decreased learning rate, memory power and vision are also observed.

Renal System

With decreased blood flow and functioning nephrons glomerular filteration and tubular reabsorption lessens and wastes may sometimes are not excreted properly.

Skeletal Changes

Demineralisation of bone has been observed in most of the aged persons which is called osteoporosis.

The recommended daily allowances for old age people are 25% less than normal individuals who are doing light work. Balanced diets for adult man and women are given in Table 31.1.

The basic principles of nutrition in old age to be considered are 1) ability to digest different foods 2) likes and dislikes, 3) Protein intake to maintain positive nitrogen balance, 4) variety in diet. 5) inclusion of soft dietary fibre to avoid constipation, 6) adequate caloric intake, 7) adequate calcium and iron intake to avoid obsteoporosis and anemia, 8) adequate water to maintain normal urine and 9) adequate vitamins to avoid vitamin deficiencies.

Foods served attractively, leisurely meals, meals with near and dear and avoiding strong flavours make the meal time of elders enjoyable.

Table 31.1 : Balanced Diets for Adult Man and Woman

Food Item	Adult man		Adult woman	
	Vegetarian	*Non-Vegetarian*	*Vegetarian*	*Non-Vegetarian*
	g	g	g	g
Cereals	400	400	300	300
Pulses	70	55	60	45
Green leafy Vegetables	100	100	125	125
Other Vegetables	75	75	75	75
Roots and Tubers	75	75	50	50
Fruits	30	30	30	30
Milk	200	100	200	100
Fats and Oils	35	40	30	35
Meat and Fish	---	30	--	30
Eggs	--	30	--	30
Sugars and Jaggery	30	30	--	30

32

Nutrition of Pregnant and Lactating Woman

Pregnancy and lactation lays considerable stress on woman. Nutritional needs during this period increase. But the societies framed some rigid rules for pregnant woman including the foods she could eat and foods she should not even touch. These superstitions make the pregnant and lactating woman receive deficient diseases and lead to complications. Semi-starvation of mother with a view of smaller baby and easy delivery is false. Restriction of salt and fluids to reduce incidence of toxemia and theory of maternal organism are proved to be false.

Neonatal mortality also increases with poor nourishment of the expectant mother. If mother has one or more of the following factors neonatal mortality or low birth weight infant may be the result.

1. Mother under 17 years
2. Small stature
3. Poor nutritional status
4. Low body weight
5. Low gain in weight during pregnancy
6. Smoking, alcoholism, etc.

7. Complications of pregnancy
8. Infections
9. Unfavourable social environment

Mother in a good nutritional state prior to conception and that the status is maintained all through pregnancy have few complications in pregnancy, parturition and have healthy babies. The mothers protein intake correlates well with infants weight, length and physical condition. Eclampsia was not found in women who had good diets all through the pregnancy. Under weight women produce smaller babies and premature babies. Overweight women had more still births. Pregnant adolescents are medically, nutritionally and socially at risk. Anemia, eclampsia, prenuature and prolonged labour and maternal death are common in such cases.

CHANGES DURING PREGNANCY

Pregnancy can be conveniently divided into three stages. In the first stage the fertilized Ovum becomes implanted in endometrium of the uterus where rapid cell proliferation occurs. The uterine glands and outer layers of germ plasm nourish the embryo and placenta begins to develop. This stage extends over a period of 2 weeks. In the second stage all the major organs like heart, liver, lungs, kidneys and skeleton forms. This stage is about 2 to 8 weeks. From eighth week to parturition rapid growth of the fetus, production of milk and preparation for labour takes place. Hyperplasia and hypertrophy occur with rate varying from organ to organ.

The placenta is the organ by which the fetus is attached by means of the umbilical cord and maintains connection with mother. Water, oxygen and electrolytes diffuse from maternal circulation to fetal circulation through placental membrane. Glucose and amino acid require active transport from maternal circilation to fetal circulation. All substances are not filtered through this membrane. Undernourishment leads to small placenta and so is the transfer of nutrients due to which the baby born will be small.

Progesteron is a hormone secreted by corpus luteum which brings about increased secretion by the endometrium as well as increase in lipid and glycogen stores of the body. It also inhibits contraction of uterine muscles and prevents expulsion of embryo. Progesteron with estrogen stimulates growth of mammary glands and inhibits lactogenic function of pitutary until the birth of infant.

The total blood volume increases by 1/3rd by the end of pregnancy. As the volume of blood increases concentration of serum albumin, hemoglobin and other constituents of blood decreases. Pregnant women have cravings and aversions. Especially it is found in first half of the pregnancy. Strong flavours, coffee, meat, poultry, etc. produce nausea and induce vomitings. Some have cravings for ice cream, sweets, fruits, etc. Pica is found in some women. Pica is appetite for abnormal non-food substances like chalk, mud, clay, starch, etc.

Basal metabolism increases during pregnancy which averages 150 K cals per day during the second half of the pregnancy. Gastric tone, motility and secretion are also reduced slightly. The glomerular filteration rate is increased to clear various substances like creatinine, urea, uric acid etc. Water excretion is high in mid pregnancy than in advanced pregnancy due to stress on bladder frequent urination is seen. The average weight gain at the end of prenancy would be 10 to 12 kg. Table 32.1 gives average components of weight gain in pregnancy.

Table 32.1 : Average Components of Weight Gain in Pregnancy*

	Cumulative gain (kg) at end of each trimester		
	First	*Second*	*Third*
Fetus	Negligible	1.0	3.4
Placenta	Negligible	0.3	0.6
Amniotic fluid	Negligible	0.4	1.0
Increased uterine size	0.3	0.8	1.0
Increased breast size	0.1	0.3	0.5
Increased blood volume	0.3	1.3	1 5
Increased extracellular fluid	0	0	1.5
Total :	0.7	4.1	9.5

* Pitkin RM, et al. "Maternal Nutrition—A Selective Review of Clinical Topics", Obstet. Gynecol., 1972; 40; 777.

Recommended dietary allowances for pregnant and lactating woman are given in Table 32.2. Nursing mothers produce 20 to 30 ounces of milk each day. The energy needs to convert food energy to milk energy is 80 to 90 per cent efficient. 100 ml of breast milk supplies 67 to 77 K cals. Thus 850 ml of milk production needs 750 K cals. Fot deposites furnish 200 to 300 K cals for first 3 months of lactation. Thus, an additional allowance of 500 K cal to diet is recommended for a nursing mother. 100 ml of Kuman milk contains 1.2 gm protein. Thus 850 ml has 10 g protein. Conversion of dietary protein of milk protein is about 70 per cent. Thus an additional allowance of 20 g protein is needed for every nursing mother. Table 32.3 gives the balanced diets for pregnant and lactating mothers.

Table 32.2 : Recommended Dietary Allowances for Pregnant and Lectating Women (I.C.M.R., 1981)

Nutrients	Women (Ordinary)				Lactation	
	Sedent-ary	Moder-ate work	Heavy work	Pregnancy (Second half)	0–6 mon-ths	7–12 mon-ths
Calories (Kcal)	1900	2200	3000	+300	+550	+400
Proteins (g)	45	45	45	+14	+25	+25
Calcium (g)	0.4 to 0.5	0.4 to 0.5	0.4 to 0.5	1.0	1.0	1.0
Iron (mg)	32	32	32	40	32	32
Retinol (μg) or β-Carotene (μg)	750 3000	750 3000	750 3000	750 3000	1150 4600	1150 4600
Thiamine (mg)	1.0	1.1	1.5	+0.2	+0.3	+0.2
Riboflavin (mg)	1.1	1.3	1.8	+0.2	+0.3	+0.2
Nicotinio acid (mg)	12	--	--	+1.2	+4	+3
Vitamin B_6 (mg)	2.0	2.0	2.0	2.5	2.5	2.5
Ascorbic acid (mg)	40	40	40	40	80	80
Folic acid (μg)	100	100	100	300	150	150
Vitamin B_{12} (μg)	1	1	1	1.5	1.5	1.5
Vitamin D (I. U.0	200	200	200	400	200	200

Table 32.3 : Balanced Diets for Adult Woman

	Sedentary work		Moderate work		Heavy work		Additional Allowances During	
	V (gm)	NV (gm)	V (gm)	NV (gm)	V (gm)	NV (gm)	P (gm)	L (gm)
Cereals	300	300	350	350	475	475	50	100
Pulses	60	45	70	55	70	55		10
Green Leafy Vegetables	125	125	125	125	125	125	25	25
Other Vegetables	75	75	75	75	100	100	--	--
Roots and Tubers	50	50	75	75	100	100	--	--
Fruits	30	30	30	30	30	30	--	--
Milk	200	100	200	100	200	100	125	125
Fats and Oils	30	35	35	40	40	45	--	15
Sugar and Jaggery	30	30	30	30	40	40	10	20
Meat and Fish	--	30	--	30	--	30	--	--
Eggs	--	30	--	30	--	30	--	--
Ground nuts	--	--	--	--	40*	40*	--	--

* An additional 25 gm. of fats and oils can be included in place of groundnuts.

V-Vegetarian NV-Non Vegetarian P-Pregnancy L-Lactation

Appendices

Table 1 : Nutritive Values of Common Foods

All the Values are per 100 gms. of Edible Portion

Name of the Foodstuff	Moisture	Protein (N×6.25)	Fat	Minerals	Fibre	Carbo hydrates	Energy	Calcium	Phosphorus	Iron
	g	g	g	g	g	g	Kcal.	mg.	mg.	mg.
(1)	(2)	(3)	(4)	(5)	(6)	(7)	(8)	(9)	(10)	(11)
CEREAL GRAINS AND PRODUCTS										
BAJRA	12.4	11.6	5.0	2.3	1.2	67.5	361	42	296	8.0
BARLEY	12.5	11.5	1.3	1.2	3.9	69.6	336	26	215	1.67
ITALIAN MILLET	11.2	12.3	4.3	3.3	8.0	60.9	331	31	290	2.8
JOWAR	11.9	10.4	1.9	1.6	1.6	72.6	349	25	222	4.1
MAIZE, dry	14.9	11.1	3.6	1.5	2.7	66.2	342	10	348	2.3
MAIZE, tender	67.1	4.7	0.9	0.8	1.9	24.6	125	9	121	1.1
PANIVARAGU	11.9	12.5	1.1	1.9	2.2	70.4	341	14	206	0.8
RAGI	13.1	7.3	1.3	2.7	3.6	72.0	328	344	283	3.9
RICE, paraboiled, handpounded	12.6	8.5	0.6	0.9	--	77.4	349	10	280	2.8
RICE, paraboiled, milled	13.3	6.4	0.4	0.7	0.2	79.0	346	9	143	1.0
RICE, raw, handpounded	13.3	7.5	1.0	0.9	0.6	76.7	346	10	190	3.2
RICE, raw, milled	13.7	6.8	0.5	0.6	0.2	78.2	345	10	160	0.7
RICE, bran	11.0	13.5	16.2	6.6	4.3	48.4	393	67	1410	35.0
RICE, flakes	12.2	6.6	1.2	2.0	0.7	77.3	346	20	238	20.0
RICE, puffed	14.7	7.5	0.1	3.8	0.3	73.6	325	23	150	6.6
SAMAI	11.5	7.7	4.7	1.5	7.6	67.0	341	17	220	9.3

(Contd.)

Table 1 : (Contd.)

All the Values are per 100 gms. of Edible Portion

Name of the Foodstuff	Mois-ture g	Protein (N×6.25) g	Fat g	Mine-rals g	Fibre g	Carbo hydrates g	Energy Kcal.	Cal-cium mg.	Phos-phorus mg.	Iron mg.
(1)	(2)	(3)	(4)	(5)	(6)	(7)	(8)	(9)	(10)	(11)
SANWA MILLET	11.9	6.2	2.2	4.4	9.8	65.5	307	20	280	5.0
VARAGU	12.8	8.3	1.4	2.6	9.0	65.9	309	27	188	0.5
WHEAT, bulgar (parboiled)	9.8	8.2	1.6	1.5	1.7	77.2	356	37	298	4.9
WHEAT, whole	12.8	11.8	1.5	1.5	1.2	71.2	346	41	306	5.3
WHEAT, flour (whole)	12.2	12.1	1.7	2.7	1.9	69.4	341	48	355	4.9
WHEAT, flour (refined)	13.3	11.0	0.9	0.6	0.3	73.9	348	23	121	2.7
WHEAT, germ	5.2	29.2	7.4	3.5	1.4	53.3	397	40	846	6.0
WHEAT, semolina	--	10.4	0.8	--	0.2	74.8	348	16	102	1.6
WHEAT, vermicelli	11.7	8.7	0.4	0.7	0.2	78.3	352	22	92	2.0
WHEAT, bread (brown)	39.0	8.8	1.4	--	1.2	49.0	244	18	--	2.2
WHEAT, bread (white)	39.0	7.8	0.7	--	0.2	51.9	245	11	--	1.1
PULSES AND LEGUMES										
BENGAL GRAM, whole	9.8	17.1	5.3	3.0	3.9	60.9	360	202	312	4.6
BENGAL GRAM, dhal	9.9	20.8	5.6	2.7	1.2	59.8	372	56	331	5.3
BENGAL GRAM, roasted	10.7	22.5	5.2	2.5	1.0	58.1	369	58	340	9.5
BLACK GRAM, dhal	10.9	24.0	1.4	3.2	0.9	59.6	347	154	385	3.8
COW PEA	13.4	24.1	1.0	3.2	3.8	54.5	323	77	414	8.6
FIELD BEAN, dry	9.6	24.9	0.8	3.2	1.4	60.1	347	60	433	2.7

(Contd.)

Table 1 : (Contd.)

All the Values are per 100 gms. of Edible Portion

Name of the Foodstuff	Moisture g	Protein (N×6.25) g	Fat g	Minerals g	Fibre g	Carbo hydrates g	Energy Kcal.	Calcium mg.	Phosphorus mg.	Iron mg.
(1)	(2)	(3)	(4)	(5)	(6)	(7)	(8)	(9)	(10)	(11)
GREEN GRAM, whole	10.4	24.0	1.3	3.5	4.1	56.7	334	124	326	4.4
GREEN GRAM, dhal	10.1	24.5	1.2	3.5	0.8	59.9	348	75	405	3.9
HORSE GRAM, whole	11.8	22.0	0.5	3.2	5.3	57.2	321	287	311	6.77
KHESARI, dhal	10.0	28.2	0.6	2.3	2.3	56.6	345	90	317	6.3
LENTIL	12.4	25.1	0.7	2.1	0.7	59.0	343	69	293	7.58
MOTH BEANS	10.8	23.6	1.1	3.5	4.5	56.5	330	202	230	9.5
PEAS green	72.9	7.2	0.1	0.8	4.0	15.9	93	20	139	1.5
PEAS dry	16.0	19.7	1.1	2.2	4.5	56.5	315	75	298	7.05
PEAS, roasted	10.1	22.9	1.4	2.4	4.4	58.8	340	81	345	6.4
RAJMAH	12.0	22.9	1.3	3.2	(4.8)	60.6	346	260	410	5.1
RED GRAM, dhal	13.4	22.3	1.7	3.5	1.5	57.6	335	73	304	2.7
RED GRAM (tender)	65.1	9.8	1.0	1.0	6.2	16.9	116	57	164	1.1
SOYABEAN	8.1	43.2	19.5	4.6	3.7	20.9	432	240	690	10.4
LEAFY VEGETABLES										
AGATHI	73.1	8.4	1.4	3.1	2.2	11.8	93	1130	80	3.9
AMARNATH caudatus	90.0	3.0	0.7	3.3	1.0	2.0	26	200	40	..
AMARNATH gangeticus (tender)	85.7	4.0	0.5	2.7	1.0	6.1	45	397	83	3.49

(Contd.)

Table 1 : (Contd.)

All the Values are per 100 gms. of Edible Portion

Name of the Foodstuff	Moisture g	Protein (N×6.25) g	Fat g	Minerals g	Fibre g	Carbo hydrates g	Energy Kcal.	Calcium mg.	Phosphorus mg.	Iron mg.
(1)	(2)	(3)	(4)	(5)	(6)	(7)	(8)	(9)	(10)	(11)
AMARNATH gangeticus (stem)	92.5	0.9	0.1	1.8	1.2	3.5	19	260	30	1.8
AMARNATH paniculatus	78.6	5.9	1.0	3.8	2.1	8.6	67	530	60	18.4
AMARNATH polygonoides	90.0	2.8	0.3	2.1	--	4.8	33	251	55	27.3
AMARNATH spinosus	85.0	3.0	0.3	3.6	1.1	7.0	43	800	50	22.9
AMARNATH species (Charavarthikeerai)	80.6	4.5	0.6	4.2	1.6	8.5	57	321	71	18.0
AMARNATH species (Koyakeerai)	88.0	2.8	0.5	1.2	2.2	5.3	37	292	51	2.5
AMARNATH tristis	87.0	2.8	0.5	1.2	2.2	5.3	37	292	51	2.5
AMARNATH viridis	81.8	5.2	0.3	2.8	6.1	3.8	38	330	52	18.7
AMBAT CHUKA	95.2	1.6	0.3	0.9	0.6	1.4	15	63	17	0.75
BATHUA LEAVES	89.6	3.7	0.4	2.6	0.8	2.9	30	150	80	4.2
BEET GREENS	86.4	3.4	0.8	2.2	0.7	6.5	46	380	30	16.2
BENGAL GRAM LEAVES	73.4	7.0	1.4	2.1	2.0	14.1	97	340	120	23.8
BETEL LEAVES	85.4	3.1	0.8	2.3	2.3	6.1	44	230	40	10.6
BOTTLE GOURD LEAVES	87.9	2.3	0.7	1.7	1.3	6.1	39	80	59	--
BROAD BEAN LEAVES	77.6	5.6	0.3	1.3	3.7	11.5	71	111	149	--
BURSSELS SPROUTS	85.5	4.7	0.5	1.0	1.2	7.1	52	43	82	1.8

(Contd.)

Table 1 : (Contd.)

All the Values are per 100 gms. of Edible Portion

Name of the Foodstuff	Moisture	Protein (N×6.25)	Fat	Minerals	Fibre	Carbo hydrates	Energy	Calcium	Phosphorus	Iron
	g	g	g	g	g	g	Kcal.	mg.	mg.	mg.
(1)	(2)	(3)	(4)	(5)	(6)	(7)	(8)	(9)	(10)	(11)
CABBAGE	91.9	1.8	0.1	0.6	1.0	4.6	27	39	44	0.8
CARROT LEAVES	76.6	5.1	0.5	2.8	1.9	13.1	77	340	110	8.8
CAULIFLOWER GREENS	80.0	5.9	1.3	3.2	2.0	7.6	66	626	107	40.0
CELERY LEAVES	88.0	6.3	0.6	2.1	1.4	1.6	37	230	140	6.3
CELERGY STALK	93.5	0.8	0.1	0.9	1.2	3.5	18	30	38	4.8
CHEKKUR MANIS	73.6	6.8	3.2	3.4	1.4	11.6	103	570	200	28.0
COLOCASIA LEAVES (black variety)	78.8	6.8	2.0	2.5	1.8	8.1	77	460	125	0.98
COLOCASIA LEAVES (green variety)	82.7	3.9	1.5	2.2	2.9	6.8	56	227	82	10.0
COLOCASIA LEAVES (dried)	9.3	13.7	5.9	12.8	16.0	42.3	277	1546	308	--
CORIANDER LEAVES	86.3	3.3	0.6	2.3	1.2	6.3	44	184	71	1.42
COW PEA LEAVES	89.0	3.4	0.7	1.6	1.2	4.1	38	290	58	20.1
CURRY LEAVES	63.8	6.1	1.0	4.0	6.4	18.7	108	830	57	0.93
DRUMSTICK LEAVES	75.9	6.7	1.7	2.3	0.9	12.5	92	440	70	0.85
FENUGREEK LEAVES	86.1	4.4	0.9	1.5	1.1	6.0	49	395	51	1.93
FETID CASSIA (fresh)	84.9	5.0	0.8	1.7	2.1	5.5	49	520	39	12.4

(Contd.)

Table 1 : (Contd.)

All the Values are per 100 gms. of Edible Portion

Name of the Foodstuff	Moisture	Protein (N×6.25)	Fat	Minerals	Fibre	Carbohydrates	Energy	Calcium	Phosphorus	Iron
	g	g	g	g	g	g	Kcal.	mg.	mg.	mg.
(1)	(2)	(3)	(4)	(5)	(6)	(7)	(8)	(9)	(10)	(11)
FETID CASSIA (dri..	9.7	20.7	3.9	11.8	10.4	43.5	292	3200	292	--
GARDEN CRESS	82.3	5.8	1.0	2.2	--	8.7	67	360	110	28.6
GARDEN SORREL (sepals)	91.9	0.6	0.2	0.9	1.3	5.1	25	130	20	1.7
GOGU	86.4	1.7	1.1	0.9	--	9.9	56	172	40	2.28
IPOMOEA STEMS	93.7	0.9	0.2	1.8	--	3.4	19	80	30	0.8
IPOMOEA LEAVES	90.3	2.9	0.4	2.1	1.2	3.1	28	110	46	3.9
KNOL-KHOL GREENS	86.7	3.5	0.4	1.2	1.8	6.4	43	740	50	13.3
KUPPAMENI	80.5	6.7	1.4	3.1	2.3	6.0	64	667	99	17.3
LETTUCE	93.4	2.1	0.3	1.2	0.5	2.5	21	50	28	2.4
LETTUCE TREE LEAVES, mature	81.7	5.1	0.4	2.6	--	10.2	65	320	80	2.6
LELUCE TREE LEAVES, tender	90.2	3.6	0.2	2.2	0.6	3.2	29	170	60	3.6
MANATHAKKALI LEAVES	82.1	5.9	1.0	2.1	--	8.9	68	410	70	20.5
MAYALU	90.8	2.8	0.4	1.8	--	4.2	32	200	35	10.0
MINT	84.9	4.8	0.6	1.9	2.0	5.8	48	200	62	15.6
MODAKANTHAN KEERAI	83.3	4.7	0.6	2.3	--	9.1	61	--	--	--
MUKARRATE KEERAI	84.5	6.1	0.9	1.3	--	7.2	61	667	99	18.4
MUSTARD LEAVES	89.8	4.0	0.6	1.6	0.8	3.2	34	155	26	16.3
NEERINGI	79.1	7.2	0.5	4.6	--	8.6	68	1550	82	9.2

(Contd.)

Table 1 : (Contd.)

All the Values are per 100 gms. of Edible Portion

Name of the Foodstuff	Moisture	Protein (N×6.25)	Fat	Minerals	Fibre	Carbo hydrates	Energy	Calcium	Phosphorus	Iron
	g	g	g	g	g	g	Kcal.	mg.	mg.	mg.
(1)	(2)	(3)	(4)	(5)	(6)	(7)	(8)	(9)	(10)	(11)
PARSLEY	74.6	5.9	1.0	3.2	1.8	13.5	87	390	175	17.9
PARUPPU KEERAI	90.5	2.4	0.6	2.3	1.3	2.9	27	111	45	14.8
PONNANGANNI	77.4	5.0	0.7	2.5	2.8	11.6	73	510	60	1.63
PUMPKIN LEAVES	81.9	4.6	0.8	2.7	2.1	7.9	57	392	112	--
RADISH LEAVES	90.8	3.8	0.4	1.6	1.0	2.4	28	265	59	0.09
RADISH LEAVES table	89.1	3.9	0.6	1.6	0.6	4.2	38	310	60	18.0
RAPE stem	91.4	3.1	0.1	1.4	--	4.0	29	100	100	1.2
RAPE LEAVES	84.9	5.1	0.4	2.5	1.2	5.9	48	370	110	12.5
RAPE LEAVES (dried)	7.4	27.0	2.9	15.3	6.7	40.7	297	3095	500	--
SAFFLOWER LEAVES	91.1	2.5	0.6	1.3	--	4.5	33	185	35	5.7
SHEPU	88.0	3.0	0.5	2.2	1.1	5.2	37	190	42	17.4
SPINACH	92.1	2.0	0.7	1.7	0.6	2.9	26	73	21	1.14
SPINACH stalks	93.4	0.9	0.1	1.8	--	3.8	20	90	20	1.6
SUSNI SAG	86.9	3.7	1.4	2.1	1.3	4.6	46	53	91	--
TAMARIND LEAVES, tender	70.5	5.8	2.1	1.5	1.9	18.2	115	101	140	0.30
TURNIP GREENS	81.9	4.0	1.5	2.2	1.0	9.4	67	710	60	28.4

(Contd.)

Table 1 : (Contd.)

All the Values are per 100 gms. of Edible Portion

Name of the Foodstuff	Moisture g	Protein (N×6.25) g	Fat g	Minerals g	Fibre g	Carbo hydrates g	Energy Kcal.	Calcium mg.	Phosphorus mg.	Iron mg.
(1)	(2)	(3)	(4)	(5)	(6)	(7)	(8)	(9)	(10)	(11)
ROOTS AND TUBERS										
ARROW ROOT FLOUR	16.5	0.2	0.1	0.1	--	83.1	334	10	20	1.0
BANANA RHIZOME	85.1	0.4	0.2	1.4	1.1	11.8	51	25	10	1.1
BEET ROOT	87.7	1.7	0.1	0.8	0.9	8.8	43	18.3	55	1.19
CARROT	86.0	0.9	0.2	1.1	1.2	10.6	48	80	530	1.03
COLOCASIA	73.1	3.0	0.1	1.7	1.0	21.1	97	40	140	0.42
KHAMALU	79.6	1.3	0.1	0.8	0.1	18.1	79	16	31	0.5
MANGO GINGER	85.0	1.1	0.7	1.4	1.3	10.5	53	25	90	2.6
ONION big	86.6	1.2	0.1	0.4	0.6	11.1	50	46.9	50	0.60
ONION small	84.3	1.8	0.1	0.6	0.6	12.6	59	40	60	1.2
PARSNIP	72.4	1.3	0.3	1.1	1.7	23.2	101	50	40	0.5
POTATO	74.7	1.6	0.1	0.6	0.4	22.6	97	10	40	0.48
RADISH pink	90.8	0.6	0.3	0.9	0.6	6.8	32	50	20	0.37
RADISH rat-tailed	92.3	1.3	0.3	0.7	1.1	4.3	25	78	24	--
RADISH table	94.9	0.5	0.1	0.7	0.6	3.2	16	20	20	1.0
RADISH white	94.4	0.7	0.1	0.6	0.8	3.4	17	35	22	0.4
SWEET POTATO	68.5	1.2	0.3	1.0	0.8	28.2	120	46	50	0.21
TAPIOCA	59.4	0.7	0.2	1.0	0.6	38.1	157	50	40	0.9

(Contd.)

Table 1 : (Contd.)

All the Values are per 100 gms. of Edible Portion

Name of the Foodstuff	Moisture g	Protein (N×6.25) g	Fat g	Minerals g	Fibre g	Carbohydrates g	Energy Kcal.	Calcium mg.	Phosphorus mg.	Iron mg.
(1)	(2)	(3)	(4)	(5)	(6)	(7)	(8)	(9)	(10)	(11)
TAPIOCA chips dried	12.0	1.3	0.3	2.0	1.8	82.6	338	91	70	3.6
TURNIP	91.6	0.5	0.2	0.6	0.9	6.2	29	30	40	0.4
YAM, elephant	78.7	1.2	0.1	0.8	0.8	18.4	79	50	34	0.6
YAM, ordinary	69.9	1.4	0.1	1.6	1.0	26.0	111	35	20	1.19
YAM, wild	70.4	2.5	0.3	1.4	1.0	24.4	110	20	74	1.0
OTHER VEGETABLES										
ASH GOURD	96.5	0.4	0.1	0.3	0.8	1.9	10	30	20	0.8
BEANS, scarlet runner	58.3	7.4	1.0	1.6	1.9	29.8	158	50	160	2.6
BITTER, GOURD	92.4	1.6	0.2	0.8	0.8	4.2	25	20	70	0.61
BITTER GOURD small	83.2	2.1	1.0	1.4	1.7	10.6	60	23	38	2.0
BOTTLE GOURD	96.1	0.2	0.1	0.5	0.6	2.5	12	20	10	0.46
BRINJAL	92.7	1.4	0.3	0.3	1.3	4.0	24	18	47	0.38
BROAD BEANS	85.4	4.5	0.1	0.8	2.0	7.2	48	50	64	1.4
CAULIFLOWER	90.8	2.6	0.4	1.0	1.2	4.0	30	33	57	1.23
CHO-CHO-MARROW	92.5	0.7	0.1	0.4	0.6	5.7	27	140	30	0.6
CLUSTER BEANS	81.0	3.2	0.4	1.4	3.2	10.8	16	130	57	1.08
COLOCASIA STEM	94.0	0.3	0.3	1.2	0.6	3.6	18	60	20	0.5
COWPEA PODS	85.3	3.5	0.2	0.9	2.0	8.1	48	72	59	2.5

(Contd.)

Table 1 : (Contd.)

All the Values are per 100 gms. of Edible Portion

Name of the Foodstuff	Moisture g	Protein (N×6.25) g	Fat g	Minerals g	Fibre g	Carbo hydrates g	Energy Kcal.	Calcium mg.	Phosphorus mg.	Iron mg.
(1)	(2)	(3)	(4)	(5)	(6)	(7)	(8)	(9)	(10)	(11)
CUCUMBER	96.3	0.4	0.1	0.3	0.4	2.5	13	10	25	0.60
DOUBLE BEANS	73.8	8.3	0.3	1.0	4.3	12.3	85	40	140	2.3
DRUMSTICK	86.9	2.5	0.1	2.0	4.8	3.7	26	30	110	0.18
DRUMSTICK flowers	85.9	3.6	0.8	1.3	1.3	7.1	50	51	90	--
FIELD BEANS, tender	86.1	3.8	0.7	0.9	1.8	6.7	48	210	68	0.83
FIGS, red (Ficus cunia)	79.4	1.2	0.6	1.6	6.4	10.8	53	187	39	--
FRENCH BEANS	91.4	1.7	0.1	0.5	1.8	4.5	26	50	28	0.61
GHOSALA	93.2	1.2	0.2	0.5	2.0	2.9	18	36	19	1.1
GIANT CHILLIES (capsicum)	92.4	1.3	0.3	0.7	1.0	4.3	24	10	30	0.567
JACK, tender	84.0	2.6	0.3	0.9	2.8	9.4	51	20	40	1.7
JACK FRUIT, seeds	64.5	6.6	0.4	1.2	1.5	25.8	133	50	97	1.5
KANKODA	84.1	3.1	1.0	1.1	3.0	7.7	52	33	42	4.6
KARONDA fresh	91.0	1.1	2.9	0.6	1.5	2.9	42	21	28	--
KARONDA dry	18.2	2.3	9.6	2.8	--	67.1	364	160	60	39.1
KHEKSA	90.4	0.6	0.1	0.9	1.6	6.4	29	27	38	--
KOVAI	93.5	1.2	0.1	0.5	1.6	3.1	18	40	30	0.38
KNOL-KHOL	92.7	1.1	0.2	0.7	1.5	3.8	21	20	35	1.54

(Contd.)

Table 1 : (Contd.)

All the Values are per 100 gms. of Edible Portion

Name of the Foodstuff	Moisture g	Protein (N×6.25) g	Fat g	Minerals g	Fibre g	Carbohydrates g	Energy Kcal.	Calcium mg.	Phosphorus mg.	Iron mg.
(1)	(2)	(3)	(4)	(5)	(6)	(7)	(8)	(9)	(10)	(11)
LADIES FINGERS	89.6	1.9	0.2	0.7	1.2	6.4	35	66	56	0.35
LAKUCH, raw	89.4	1.6	1.2	1.1	2.8	13.9	73	67	25	--
LEEKS	78.9	1.8	0.1	0.7	1.3	17.2	77	50	70	2.3
LOTUS STEM, dry	9.5	4.1	1.3	8.7	25.0	51.4	234	405	128	60.6
MANGO, green	87.5	0.7	0.1	0.4	1.2	10.1	44	10	19	0.33
ONION STALKS	87.6	0.9	0.2	0.8	1.6	8.9	41	50	50	7.43
PAPAYA, green	92.0	0.7	0.2	0.5	0.9	5.7	27	28	40	0.9
PARWAR	92.0	2.0	0.3	0.5	3.0	2.2	20	30	40	1.7
PINK BEANS	86.8	3.1	0.4	0.6	2.1	7.0	44	54	70	1.5
PLANTAIN flower	89.9	1.7	0.7	1.3	1.3	5.1	34	32	42	1.6
PLANTAIN green	83.2	1.4	0.2	0.5	0.7	14.0	64	10	29	6.27
PLANTAIN stem	88.3	0.5	0.1	0.6	0.8	9.7	42	10	10	1.1
PUMPKIN fruit	92.6	1.4	0.1	0.6	0.7	4.6	25	10	30	0.11
PUMPKIN flowers	89.1	2.2	0.8	1.4	0.7	5.8	39	120	60	--
RIDGE GOURD	95.2	0.5	0.1	0.3	0.5	3.4	17	18	26	0.39
SNAKE GOURD	94.6	0.5	0.3	0.5	0.8	3.3	18	26	20	1.51
SUNDAKAI, dry	12.3	8.3	1.7	5.1	17.6	55.0	269	390	180	22.2
SWORD BEANS	87.2	2.7	0.2	0.6	1.5	7.8	44	60	40	2.0

(Contd.)

Table 1 : (Contd.)

All the Values are per 100 gms. of Edible Portion

Name of the Foodstuff	Moisture g	Protein (N×6.25) g	Fat g	Minerals g	Fibre g	Carbo hydrates g	Energy Kcal.	Calcium mg.	Phosphorus mg.	Iron mg.
(1)	(2)	(3)	(4)	(5)	(6)	(7)	(8)	(9)	(10)	(11)
TINDA, tender	93.5	1.4	0.2	0.5	1.0	3.4	21	25	24	0.9
TOMATO, green	93.1	1.0	0.1	0.6	0.7	3.6	23	20	36	1.8
VEGETABLE MARROW	94.8	0.5	0.1	0.3	0.8	3.5	17	10	30	0.6
WATER CHESTNUT, fresh	70.0	4.7	0.3	1.1	0.6	23.3	115	20	150	1.35
WATER CHESTNUT, dry	13.8	13.4	0.8	3.1	--	68.9	330	70	440	2.4
NUTS AND OILSEEDS										
ALMOND	5.2	20.8	58.9	2.9	1.7	10.5	655	230	490	5.09
ARECANUT	31.3	4.9	4.4	1.0	11.2	47.2	249	50	130	1.5
AVOCADOPEAR (nut)	63.7	2.5	0.7	1.1	--	32.0	144	20	80	1.2
CASHEWNUT	5.9	21.2	46.9	2.4	1.3	22.3	596	50	450	5.81
CHILGOZA	4.0	13.9	49.3	2.8	1.0	29.0	615	91	494	3.6
COCONUT dry	4.3	6.8	62.3	1.6	6.6	18.4	662	400	210	7.8
COCONUT fresh	36.3	4.5	41.6	1.0	3.6	13.0	444	10	240	1.7
COCONUT tender	90.8	0.9	1.4	0.6	--	6.3	41	10	30	0.9
COCONUT milk	42.8	3.4	41.0	0.9	0	11.9	430	15	140	1.6
COCONUT water	93.8	1.4	0.1	0.3	0	4.4	24	24	10	0.1
COCONUT meal, deoiled	8.7	23.8	2.8	7.0	9.8	47.9	312	112	646	69.4
GARDEN CRESS SEEDS	3.2	25.3	24.5	6.4	7.6	33.0	454	377	723	100.0

(Contd.)

Table 1 : (Contd.)

All the Values are per 100 gms. of Edible Portion

Name of the Foodstuff	Moisture g	Protein (N×6.25) g	Fat g	Minerals g	Fibre g	Carbo hydrates g	Energy Kcal.	Calcium mg.	Phosphorus mg.	Iron mg.
(1)	(2)	(3)	(4)	(5)	(6)	(7)	(8)	(9)	(10)	(11)
GINGELLY SEEDS	5.3	18.3	43.3	5.2	2.9	25.0	563	1450	570	9.3
GROUND NUT	3.0	25.3	40.1	2.4	3.1	26.1	567	90	350	2.5
GROUND NUT roasted	1.7	26.2	39.8	2.5	3.1	26.7	570	77	370	3.1
GROUND NUT cake	7.2	40.9	7.4	2.5	3.2	38.8	386	213	548	--
LINSEED SEEDS	6.5	20.3	37.1	2.4	4.8	28.9	530	170	370	2.7
MUSTARD SEEDS	8.5	20.0	39.7	4.2	1.8	23.8	541	490	700	7.9
NIGER SEEDS	4.2	23.9	39.0	4.9	10.9	17.1	515	300	224	56.7
PISTACHIO NUT	5.6	19.8	53.5	2.8	2.1	16.2	626	140	430	7.7
PIYAL SEEDS	3.0	19.0	59.1	3.0	3.8	12.1	656	279	528	8.5
SAFFLOWER SEEDS	5.5	13.5	25.6	2.6	34.9	17.9	356	236	823	4.6
SUNFLOWER SEEDS	5.5	19.8	52.1	3.7	1.0	17.9	620	280	670	5.0
WALNUT	4.5	15.6	64.5	1.8	2.6	11.0	687	100	380	2.64
WATER MELON SEEDS (kernal)	4.3	34.1	52.6	3.7	0.8	4.5	628	100	937	7.4
CONDIMENTS ANL SPICES										
ARISITHIPPILI	12.5	13.2	4 7	6.0	5.2	58.4	329	460	325	13.50
ASAFOETIDA	16.0	4.0	1.1	7.0	4.1	67.8	297	690	50	39.4
CARDAMOM	20.0	10.2	2.2	5.4	20.1	42.1	229	130	160	4.6

(Contd.)

Table 1 : (Contd.)

All the Values are per 100 gms. of Edible Portion

Name of the Foodstuff	Moisture g	Protein (N×6.25) g	Fat g	Minerals g	Fibre g	Carbohydrates g	Energy Kcal.	Calcium mg.	Phosphorus mg.	Iron mg.
(1)	(2)	(3)	(4)	(5)	(6)	(7)	(8)	(9)	(10)	(11)
CHILLIES dry	10.0	15.9	6.2	6.1	30.2	31.6	246	160	370	2.3
CHILLIES green	85.7	2.9	0.6	1.0	6.8	3.0	29	30	80	4.4
CLOVES dry	25.2	5.2	8.9	5.2	9.5	46.0	286	740	100	11.7
CLOVES green	65.5	2.3	5.9	2.2	--	24.1	159	310	40	2.1
CORIANDER	11.2	14.1	16.1	4.4	32.6	21.6	288	630	393	7.1
CUMIN SEEDS	11.9	18.7	15.0	5.8	12.0	36.6	356	1080	511	11.7
FENUGREEK SEEDS	13.7	26.2	5.8	3.0	7.2	44.1	333	160	370	6.5
GARLIC dry	62.0	6.3	0.1	1.0	0.8	29.8	145	30	310	1.2
GINGER fresh	80.9	2.3	0.9	1.2	2.4	12.3	67	20	60	3.5
LIME PEEL	66.5	1.8	0.5	1.8	--	29.4	129	710	60	2.7
MACE	15.9	6.5	24.4	1.6	3.8	47.8	437	180	100	12.3
MANGO POWDER	6.8	2.8	7.8	4.9	13.7	64.0	337	180	16	45.2
NUTMEG fruit	14.3	7.5	36.4	1.7	11.6	28.5	472	120	240	2.03
NUTMEG rind	86.8	1.0	0.4	0.6	--	11.2	52	40	10	2.0
OMUM	7.4	17.1	21.8	7.9	21.2	24.6	363	1525	443	12.5
PEPPER DRY (black)	18.2	11.5	6.8	4.4	14.9	49.2	304	460	198	12.4
PEPPER GREEN	70.6	4.8	2.7	1.8	6.4	13.7	98	270	70	2.4
PIPPALI	12.2	6.4	2.3	4.8	8.5	65.8	310	1230	190	62.1

(Contd.)

Table 1 : (Contd.)

All the Values are per 100 gms. of Edible Portion

Name of the Foodstuff	Moisture g	Protein (N×6.25) g	Fat g	Minerals g	Fibre g	Carbo hydrates g	Energy Kcal.	Calcium mg.	Phosphorus mg.	Iron mg.
(1)	(2)	(3)	(4)	(5)	(6)	(7)	(8)	(9)	(10)	(11)
POPPY SEEDS	4.3	21.7	19.3	9.9	8.0	36.8	408	1584	432	15.9
TAMARIND PULP	20.9	3.1	0.1	2.9	5.6	67.4	283	170	110	17.0
TURMERIC	13.1	6.3	5.1	3.5	2.6	69.4	349	150	282	67.8
FRUITS										
AMBADA	90.3	0.7	3.0	0.5	1.0	4.5	48	36	11	3.9
AMLA	81.8	0.5	0.1	0.5	3.4	13.7	58	50	20	1.2
APPLE	84.6	0.2	0.5	0.3	1.0	13.4	59	10	14	0.660
APRICOT fresh	85.3	1.0	0.3	0.7	1.1	11.6	53	20	25	2.2
APRICOT dry	19.4	1.6	0.7	2.8	2.1	73.4	306	110	70	4.6
AVOCADO PEAR	73.6	1.7	22.8	1.1	--	0.8	215	10	80	0.7
BAEL FRUIT	61.5	1.8	0.3	1.7	2.9	31.8	137	85	50	0.6
BANANA, ripe	70.1	1.2	0.3	0.8	0.4	27.2	116	17	36	0.36
BANYAN TREE FIGS	74.1	1.7	2.0	1.0	8.5	11.8	72	364	43	--
BILIMBI	94.4	0.5	0.3	0.3	1.0	3.5	19	15	10	1.2
BREAD FRUIT	79.5	1.5	0.2	0.9	2.1	15.8	71	40	30	0.5
BULLOCK'S HEART	76.8	1.4	0.2	0.7	5.2	15.7	70	10	10	0.6
CAPE GOOSEBERRY	82.9	1.8	0.2	0.8	3.2	11.1	53	10	67	2.0
CASHEW FRUIT	86.3	0.2	0.1	0.2	0.9	12.3	51	10	10	0.2

(Contd.)

Table 1 : (Contd.)

All the Values are per 100 gms. of Edible Portion

Name of the Foodstuff	Moisture g	Protein (N×6.25) g	Fat g	Minerals g	Fibre g	Carbo hydrates g	Energy Kcal.	Calcium mg.	Phosphorus mg.	Iron mg.
(1)	(2)	(3)	(4)	(5)	(6)	(7)	(8)	(9)	(10)	(11)
CHERRIES, red	83.4	1.1	0.5	0.8	0.4	13.8	64	24	25	0.57
CURRANTS, black	18.4	2.7	0.5	2.2	1.0	75.2	316	130	110	8.5
DATES dried	15.3	2.5	0.4	2.1	3.9	75.8	317	120	50	7.3
DATES fresh	59.2	1.2	0.4	1.7	3.7	33.8	144	22	38	0.96
FIGS (Ficus carcia)	88.1	1.3	0.2	0.6	2.2	7.6	37	80	30	1.0
GRAPES blue variety	82.2	0.6	0.4	0.9	2.8	13.1	58	20	23	0.5
GRAPES pale green variety	79.2	0.5	0.3	0.6	2.9	16.5	71	20	30	0.52
GRAPE FRUIT marsh's seedless	88.5	1.0	0.1	0.4	--	10.0	45	30	30	0.2
GRAPE FRUIT triumph	92.0	0.7	0.1	0.2	--	7.0	32	20	20	0.2
GUAVA, country	81.7	0.9	0.3	0.7	5.2	11.2	51	10	28	0.27
GUAVA, hill	85.3	0.1	0.2	0.6	4.8	9.0	38	50	20	1.2
HARFAROWRIE	91.2	0.7	0.6	0.5	1.1	5.9	32	6	6	--
JACK FRUIT	76.2	1.9	0.1	0.9	1.1	19.8	88	20	41	0.56
JAMB, safed	93.5	0.1	0.4	0.1	2.2	3.7	19	17	3	0.1
JAMBU FRUIT	83.7	0.7	0.3	0.4	0.9	14.0	62	15	15	0.43
KORUKKAPALLI	79.2	2.7	0.4	0.7	1.0	16.0	78	14	49	1.0
LAKUCH	82.1	0.7	1.1	0.8	2.0	13.3	66	50	20	0.5

(Contd.)

Table 1 : (Contd.)

All the Values are per 100 gms. of Edible Portion

Name of the Foodstuff	Moisture g	Protein (N×6.25) g	Fat g	Minerals g	Fibre g	Carbohydrates g	Energy Kcal	Calcium mg.	Phosphorus mg.	Iron mg.
(1)	(2)	(3)	(4)	(5)	(6)	(7)	(8)	(9)	(10)	(11)
LEMON	85.0	1.0	0.9	0.3	1.7	11.1	57	70	10	0.26
LEMON SWEET	90.5	0.7	0.3	0.5	0.7	7.3	35	30	20	0.7
LICHI	84.1	1.1	0.2	0.5	0.5	13.6	61	10	35	0.7
LICHIES, bastard	83.9	1.4	0.3	0.8	0.5	13.1	61	15	35	--
LIME	84.6	1.5	1.0	0.7	1.3	10.9	59	90	20	0.3
LIME, sweet malta	90.3	0.7	0.2	0.4	0.6	7.8	36	30	20	1.0
LIME, sweet musambi	88.4	0.8	0.3	0.7	0.5	9.3	43	40	30	0.7
LOQUAT	88.2	0.6	0.3	0.5	0.8	9.6	43	30	20	1.3
MAHUA, ripe	73.6	1.4	1.6	0.7	--	22.7	111	45	22	0.23
MANGO, ripe	81.0	0.6	0.4	0.4	0.7	16.9	74	14	16	1.3
MANGOSTEEN	84.9	0.5	0.1	0.2	--	14.3	60	10	20	0.2
MELON, musk	95.2	0.3	0.2	0.4	0.4	3.5	17	32	14	1.4
MELON, water	95.8	0.2	0.2	0.3	0.2	3.3	16	11	12	7.9
MULBERRY	86.5	1.1	0.4	0.6	1.1	10.3	49	70	30	2.3
ORANGE	87.6	0.7	0.2	0.3	0.3	10.9	48	26	20	0.32
ORANGE juice	97.7	0.2	0.1	0.1	--	1.9	9	5	9	0.7
PALMYRA FRUIT ripe (mesocarp)	77.2	0.7	0.2	0.7	0.5	20.7	87	9	33	--

(Contd.)

Table 1 : (Contd.)

All the Values are per 100 gms. of Edible Portion

Name of the Foodstuff	Moisture g	Protein (N×6.25) g	Fat g	Minerals g	Fibre g	Carbo hydrates g	Energy Kcal.	Calcium mg.	Phosphorus mg.	Iron mg.
(1)	(2)	(3)	(4)	(5)	(6)	(7)	(8)	(9)	(10)	(11)
PALMYRA FRUIT tender	92.3	0.6	0.1	0.2	0.3	6.5	29	10	20	0.5
PAPAYA, ripe	90.8	0.6	0.1	0.5	0.8	7.2	32	17	13	0.5
PASSION FRUIT	76.3	0.9	0.1	0.7	9.6	12.4	54	10	60	2.0
PASSION FRUIT juice	89.0	1.2	0.2	0.7	1.2	7.7	37	10	30	0.7
PEACHES	86.0	1.2	0.3	0.8	1.2	10.5	50	15	41	2.4
PEARS	86.0	0.6	0.2	0.3	1.0	11.9	52	8	15	0.5
PERSIMMON	80.0	0.7	0.2	0.3	0.9	17.9	76	15	10	0.3
PHALSA	80.8	1.3	0.9	1.1	1.2	14.7	72	129	39	3.1
PINE APPLE	87.8	0.4	0.1	0.4	0.5	10.8	46	20	9	2.42
PLUM	86.9	0.7	0.5	0.4	0.4	11.1	52	10	12	0.6
POMEGRANATE	78.0	1.6	0.1	0.7	5.1	14.5	65	10	70	1.79
PRUNES	85.3	0.5	0.3	0.6	0.5	12.8	56	10	18	..
PUMMELO	88.0	0.6	1.0	0.5	0.6	10.2	44	30	30	0.3
QUINCE	85.7	0.3	0.1	0.3	1.7	11.9	50	10	20	0.4
RAISINS	20.2	1.8	0.3	2.0	1.1	74.6	308	87	80	7.7
RASPBERRY	84.8	1.0	0.6	0.9	1.0	11.7	56	40	110	2.3
ROSE APPLE	89.1	0.7	0.2	0.3	1.2	8.5	39	10	30	0.5
SAPOTA	73.7	0.7	1.1	0.5	2.6	21.4	98	28	27	1.25

(Contd.)

Table 1 : (Contd.)

All the Values are per 100 gms. of Edible Portion

Name of the Foodstuff	Moisture g	Protein (N×6.25) g	Fat g	Minerals g	Fibre g	Carbohydrates g	Energy Kcal.	Calcium mg.	Phosphorus mg.	Iron mg.
(1)	(2)	(3)	(4)	(5)	(6)	(7)	(8)	(9)	(10)	(11)
SEETHAPHAL	70.5	1.6	0.4	0.9	3.1	23.5	104	17	47	4.31
STRAWBERRY	87.8	0.7	0.2	0.4	1.1	9.8	44	30	30	1.8
TOMATO, ripe	94.0	0.9	0.2	0.5	0.8	3.6	20	48	20	0.64
TOMATILLO	91.7	0.7	0.6	0.6	0.6	5.8	31	7	40	1.4
TREE TOMATO	86.2	1.5	0.2	1.2	4.2	6.7	35	12	46	1.0
WOOD APPLE	64.2	7.1	3.7	1.9	5.0	18.1	134	130	110	0.48
ZIZYPHUS	81.6	0.8	0.3	0.3	--	17.0	74	4	9	0.50
FISHES AND OTHER SEA FOODS										
AIR	78.1	15.9	1.3	1.2	--	3.5	89	380	180	0.7
ANCHOVY	69.3	19.3	9.6	1.6	--	0.2	164	143	174	1.5
BACHA	68.8	18.1	5.6	1.4	--	6.1	147	520	180	0.7
BAM	74.8	16.1	0.9	1.3	--	6.9	100	330	240	0.8
BASPATA MACHLI	76.1	18.2	4.4	1.4	--	0	112	175	225	--
BATA, small varieties	79.0	14.3	2.5	2.0	--	2.2	89	790	200	1.1
BELEY	79.7	14.5	0.6	2.3	--	2.9	75	370	330	1.0
BHAGON fresh	70.6	14.8	8.8	2.0	--	3.8	154	182	190	1.2
BHAGON dried	17.9	61.5	2.3	16.5	--	1.8	274	6235	207	9.3
BHANGAN BATA	67.3	19.4	4.4	2.2	--	6.7	144	580	310	1.1

(Contd.)

Table 1 : (Contd.)

All the Values are per 100 gms. of Edible Portion

Name of the Foodstuff	Moisture g	Protein (N×6.25) g	Fat g	Minerals g	Fibre g	Carbo hydrates g	Energy Kcal.	Calcium mg.	Phosphorus mg.	Iron mg.
(1)	(2)	(3)	(4)	(5)	(6)	(7)	(8)	(9)	(10)	(11)
BHEKTI fresh	79.9	14.9	0.8	1.4	--	3.0	79	480	350	3.1
BHEKTI dried	20.1	60.2	2.0	15.9	--	1.8	266	939	347	15.0
BHOLA	78.1	15.2	1.1	1.9	--	3.7	86	550	580	0.4
BIG JAWED JUMPER	73.3	19.4	5.8	1.4	--	0.1	130	214	306	3.4
BOAL	73.3	15.4	2.7	1.3	--	7.6	116	160	490	0.6
BOMBAY DUCK, dried	16.7	61.7	4.0	15.1	--	2.5	293	1389	240	19.1
BLUE MUSSEL	81.5	9.9	2.0	3.0	--	3.6	72	1134	286	8.0
CAT FISH	77.1	21.4	--	--	--	--	86	10	230	--
CHELA	77.5	14.6	4.3	2.1	--	1.5	103	590	340	2.0
CHELA dried	4.7	64.8	17.0	13.4	--	0.1	413	3590	2342	--
CHINGRI small dried	17.9	62.4	3.9	13.9	--	1.9	292	3539	354	27.9
CHINGRI goda, dried	14.9	60.0	3.2	17.3	--	4.6	287	3847	828	49.6
CHITAL	75.0	18.6	2.3	1.0	--	3.1	108	180	250	3.0
CRAB muscle	83.5	8.9	1.1	3.2	--	3.3	59	1370	150	21.2
CRAB small	65.3	11.2	9.8	4.6	--	9.1	169	1606	253	--
FOLUI	73.0	19.0	1.0	2.5	--	3.7	109	590	450	1.7
GHOL	69.7	18.4	0.9	--	--	--	82	90	150	2.1
GOGGLER	76.9	18.7	1.6	1.8	--	1.0	93	437	349	8.2

(Contd.)

Table 1 : (Contd.)

All the Values are per 100 gms. of Edible Portion

Name of the Foodstuff	Mois-ture g	Protein (N×6.25) g	Fat g	Mine-rals g	Fibre g	Carbo hydrates g	Energy Kcal.	Cal-cium mg.	Phos-phorus mg.	Iron mg.
(1)	(2)	(3)	(4)	(5)	(6)	(7)	(8)	(9)	(10)	(11)
HERRING, Indian	72.8	20.3	3.2	1.5	--	2.2	119	429	305	9.3
HERRING ox-eyed	73.7	20.7	2.2	1.6	--	0.8	106	429	131	6.3
HILSA	53.7	21.8	19.4	2.2	--	2.9	273	180	280	2.1
HORSE MACKEREL	76.9	21.2	1.6	1.3	--	0	99	357	262	2.0
INDIAN WHITING	77.1	19.2	0.6	1.5	--	1.6	89	71	262	2.2
JEW FISH (kora)	78.3	18.8	0.8	1.9	--	0.2	83	286	305	4.4
JEW FISH (pallikora)	77.0	20.0	2.2	1.6	--	--	100	214	262	4.8
KALABASU	81.0	14.7	1.0	1.3	--	2.0	76	320	380	0.8
KATLA	73.7	19.5	2.4	1.5	--	2.9	111	530	235	0.9
KHORSULA	75.3	16.3	5.1	1.8	--	1.5	117	410	160	0.6
KHOYRA fresh	72.0	18.0	3.0	1.8	--	5.2	120	590	220	0.7
KHOYRA dried	17.3	58.9	6.2	16.4	--	1.2	296	--	--	--
KOI	70.0	14.8	8.8	2.0	--	4.4	156	410	390	1.4
KOOCHA MACHLI	76.7	18.7	0.8	1.4	--	2.4	92	185	119	--
LATA	74.0	19.4	0.6	2.6	--	3.4	97	610	530	1.3
LOBSTER	77.3	20.5	0.9	1.4	--	0	90	16	279	--
MACKEREL	77.3	18.9	1.7	1.6	--	0.5	93	429	305	4.5
MAGUR	78.5	15.0	1.0	1.3	--	4.2	86	210	290	0.7

(Contd.)

Table 1 : (Contd.)

All the Values are per 100 gms. of Edible Portion

Name of the Foodstuff	Moisture g	Protein (N×6.25) g	Fat g	Minerals g	Fibre g	Carbohydrates g	Energy Kcal.	Calcium mg.	Phosphorus mg.	Iron mg.
(1)	(2)	(3)	(4)	(5)	(6)	(7)	(8)	(9)	(10)	(11)
MAHASOLE	70.3	25.2	2.3	1.2	--	1.0	126	130	280	3.8
MANDELI, dried	31.1	52.5	5.4	--	--	--	259	143	259	11.9
MRIGAL	75.0	19.5	0.8	1.5	--	3.2	98	350	280	1.1
MULLET	69.9	19.1	7.8	1.1	--	2.1	155	357	175	4.4
MUSHI dried	9.6	67.0	4.9	--	--	--	312	541	507	2.7
MUSSEL, fresh water	79.5	14.5	1.6	2.3	--	2.1	81	592	406	--
MUTIJELLA, dried	19.2	63.6	2.4	11.8	--	3.0	288	7240	834	1.0
OIL SARDINE	76.5	19.6	2.0	1.8	--	0.1	97	357	349	6.1
PABDA	73.0	19.2	2.1	1.1	--	4.6	114	310	210	1.3
PANGAS	72.3	14.2	10.8	1.0	--	1.7	161	180	130	0.5
PARSEY fresh	70.8	17.5	5.9	1.5	--	4.3	140	850	490	2.7
PARSEY dried	11.8	65.0	4.4	15.8	--	3.0	312	2231	396	17.4
POMFRETS, black	74.5	20.3	2.6	1.1	--	1.5	111	286	306	2.3
POMFRETS, white	78.4	17.0	1.3	1.5	--	1.8	87	200	290	0.9
PRAWN	77.4	19.1	1.0	1.7	--	0.8	89	323	278	5.3
PUTI	75.0	18.1	2.4	1.4	--	3.1	106	110	96	1.0
RAVAS	71.4	22.2	1.1	2.0	--	3.3	112	405	335	2.0
RAY	75.3	20.9	0.5	1.2	--	2.1	97	214	262	5.3
RIBBON FISH fresh	76.6	18.1	3.2	1.5	--	0.6	104	214	218	13.9

(Contd.)

Table 1 : (Contd.)

All the Values are per 100 gms. of Edible Portion

Name of the Foodstuff	Mois-ture	Protein (N×6.25)	Fat	Mine-rals	Fibre	Carbo hydrates	Energy	Cal-cium	Phos-phorus	Iron
	g	g	g	g	g	g	Kcal.	mg.	mg.	mg.
(1)	(2)	(3)	(4)	(5)	(6)	(7)	(8)	(9)	(10)	(11)
RIBBON FISH dried	6.7	76.1	8.7	--	--	--	383	739	700	4.2
ROHU	76.7	16.6	1.4	0.9	--	4.4	97	650	175	1.0
SARDINE	78.1	21.0	1.9	1.7	--	--	101	90	360	2.5
SARPUTI	70.2	16.5	9.5	1.5	--	2.3	161	220	120	0.5
SHARK	76.0	21.6	0.4	1.2	--	0.8	93	357	262	1.4
SHRIMP (small, dried)	6.0	68.1	8.5	17.4	--	--	349	4384	1160	--
SEER	72.7	22.5	4.0	1.5	--	--	126	71	572	5.4
SILVER BELLY	76.4	19.2	1.6	3.2	--	0	91	715	741	2.2
SINGHALA	61.0	20.9	3.1	1.1	--	13.9	167	93	152	1.8
SINGHI	68.0	22.8	0.6	1.7	--	6.9	124	670	650	2.3
SOLE	78.0	16.2	2.3	1.3	--	2.2	94	140	95	0.5
SOLE (malabar)	78.0	19.5	4.7	3.1	--	--	120	1072	524	0.5
SURMAI fresh	63.0	19.9	1.4	--	--	--	92	92	161	2.0
SURMAI dried	43.3	38.6	6.2	--	--	--	210	148	172	4.4
TAPRA (dried)	12.6	62.3	9.0	15.1	--	1.0	334	771	552	19.3
TAPSI (dried)	16.2	58.5	12.1	17.2	--	--	343	1597	595	41.2
TARTOOR	78.3	18.2	0.2	2.1	--	1.2	79	1072	218	4.9
TENGRA fresh	70.0	19.2	6.4	2.1	--	2.3	144	270	170	2.0

(Contd.)

Table 1 : (Contd.)

All the Values are per 100 gms. of Edible Portion

Name of the Foodstuff	Moisture g	Protein (N×6.25) g	Fat g	Minerals g	Fibre g	Carbo hydrates g	Energy Kcal.	Calcium mg.	Phosphorus mg.	Iron mg.
(1)	(2)	(3)	(4)	(5)	(6)	(7)	(8)	(9)	(10)	(11)
TENGRA dried	13.8	54.9	3.9	27.5	--	--	255	843	400	--
TUNNY	71.9	23.8	1.6	1.8	--	0.9	113	429	349	6.8
WHITE BAIT	79.1	14.5	1.4	2.5	--	2.5	81	643	437	3.8
MEAT AND POULTRY										
BEEF meal	8.2	79.2	10.3	1.6	0.5	0.2	410	68	324	18.8
BEEF muscle	74.3	22.6	2.6	1.0	--	--	114	10	190	0.8
BUFFALO MEAT	78.7	19.4	0.9	1.0	--	--	86	3	189	--
DUCK	72.3	21.6	4.8	1.2	--	0.1	130	4	235	--
EGG, duck	71.0	13.5	13.7	1.0	--	0.8	181	70	260	2.5
EGG, hen	73.7	13.3	13.3	1.0	--	--	173	60	220	2.1
EGG, turtle	76.0	12.2	6.7	1.5	--	3.6	124	93	299	--
FINCH	68.8	26.6	3.0	1.7	--	--	133	90	347	--
FOWL	72.2	25.9	0.6	1.3	--	--	109	25	245	--
GOAT MEAT (lean)	74.2	21.4	3.6	1.1	--	--	118	12	193	--
GREY QUAIL	75.0	21.9	1.7	1.4	--	--	103	22	282	--
LIVER GOAT	76.3	20.0	3.0	1.3	--	--	107	17	279	--
LIVER SHEEP	70.4	19.3	7.5	1.5	--	1.3	150	10	380	6.3
MUTTON, muscle	71.5	18.5	13.3	1.3	--	--	194	150	150	2.5

(Contd.)

Table 1 : (Contd.)

All the Values are per 100 gms. of Edible Portion

Name of the Foodstuff	Moisture g	Protein (N×6.25) g	Fat g	Minerals g	Fibre g	Carbo hydrates g	Energy Kcal.	Calcium mg.	Phosphorus mg.	Iron mg.
(1)	(2)	(3)	(4)	(5)	(6)	(7)	(8)	(9)	(10)	(11)
PIGEON	70.4	23.3	4.9	1.4	--	--	137	12	290	--
PORK, muscle	77.4	18.7	4.4	1.0	--	--	114	30	200	2.2
RUFF AND REEVE	70.3	25.9	2.3	1.5	--	--	124	3	321	--
SNAIL, small	78.9	12.6	1.0	3.8	--	3.7	74	1321	147	--
SNAIL, big	74.1	10.5	0.6	2.4	--	12.4	97	870	116	--
TURTLE'S MEAT	79.4	16.5	1.5	1.1	--	1.5	86	7	162	--
VENISON	75.3	21.0	0.6	1.2	--	1.9	97	3	233	--
MILK AND MILK PRODUCTS										
MILK ass's	89.9	2.1	1.5	--	6.5	48.0	80	--	--	
MILK buffalo's	81.0	4.3	6.5	0.8	--	5.0	117	210	130	0.2
MILK Cow's	87.5	3.2	4.1	0.8	--	4.4	67	120	90	0.2
MILK goat's	86.8	3.3	4.5	0.8	--	4.6	72	170	120	0.3
MULK human	88.0	1.1	3.4	0.1	--	7.4	65	28	11	--
CURDS (cow's milk)	89.1	3.1	4.0	0.8	--	3.0	60	149	93	0.2
BUTTER MILK	97.5	0.8	1.1	0.1	--	0.5	15	30	30	0.1
SKIMMED MILK, liquid	92.1	2.5	0.1	0.7	--	4.6	29	120	90	0.2
CHANNA, cow's milk	57.1	18.3	20.8	2.6	--	1.2	265	208	138	--
CHANNA, buffalo's milk	54.1	13.4	23.0	1.6	--	7.9	292	480	277	--

(Contd.)

Table 1 : (Contd.)

All the Values are per 100 gms. of Edible Portion

Name of the Foodstuff	Moisture g	Protein (N×6.25) g	Fat g	Minerals g	Fibre g	Carbohydrates g	Energy Kcal.	Calcium mg.	Phosphorus mg.	Iron mg.
(1)	(2)	(3)	(4)	(5)	(6)	(7)	(8)	(9)	(10)	(11)
CHEESE	40.3	24.1	25.1	4.2	--	6.3	348	790	520	2.1
KHOA (buffalo's milk)	30.6	14.6	31.2	3.1	--	20.5	421	650	420	5.8
KHOA (Skimmed buffalo milk)	46.1	22.3	1.6	4.3	--	25.7	206	990	650	2.7
KHOA (whole cow milk)	25.2	20.0	25.9	4.0	--	24.9	413	956	613	--
SKIMMED MILK POWDER (cow's milk)	4.1	38.0	0.1	6.8	--	51.0	357	1370	1000	1.4
WHOLE MILK POWDER (cow's milk)	3.5	25.8	26.7	6.0	--	38.0	496	950	730	0.6
FATS AND EDIBLE OILS										
BUTTER	19.0	--	81.0	2.5	--	--	729	--	--	--
GHEE (cow)	--	--	100.0	--	--	--	900	--	--	--
GHEE (buffalo)	--	--	100.0	--	--	--	900	--	--	--
HYDROGENATED OIL (fortified)	--	--	100.0	--	--	--	900	--	--	--
COOKING OIL (Groundnut, Gingelly, Palmolein, Mustard, Coconut, etc.)	--	--	100.0	--	--	--	900	--	--	--

(Contd.)

Table 1 : (Contd.)

All the Values are per 100 gms. of Edible Portion

Name of the Foodstuff	Moisture g	Protein (N×6.25) g	Fat g	Minerals g	Fibre g	Carbohydrates g	Energy Kcal.	Calcium mg.	Phosphorus mg.	Iron mg.
(1)	(2)	(3)	(4)	(5)	(6)	(7)	(8)	(9)	(10)	(11)
SUGARS										
SUGAR CANE	0.4	0.1	0	0.1	--	99.4	398	12	1	0.155
HONEY	20.6	0.3	0	0.2	--	79.5	319	5	16	0.696
JAGGERY (cane)	3.9	0.4	0.1	0.6	--	95.0	383	80	40	2.64
JAGGERY (coconut palm)	10.3	1.0	0.2	5.0	--	83.5	340	1638	62	--
JAGGERY (date palm)	9.6	1.5	0.3	2.6	--	86.1	353	363	62	--
JAGGERY (fan palm)	8.6	1.0	0.1	1.8	--	98.5	359	225	44	--
JAGGERY (sago palm)	9.2	2.3	0.1	3.7	--	84.7	349	1252	372	--
SAGO	12.2	0.2	0.2	0.3	--	87.1	351	10	10	1.3
BEVERAGES (Alcoholic)										
PACHWAI (Assam)	88.2	3.0	1.8	0.6	0.6	5.8	51	12	100	4.5
TODDY, fermented	97.6	0.1	0.3	0.2	--	1.8	38	--	--	--
TODDY, sweet	84.7	0.1	0.3	0.7	--	14.3	59	150	10	0.3
BEVERAGES (non-Alcoholic)										
NEERA	--	0.4	--	0.5	--	10.9	45	0	140	0.1
SUGAR CANE JUICE	90.2	0.1	0.2	0.4	--	9.1	39	10	10	0.1

Table 2 : Vitamin Content : Common Foods (*All the Values are per 100 gms. of Edible Portion*)

Name of the foodstuff	Carotene µg	Thiamine mg	Riboflavin mg	Niacin mg	Total B6 mg	Folic Acid (µg) Free	Folic Acid (µg) Total	Vitamin C mg	Choline
(1)	(2)	(3)	(4)	(5)	(6)	(7)	(8)	(9)	(10)
CEREAL GRAINS AND PRODUCTS									
BAJRA	132	0.33	0.25	2.3	--	14.7	45.5	0	--
BARLEY	10	0.47	0.20	5.4	--	--	--	0	--
ITALIAN MILLET	32	0.59	0.11	3.2	--	4.2	15.0	0	--
JOWAR	47	0.37	0.13	3.1	(0.21)	14.0	20.0	0	--
MAIZE, dry	90	0.42	0.10	1.8	--	14.0	20.0	0	--
MAIZE, tender	32	0.11	0.17	0.6	--	--	--	6	--
PANIVARAGU	0	0.20	0.18	2.3	--	--	--	0	748
RAGI	42	0.42	0.19	1.1	--	5.2	18.3	0	--
RICE, parboiled, hand pounded	9	0.27	0.12	4.0	--	--	--	0	--
RICE, parboiled, milled	--	0.21	0.05	3.8	(0.24)	8.9	11.0	0	--
RICE, raw, hand pounded	2	0.21	0.16	3.9	--	--	--	0	77
RICE, raw, milled	0	0.06	0.06	1.9	--	4.1	8.0	0	--
RICE, bran	--	2.70	0.48	(29.8)	--	--	--	0	--
RICE, flakes	0	0.21	0.05	4.0	--	--	--	0	--
RICE, puffed	0	0.21	0.01	4.1	--	--	--	0	--
SAMAI	0	0.30	0.09	3.2	--	2.2	9.0	0	--
SANWA MILLET	0	(0.33)	(0.10)	4.2	--	--	--	0	--
VARAGU	0	0.33	0.09	2.0	--	7.4	23.1	0	--

(Contd.)

Table 2 : (Contd.)

Name of the foodstuff	Carotene µg	Thiamine mg	Riboflavin mg	Niacin mg	Total B6 mg	Folic Acid (µg)		Vitamin C mg	Choline
						Free	Total		
(1)	(2)	(3)	(4)	(5)	(6)	(7)	(8)	(9)	(10)
WHEAT, bulgar	--	(0.74)	0.11	4.8	--	--	--	0	206
WHEAT, whole	64	0.45	0.17	5.5	(0.57)	142	36.6	0	--
WHEAT, flour (Whole)	29	0.49	0.17	4.3	--	12.1	35.8	0	--
WHEAT, flour (refined)	25	0.12	0.07	2.4	--	--	--	0	--
WHEAT, germ	--	1.40	0.54	2.9	--	--	--	0	--
WHEAT, semolina	--	0.12	0.03	1.6	--	--	--	0	--
WHEAT, vermicelli	0	0.19	0.05	1.8	--	--	--	0	--
WHEAT, bread, (brown)	--	0.21	--	2.5	--	--	--	--	--
WHEAT, bread, (white)	--	0.07	--	0.07	--	--	--	--	--
PULSES AND LEGUMES									
BENGAL GRAM, whole	189	0.30	0.15	2.9	--	34.0	186.0	3	194
BENGAL GRAM, dhal	129	0.48	0.18	2.4	--	32.0	147.5	1	--
BENGAL GRAM, roasted	113	0.20	--	1.3	--	22.0	139.0	0	--
BLACK GRAM, dhal	38	0.42	0.20	2.0	--	24.0	132.0	0	206
COWPEA	12	0.51	0.20	1.3	--	69.0	133.0	0	202
FIELD BEAN, dry	0	0.52	0.16	1.8	--	--	--	0	352
GREEN GRAM, whole	94	0.47	0.27	2.1	--	--	--	0	167
GREEN GRAM, dhal	49	0.47	0.21	2.4	--	24.5	140.0	0	--
HORSE GRAM	71	0.42	0.20	1.5	--	--	--	1	--

(Contd.)

Table 2 : (Contd.)

Name of the foodstuff	Carotene µg	Thiamine mg	Riboflavin mg	Niacin mg	Total B6 mg	Folic Acid (µg) Free	Folic Acid (µg) Total	Vitamin C mg	Choline
(1)	(2)	(3)	(4)	(5)	(6)	(7)	(8)	(9)	(10)
KHESARI, dhal	120	0.39	0.17	2.9	--	--	--	0	--
LENTIL	270	0.45	0.20	2.6	--	14.5	36.0	0	299
MOTH BEANS	9	0.25	0.09	1.5	--	--	--	2	--
PEAS	83	0.25	0.01	0.8	--	--	--	9	20
PEAS, dry	39	0.47	0.19	3.4	--	4.6	7.5	0	235
PEAS, roasted	18	0.47	0.21	3.5	--	--	--	0	--
RED GRAM, dhal	132	0.45	0.19	2.9	(0.54)	19.0	103.0	0	183
RED GRAM, tender	469	0.32	0.33	3.0	--	--	--	25	72
SOYABEAN	426	0.73	0.39	3.2	--	8.65	100.0	--	--
LEAFY VEGETABLES									
AGATHI	5,400	0.21	0.09	1.2	--	--	--	169	--
AMARNATH, tender gangeticus	5,520	0.03	0.30	1.2	--	41.0	149.0	99	31
AMARNATH, stem gangeticus	255	0.01	0.18	0	--	--	--	10	--
AMARNATH, paniculatus	14,190	0.01	0.24	1.1	--	--	--	81	--
AMARNATH, spinosus	3,564	0	--	--	--	--	--	33	--
AMARNATH, viridis	--	--	--	--	--	--	--	179	--
AMBAT CHUKA	3,660	0.03	0.06	0.2	--	40.0	125.0	12	--
BATHUA LEAVES	1,740	0.01	0.14	0.6	--	--	--	35	--
BEET GREENS	5,862	0.26	0.56	3.3	--	--	--	70	--

(Contd.)

Table 2 : (Contd.)

Name of the foodstuff	Carotene μg	Thiamine mg	Riboflavin mg	Niacin mg	Total B6 mg	Folic Acid (μg) Free	Total	Vitamin C mg	Choline
(1)	(2)	(3)	(4)	(5)	(6)	(7)	(8)	(9)	(10)
BETEL LEAVES	5,760	0.07	0.03	0.7	--	--	--	5	--
BRUSSELS SPROUTS	126	0.05	0.16	0.4	--	--	--	72	--
CABBAGE	120	0.06	0.09	0.4	--	13.3	23.0	124	120
CARROT LEAVES	5,70	0.04	0.37	2.1	--	--	--	79	--
CELLERY LEAVES	3,990	0	0.11	1.2	--	--	--	62	--
CELERY STALK	520	0.12	0.05	0.3	--	--	--	6	--
CHEKKUR MANIS	5,706	0.48	0.32	2.6	--	--	--	247	--
COLOCASIA LEAVES (black variety)	12,000	0.06	0.45	1.9	--	--	--	63	--
COLOCASIA LEAVES (green variety)	10,278	0.22	0.26	1.1	--	--	--	12	--
CORIANDER LEAVES	6,918	0.05	0.06	0.8	--	--	--	135	--
COW PEA LEAVES	6,918	0.05	0.18	0.6	--	--	--	4	--
CURRY LEAVES	7,560	0.08	0.21	2.3	--	23.5	93.9	4	--
DRUMSTICK LEAVES	6,780	0.06	0.05	0.8	--	--	--	220	--
FENUGREEK LEAVES	2,340	0.04	0.31	0.8	--	--	--	52	--
FETID CASSIA, fresh	10,152	0.08	0.19	0.8	--	--	--	82	--
GARDEN CRESS	--	0.15	--	--	--	--	--	--	--
GOGU	2,898	0.07	0.39	1.1	--	--	--	20	--

(Contd.)

Table 2 : (Contd.)

Name of the foodstuff	Carotene µg	Thiamine mg	Riboflavin mg	Niacin mg	Total B6 mg	Folic Acid (µg) Free	Folic Acid (µg) Total	Vitamin C mg	Choline
(1)	(2)	(3)	(4)	(5)	(6)	(7)	(8)	(9)	(10)
IPOMOEA LEAVES	1,980	0.05	0.13	0.6	--	--	--	37	--
KNOL-KHOL GREENS	4,146	0.25	--	3	--	--	--	157	--
KUPPAMENI	--	--	--	--	--	--	--	147	--
LETTUCE	990	0.09	0.13	0.50	--	--	--	10	178
MANATHAKKALI LEAVES	--	--	0.59	0.90	--	--	--	11	--
MAYALU	7,440	0.03	0.16	0.5	--	--	--	87	--
MINT	1,620	0.05	0.26	1.0	--	9.7	114.0	27	--
MUKARRATE KEERAI	--	--	--	--	--	--	--	27	--
MUSTARD LEAVES	2,662	0.03	--	--	--	--	--	33	--
NERRINGI	--	--	--	--	--	--	--	41	--
PARSLEY	1,920	0.04	0.18	0.5	--	--	--	281	--
PARUPPU KEERAI	2,292	0.10	0.22	0.7	--	--	--	29	--
PONNANGANNI	1,926	0	0.14	1.2	--	--	--	17	--
RADISH LEAVES	5,295	0.18	0.47	0.8	--	--	--	81	--
TABLE RADISH LEAVES	5,742	0.18	0.35	5.5	--	--	--	106	--
RAPE PLANT LEAVES	1,280	0.01	0.03	0.9	--	--	--	65	--
SAFFLOWER LEAVES	3,540	0.04	0.10	0	--	--	--	15	--
SHEPU	7,182	0.03	0.13	0.20	--	--	--	--	25
SPINACH	5,580	0.03	0.26	0.5	--	51.00	123.0	28	--

(Contd.)

Table 2 : (Contd.)

Name of the foodstuff	Carotene μg	Thiamine mg	Riboflavin mg	Niacin mg	Total B6 mg	Folic Acid (μg)		Vitamin C mg	Choline
						Free	Total		
(1)	(2)	(3)	(4)	(5)	(6)	(7)	(8)	(9)	(10)
TAMARIND LEAVES, tender	250	0.24	0.17	4.1	--	--	--	3	--
TURNIP GREENS	9,396	0.31	0.57	5.4	--	--	--	180	--
ROOTS & TUBERS									
BANANA RHIZOME	16	0	0.03	0.2	--	--	--	1	--
BEET ROOT	0	0.04	0.09	0.4	--	--	--	10	242
CARROT	1,890	0.04	0.02	0.6	--	5.0	15.0	3	168
COLOCASIA	24	0.09	0.03	0.4	--	16.0	54.0	0	--
MANGO GINGER	20	0.01	0.03	0	--	--	--	1	--
ONION, big	0	0.08	0.01	0.4	--	1.5	6.0	11	--
ONION, small	15	0.08	0.02	0.5	--	--	--	2	--
PARSNIP	18	0.06	--	0.4	--	--	--	16	--
POTATO	24	0.10	0.01	1.2	--	3.0	7.0	17	100
RADISH, pink	3	0.06	0.02	0.4	--	--	--	17	--
RADISH, table	4	0.02	0.03	1.4	--	--	--	21	--
RADISH, white	3	0.06	0.02	0.5	--	--	--	15	63
SWEET POTATO	6	0.08	0.04	0.7	--	--	--	24	--
TAPIOCO	--	0.05	0.10	0.3	--	--	--	25	--
TAPIOCA, chips, dried	0	0.23	0.10	1.4	--	--	--	0	--
TURNIP	0	0.04	0.04	0.5	--	--	--	43	137

(Contd.)

Table 2 : (Contd.)

Name of the foodstuff	Carotene µg	Thiamine mg	Riboflavin mg	Niacin mg	Total B6 mg	Folic Acid (µg)		Vitamin C mg	Choline
						Free	Total		
(1)	(2)	(3)	(4)	(5)	(6)	(7)	(8)	(9)	(10)
YAM, elephant	260	0.06	0.07	0.7	--	--	--	0	--
YAM, ordinary	78	0.07	--	0.7	--	0.9	17.5	--	--
YAM, wild	565	0.19	0.47	1.2	--	--	--	1	--
OTHER VEGETABLES									
ASH GUARD	0	0.06	0.01	0.4	--	--	--	1	--
BEANS, scarlet runner	34	0.34	0.19	0	--	--	--	27	--
BITTER GOURD	126	0.07	0.09	0.5	--	--	--	88	--
BITTER GOURD, Small	126	0.07	0.06	0.4	--	--	--	96	--
BOTTLE GOURD	0	0.03	0.01	0.2	--	--	--	0	--
BRINJAL	74	0.04	0.11	0.9	--	5.0	34.0	12	52
BROAD BEANS	9	0.08	--	0.8	--	--	--	12	5
CAULIFLOWER	30	0.04	0.10	1.0	--	--	--	56	127
CHO-CHO-MARROW	0	0	0.04	0.4	--	--	--	4	--
CLUSTER BEANS	198	0.09	0.03	0.6	--	50.0	144.0	49	--
COLOCASIA STEM	104	0.07	0.07	0.1	--	--	--	3	--
COW PEA PODS	564	0.07	0.09	0.9	--	--	--	14	--
CUCUMBER	0	0.03	0	0.2	--	12.6	14.7	7	--
DOUBLE BEANS	--	--	--	--	--	--	--	22	--
DRUM STICK	110	0.05	0.07	0.2	--	--	--	120	--

(Contd.)

Table 2 : (Contd.)

Name of the foodstuff	Carotene μg	Thiamine mg	Riboflavin mg	Niacin mg	Total B6 mg	Folic Acid (μg) Free	Folic Acid (μg) Total	Vitamin C mg	Choline
(1)	(2)	(3)	(4)	(5)	(6)	(7)	(8)	(9)	(10)
FIELD BEANS, tender	187	0.10	0.06	0.7	--	--	--	9	4
FRENCH BEANS	132	0.08	0.06	0.3	--	15.5	45.5	24	--
GHOSALA	120	0.02	0.06	0.4	--	--	--	0	--
GIANT CHILLIES (Capsicum)	427	0.55	0.05	0.1	--	--	--	137	--
JACK, tender	0	0.05	0.04	0.2	--	--	--	14	--
JACK, fruit seed	--	--	--	--	--	--	--	--	52
KANKODA	1620	0.05	0.18	0.6	--	--	--	--	--
KOVAI	156	0.07	0.08	0.7	--	18.0	59.0	15	--
KNOL-KHOL	21	0.05	0.09	0.5	--	--	--	85	--
LADIES FINGERS	52	0.07	0.10	0.6	--	25.3	105.1	13	--
LEEKS	18	0.23	--	--	--	--	--	11	--
LOTUS STEM, dry	0	0.82	1.21	1.9	--	--	--	3	--
MANGO GREEN	90	0.04	0.01	0.2	--	--	--	3	--
ONION STALKS	595	0	0.01	0.3	--	--	--	17	--
PAPAYA GREEN	0	0.01	0.01	0.1	--	--	--	12	--
PARWAR	153	0.05	0.06	0.5	--	--	--	29	--
PINK BEANS	453	0.06	0.02	0.6	--	--	--	12	--
PLANTAIN FLOWER	27	0.05	0.02	0.4	--	--	--	16	--
PLANTAIN, green	30	0.05	0.02	0.3	--	1.6	16.4	24	--

(Contd.)

Table 2 : (Contd.)

Name of the foodstuff	Carotene µg	Thiamine mg	Riboflavin mg	Niacin mg	Total B6 mg	Folic Acid (µg) Free	Folic Acid (µg) Total	Vitamin C mg	Choline
(1)	(2)	(3)	(4)	(5)	(6)	(7)	(8)	(9)	(10)
PLANTAIN, stem	0	0.02	0.01	0.2	--	--	--	7	--
PUMPKIN	50	0.06	0.04	0.5	--	3.0	13.0	2	136
RIDGE GOURD	33	--	0.01	0.2	--	--	--	5	--
SNAKE GOURD	96	0.04	0.06	0.3	--	7.5	15.5	0	--
SUNDAKAI, dry	450	--	--	--	--	--	--	0	--
SWORD BEANS	24	0.08	0.08	0.5	--	--	--	12	--
TINDA, tender	13	0.04	0.08	0.3	--	--	--	18	--
TOMATO, green	192	0.07	0.01	0.4	--	--	--	31	--
VEGETABLE MARROW	--	0.02	0	0.4	--	--	--	18	--
WATER CHEST NUT, fresh	12	0.05	0.07	0.6	--	--	--	9	--
NUTS AND OILSEEDS									
ALMOND	0	0.24	0.57	4.4	--	--	--	0	--
ARECANUT	3	--	--	--	--	--	--	--	--
CASHEWNUT	60	0.63	0.19	1.2	--	--	--	0	--
CHILGOZA	--	0.32	0.30	3.6	--	--	--	0	--
COCONUT, dry	0	0.08	0.01	3.0	--	15.3	16.5	7	--
COCONUT, fresh	0	0.05	0.10	0.8	--	11.7	12.5	1	--
COCONUT, milk	0	0.08	0.04	0.6	--	--	--	3	--
COCONUT, water	0	0.01	0	0.1	--	--	--	2	--

(Contd.)

Table 2 : (Contd.)

Name of the foodstuff	Carotene µg	Thiamine mg	Riboflavin mg	Niacin mg	Total B6 mg	Folic Acid (µg) Free	Folic Acid (µg) Total	Vitamin C mg	Choline
(1)	(2)	(3)	(4)	(5)	(6)	(7)	(8)	(9)	(10)
COCONUT, meal deoiled	0	0.13	0.57	6.0	--	--	--	5	--
GARDEN CRESS SEEDS	27	0.59	0.61	14.3	--	--	--	0	--
GINGELLY SEEDS	60	1.01	0.34	4.4	--	51.0	134.0	0	--
GROUNDNUT	37	0.90	0.13	19.9	--	16.0	20.0	0	224
GROUNDNUT, roasted	0	0.39	0.13	22.1	--	--	--	0	--
LINSEED	30	0.23	0.07	1.0	--	--	--	0	--
MUSTARD SEEDS	162	0.65	0.26	4.0	--	--	--	0	211
NIGER SEEDS	--	0.07	0.97	8.4	--	--	--	0	--
PISTACHIONUT	144	0.67	0.28	2.3	--	--	--	--	--
PIYAL SEEDS	0	0.69	0.53	1.5	--	--	--	5	--
SUNFLOWER SEEDS	0	0.86	0.20	4.5	--	--	--	1	--
WALNUT	6	0.45	0.40	1.0	--	--	--	0	--
CONDIMENTS & SPICES									
ASAFOETIDA	4	0	0.04	0.3	--	--	--	0	--
CARDAMOM	0	0.22	0.17	0.8	--	--	--	0	1550
CHILLIES, dry	345	0.93	0.43	9.5	--	--	--	50	--
CHILLIES, green	175	0.19	0.39	0.9	--	6.0	29.0	111	--
CLOVES, dry	253	0.08	0.13	0	---	--	--	0	--
CLOVES, green	72	--	--	--	--	--	--	--	--

(Contd.)

Table 2 : (Contd.)

Name of the foodstuff	Carotene µg	Thiamine mg	Riboflavin mg	Niacin mg	Total B6 mg	Folic Acid (µg) Free	Folic Acid (µg) Total	Vitamin C mg	Choline
(1)	(2)	(3)	(4)	(5)	(6)	(7)	(8)	(9)	(10)
CORIANDER	942	0.22	0.35	1.1	--	27.4	32.0	0	1077
CUMIN SEEDS	522	0.55	0.36	2.6	--	--	--	3	1065
FENUGREEK SEEDS	96	0.34	0.29	1.1	--	14.5	84.0	0	1161
GARLIC, dry	0	0.06	0.23	0.4	--	--	--	13	--
GINGER, fresh	40	0.06	0.03	0.6	--	--	--	6	--
MACE	3027	0.25	0.42	1.4	--	--	--	0	--
NUTMEG	0	0.33	0.01	1.4	--	--	--	0	--
OMUM	71	0.21	0.28	2.1	--	--	--	--	--
PEPPER, dry	1080	0.09	0.14	1.4	--	--	--	--	--
PEPPER, green	540	0.05	0.04	0.2	--	--	--	1	--
TAMARIND PULP	60	--	0.07	0.7	--	--	--	3	--
TURMERIC	30	0.03	0	2.3	--	10.0	18.0	00	--
FRUITS									
AMBADA	270	0.02	0.02	0.3	--	--	--	21	--
AMLA	9	0.03	0.01	0.2	--	--	--	600	256
APPLE	0	--	--	0	--	--	--	1	321
APRICOT, fresh	2160	0.04	0.13	0.6	--	--	--	6	--
APRICOT, dried	58	0.22	--	2.3	--	--	--	2	--
BAEL FRUIT	55	0.13	0.03	1.1	--	--	--	8	--

(Contd.)

Table 2 :(Contd.)

Name of the foodstuff	Carotene µg	Thiamine mg	Rboflavin mg	Niacin mg	Total B6 mg	Folic Acid (µg)		Vitamin C mg	Choline
						Free	Total		
(1)	(2)	(3)	(4)	(5)	(6)	(7)	(8)	(9)	(10)
BANANA RIPE	78	0.05	0.08	0.5	--	--	-	7	--
BILIMBI	18	0.09	0.04	0.6	--	--	--	32	--
BREAD FRUIT	9	0.04	0.07	--	--	--	--	21	--
BULLOCK'S HEART	67	--	0.07	0.6	--	--	--	5	--
CAPE GOOSEBERRY	1428	0.05	0.02	0.3	--	--	--	49	--
CASHEW FRUIT	23	0.02	0.05	0.4	--	--	--	180	--
CHERRIES, red	0	0.08	0.08	0.3	--	--	--	7	--
CURRANTS, black	21	0.03	0.14	0.4	--	--	--	1	--
DATES, dried	26	0.01	0.02	0.9	--	--	--	3	--
FIGS (Ficus Carcia)	162	0.06	0.05	0.6	--	--	--	5	--
GRAPES, blue variety	3	0.04	0.03	0.2	--	--	--	1	--
GRAPES, pale green variety	0	--	--	0	--	--	--	1	--
GRAPE FRUIT, Marsh's seedless	--	-.12	0.02	0.3	--	--	--	--	--
GRAPE FRUIT, triumph	--	0.12	0.02	0.3	--	--	--	31	--
GUAVA, country	0	0.03	0.03	0.4	--	--	--	212	--
GUAVA, hill	0	0.02	0.02	0.3	--	--	--	15	--
JACK FRUIT	175	0.03	0.13	0.4	--	--	--	7	--
JAMB, safed	--	0.01	0.02	0.2	--	--	--	30	--
JAMBU FRUIT	48	0.03	0.01	0.2	--	--	--	18	7

(Contd.)

Table 2 : (Contd.)

Name of the foodstuff	Carotene µg	Thiamine mg	Rboflavin mg	Niacin mg	Total B6 mg	Folic Acid (µg) Free	Folic Acid (µg) Total	Vitamin C mg	Choline
(1)	(2)	(3)	(4)	(5)	(6)	(7)	(8)	(9)	(10)
KORUKKAPALLI	0	0.22	0.06	1.6	--	--	--	108	--
LAKUCH	254	0.02	0.15	0.3	--	--	--	135	--
LEMON	0	0.02	0.01	0.1	--	--	--	39	--
LEMON SWEET	0	--	0.04	0	--	--	--	45	--
LICHI	0	0.02	0.06	0.4	--	--	--	31	--
LIME	15	0.02	0.03	0.1	--	--	--	63	--
LIME, sweet, malta	0	--	--	0	--	--	--	54	--
LIME, sweet, musambi	0	--	--	0	--	--	--	50	--
LOQUAT	559	--	--	0	--	--	--	0	--
MAHUA	307	--	--	--	--	--	--	40	--
MANGO RIPE	2743	0.08	0.09	0.9	--	--	--	16	--
MELON, musk	169	0.11	0.08	0.3	--	--	--	26	--
MELON, water	0	0.02	0.04	0.1	--	--	--	1	--
MULBERRY	57	0.04	0.13	0.5	--	--	--	12	--
ORANGE	1104	--	--	--	--	--	--	30	--
PALMYRA FRUIT, tender	0	0.01	0.01	0.2	--	--	--	4	--
PAPAYA, ripe	666	0.04	0.25	0.2	--	--	--	57	--
PASSION FRUIT	54	0.07	0.14	1.6	--	--	--	25	--
PASSION FRUIT JUICE	1968	0.01	0.02	0	--	--	--	13	--

(Contd.)

Table 2 :(Contd.)

Name of the foodstuff	Carotene µg	Thiamine mg	Rboflavin mg	Niacin mg	Total B6 mg	Folic Acid (µg) Free	Folic Acid (µg) Total	Vitamin C mg	Choline
(1)	(2)	(3)	(4)	(5)	(6)	(7)	(8)	(9)	(10)
PEACHES	0	0.02	0.03	0.5	--	--	--	6	--
PEARS	28	0.06	0.03	0.2	--	--	--	0	--
PERSIMMON	2268	0.03	0.01	0	--	--	--	33	--
PHALSA	419	--	--	0.3	--	--	--	22	--
PINEAPPLE	18	0.20	0.12	0.1	--	--	--	39	8
PLUM	166	0.04	0.1	0.3	--	--	--	5	--
POMEGRANATE	0	0.06	0.10	0.3	--	--	--	16	--
PUMMELO	120	0.03	0.03	0.2	--	--	--	20	--
QUINCE	--	0.02	0.02	0.2	--	--	--	11	--
RAISINS	2.4	0.07	0.19	0.7	--	--	--	1	--
RASPBERRY	1248	--	--	0.8	--	--	--	30	--
ROSE APPLE	141	0.01	0.05	0.4	--	--	--	3	--
SAPOTA	97	0.02	0.03	0.2	--	--	--	6	--
SEETHAPHAL	0	0.07	0.17	1.3	--	--	--	37	--
STRAWBERRY	18	0.03	0.02	0.2	--	--	--	52	--
TOMATO RIPE	351	0.12	0.06	0.4	--	14.0	30.0	27	--
TOMATILO	48	0.05	0.02	2.1	--	--	--	2	--
TREE TOMATO	324	0.11	0.06	2.1	--	--	--	0	--
WOOD APPLE	61	0.04	0.17	0.8	--	--	--	3	--

(Contd.)

Table 2 :(Contd.)

Name of the foodstuff	Carotene µg	Thiamine mg	Rbofla-vin mg	Niacin mg	Total B6 mg	Folic Acid (µg) Free	Folic Acid (µg) Total	Vitamin C mg	Choline
(1)	(2)	(3)	(4)	(5)	(6)	(7)	(8)	(9)	(10)
ZIZYPHUS	21	0.02	0.05	0.7	--	--	--	76	--
FISHES AND SEA FOODS									
AIR	--	--	--	0.5	--	--	--	11	--
BACHA	--	--	--	0.6	--	--	--	13	--
BAM	--	--	--	0.9	--	--	--	3	438
BELEY	--	--	--	0.3	--	--	--	3	388
BHANGER, fresh	--	--	--	1.8	--	--	--	12	--
BHANGAN BATA	--	--	--	0.6	--	--	--	--	--
BETKI, fresh	--	--	--	0.7	--	--	--	10	349
BHOLE	--	--	--	0.5	--	--	--	14	--
BOAL	--	--	--	1.0	--	--	--	8	108
CAT FISH	--	--	--	2.5	--	--	--	--	--
CHITAL	--	--	--	--	--	--	--	--	943
CRAB (muscle)	780	--	--	3.1	--	--	--	--	--
FOLUI	--	--	--	0.8	--	--	--	6	1018
HILSA	--	--	--	2.8	--	--	--	24	1364
HORSE MACKEREL	--	--	--	2.9	--	--	--	--	--
KALABASU	--	--	--	0.6	--	--	--	11	716
KATLA	--	--	--	0.8	--	--	--	--	611

(Contd.)

Table 2 :(Contd.)

Name of the foodstuff	Carotene µg	Thiamine mg	Rboflavin mg	Niacin mg	Total B6 mg	Folic Acid (µg) Free	Folic Acid (µg) Total	Vitamin C mg	Choline
(1)	(2)	(3)	(4)	(5)	(6)	(7)	(8)	(9)	(10)
KHOYRA, fresh	--	--	--	0.5	--	--	--	--	--
KOI	--	--	--	0.8	--	--	--	32	891
LATA	--	--	--	1.0	--	--	--	0	--
MAGUR	--	--	--	--	--	--	--	--	639
MRIGAL	--	--	--	0.7	--	9.7	16.7	--	480
MULLET	--	--	--	2.6	--	--	--	--	--
PABDA	--	--	--	--	--	--	--	--	1018
PANGAS	--	--	--	0.6	--	--	--	7	913
PARSEY, fresh	--	--	--	0.8	--	--	--	6	--
POMFRETS, white	--	--	0.15	2.6	--	--	--	--	--
PRAWN	0	0.01	0.10	4.8	--	--	--	--	542
PUTI	--	--	--	0.3	--	--	--	15	393
RIBBON FISH, fresh	--	--	--	2.1	--	--	--	--	--
ROHU	--	0.05	0.07	0.7	--	--	--	22	819
SARADINE	--	--	–2.6	--	--	--	--	--	
SARPUTI	--	--	--	--	--	--	--	14	--
SHARK	--	--	--	2.5	--	--	--	--	--
SHRIMP (small, dried)	--	--	--	--	--	15.7	18.6	--	--
SEER	--	--	--	1.2	--	--	--	--	--

(Contd.)

Table 2 :(Contd.)

Name of the foodstuff	Carotene µg	Thiamine mg	Rboflavin mg	Niacin mg	Total B6 mg	Folic Acid (µg) Free	Total	Vitamin C mg	Choline
(1)	(2)	(3)	(4)	(5)	(6)	(7)	(8)	(9)	(10)
SOLE	--	--	--	0.5	--	--	--	9	572
TENGRA, fresh	--	--	--	--	--	--	--	18	783
WHITE BAIT	--	--	--	2.3	--	--	--	--	--
MEAT AND POULTRY									
BEEF, meal	0	0.03	0.44	5.8	--	--	--	0	--
BEEF, muscle (lean meat)	0_a	0.15	0.04	6.4	--	--	--	2	--
BUFFALO MEAT	--	--	--	--	--	4.6	7.8	--	--
EGG, duck	54_b	0.12	0.26	0.2	--	80.0	80.0	--	--
EGG, hen	600_b	0.10	0.40	0.1	--	70.3	78.3	0	--
FOWL	--	--	0.14	--	--	3.2	6.8	--	--
GOAT MEAT	--	--	--	--	--	0.5	4.5	--	--
LIVER GOAT	--	--	--	--	--	61.2	176.2	--	--
LIVER SHEEP	0_C	0.36	1.70	17.6	--	65.5	188.0	20	--
MUTTON	0_D	0.18	0.14	6.8	--	1.0	5.8	--	--
PORK	0	0.54	0.09	2.8	--	--	--	2.	--
MILK AND MILK PRODUCTS §									
MILK, ass's	--	0.06	0.03	0.1	--	--	--10	--	
MILK, buffalo's	160	0.04	0.10	0.1	--	3.3	5.6	1	--
MILK, cow's	174#	0.05	0.19	0.1	--	5.6	8.5	2	--

(Contd.)

Table 2 :(Contd.)

Name of the foodstuff	Carotene µg	Thiamine mg	Rboflavin mg	Niacin mg	Total B6 mg	Folic Acid (µg) Free	Total	Vitamin C mg	Choline
(1)	(2)	(3)	(4)	(5)	(6)	(7)	(8)	(9)	(10)
MILK, goat's	182	0.05	0.04	0.3	--	0.7	1.3	1	--
MILK, human	137	0.02	0.02	--	--	1.3	--	3	--
CURDS, (cow's milk)	102	0.05	0.16	0.1	--	3.3	12.5	1	--
SKIMMED MILK, liquid	--	--	--	0.1	--	--	--	1	--
CHANNA, cow's milk	366	0.07	0.02	--	--	--	--	3	--
CHEESE	273	--	--	--	--	--	--	--	--
KHOA (whole cow's milk)	497	0.23	0.41	0.4	--	--	--	6	--
SKIMMED MILK POWDER (cow's milk)	0	0.45	1.64	1.0	--	--	--	5	--
WHOLE MILK POWDER (cow's milk)	1400	0.31	1.36	0.8	--	--	--	4	--
FATS AND EDIBLE OILS									
BUTTER	3200	--	--	--	--	--	--	--	--
GHEE (cow)	2000	--	--	--	--	--	--	--	--
GHEE (buffalo)	900	--	--	--	--	--	--	--	--
HYDROGENATED OIL (fortified)	2500	--	--	--	--	--	--	--	--

a) Contains also 18 µg of Vit. A.
b) Both contain 360 µg of Vit. A.
c) Contains also 6690 µg of Vit. A.
d) Contains also 9 µg of Vit. A.
§ These values represent I. U. of Vitamin "A"
\# Cow's milk contains in addition 6.0 µg carotene

Table 3 : Mineral and Trace Elements : Common Foods

Name of the Foodstuff	Mg.	Sod.	Pot.	Cu.	Mn.	Mo.	Zn.	Cr.	S.	Cl.
(1)	(2)	(3)	(4)	(5)	(6)	(7)	(8)	(9)	(10)	(11)
CEREAL GRAINS AND PRODUCTS										
BAJRA	137	10.9	307	1.06	1.15	0.069	3.1	0.023	147	39
BARLEY	21	--	--	1.19	1.03	--	1.2	0.016	130	91
ITALIAN MILLET	81	4.6	250	1.40	0.60	0.070	2.4	0.030	171	37
JOWAR	171	7.3	131	0.46	0.78	0.039	1.6	0.008	54	44
MAIZE, dry	139	15.9	286	0.41	0.48	0.038	2.8	0.004	114	33
MAIZE, tender	40	51.7	151	--	--	--	--	--	61	34
PANIVARAGU	153	8.2	113	1.60	0.60	--	1.4	0.020	157	19
RAGI	137	11.0	408	0.47	5.49	0.102	2.3	0.028	160	44
RICE, paraboiled hand pounded	157	--	--	0.24	1.10	0.078	1.4	0.009	--	--
RICE, paraboiled milled 5%	91	--	--	0.17	0.80	0.068	1.4	0.006	--	--
RICE, parboiled milled 10%	61	--	--	0.17	0.66	0.054	1.3	0.005	--	--
RICE, milled 5%	90	--	--	0.14	0.59	0.058	1.4	0.004	--	--
RICE, milled 10%	64	--	--	0.07	0.51	0.045	1.3	0.003	--	--
RICE, flakes	101	10.9	154	0.37	--	--	--	--	105	17
SAMAI	133	8.1	129	1.00	0.68	0.016	3.7	0.180	149	13
SANWA MILLET	82	--	--	0.60	0.96	--	3.0	0.090	--	--
VARAGU	147	4.6	144	1.60	1.10	--	0.7	0.020	136	11
WHEAT, bulgar (parboiled)	144	4.5	260	0.56	--	--	--	--	143	22
WHEAT, whole	138	17.1	284	0.68	2.29	0.051	2.7	0.012	128	47

(Contd.)

Table 3: Contd.

Name of the Foodstuff	Mg.	Sod.	Pot.	Cu.	Mn.	Mo.	Zn.	Cr.	S.	Cl.
(1)	(2)	(3)	(4)	(5)	(6)	(7)	(8)	(9)	(10)	(11)
WHEAT, flour (whole)	132	20.0	315	0.51	2.29	0.039	2.2	0.006	122	29
WHEAT, flour (refined)	54	9.3	130	0.21	0.62	0.011	0.6	0.001	115	47
WHEAT, semolina	--	21.0	83	--	--	--	--	--	--	--
WHEAT, vermicelli	42	7.9	138	0.29	--	--	--	--	145	46
PULSES AND LEGUMES										
BENGAL GRAM, whole (desi)	119	37.3	808	1.18	1.21	0.154	6.1	0.008	179	58
BENGAL GRAM, whole (kabuli)	169	--	--	1.01	0.74	--	2.9	0.032	--	--
BENGAL GRAM, dhal	130	73.2	720	1.34	1.05	0.195	1.7	0.001	160	39
BLACK GRAM, whole	154	--	--	1.05	1.01	0.810	3.3	0.012	--	--
BLACK GRAM, dhal	130	39.8	800	0.93	0.96	0.425	3.0	0.012	174	9
COW PEA	210	23.2	1131	0.87	1.34	1.890	4.6	0.029	165	10
GREEN GRAM, whole	127	28.0	843	0.39	2.47	0.304	3.0	0.014	188	12
GREEN GRAM, dhal	122	27.2	1150	0.39	1.02	0.446	2.8	0.010	214	25
HORSE GRAM	156	11.5	762	1.81	1.57	0.749	2.8	0.024	181	8
KHESARI, dhal	92	37.7	644	0.77	--	--	--	--	144	36
LENTIL, whole	80	40.1	629	1.87	1.04	0.171	2.8	0.024	104	19
LENTIL, dhal	74	--	--	1.37	0.81	--	3.1	0.20	--	--
MOTH BEANS	225	29.5	1096	0.85	--	--	--	--	180	9
PEAS, green	34	7.8	79	0.23	--	--	--	--	95	20
PEAS, dry	100	20.4	725	1.29	0.58	0.638	2.3	0.032	189	59

(Contd.)

Table 3: Contd.

Name of the Foodstuff	Mg.	Sod.	Pot.	Cu.	Mn.	Mo.	Zn.	Cr.	S.	Cl.
(1)	(2)	(3)	(4)	(5)	(6)	(7)	(8)	(9)	(10)	(11)
PEAS, roasted	122	14.7	750	1.32	--	--	--	--	200	73
RAJMAH	184	--	--	1.45	1.60	--	4.5	0.029	--	--
RED GRAM, whole	86	--	--	1.23	0.96	0.222	3.1	0.010	--	--
RED GRAM, tender	58	93.0	463	0.40	--	--	--	--	494	22
SOYA BEAN (black)	238	--	--	1.38	2.35	--	4.4	0.029	--	--
SOYA BEAN (white)	175	--	--	1.12	2.11	--	3.4	0.028	--	--
LEAFY VEGETABLES										
AMARANTHUS, Gangeticus	122	230.0	341	0.08	0.36	0.130	0.18	0.007	61	88
AMBAT CHUKA	123	--	--	0.04	0.40	--	0.27	0.006	--	--
BETAL LEAVES	447	--	--	2.32	4.47	--	3.44	0.137	--	--
BRUSSELS SPROUTS	26	7.9	477	0.07	--	--	--	--	212	22
CABBAGE	31	--	--	0.02	0.18	0.078	0.30	0.005	--	--
CELERY LEAVES	52	35.5	210	0.30	--	--	--	--	102	19
COLOCASIA LEAVES	32	--	--	0.18	--	--	--	0.011	--	72
CORIANDER LEAVES	31	58.3	256	0.14	0.50	1.120	0.32	0.014	49	43
CURRY LEAVES	44	--	--	0.10	0.15	--	0.20	0.006	81	198
DRUM STICK LEAVES	42	--	259	0.07	0.37	--	0.16	0.010	137	423
FENUGREEK LEAVES	33	76.1	31	0.10	0.23	0.400	0.36	0.006	167	165
GOGU	66	--	--	0.08	0.30	--	0.27	0.005	60	19
LETTUCE	30	58.0	33	0.08	--	--	--	--	27	23
MINT	60	--	--	0.18	0.57	--	0.44	0.008	84	34

(Contd.)

Table 3: Contd.

Name of the Foodstuff	Mg.	Sod.	Pot.	Cu.	Mn.	Mo.	Zn.	Cr.	S.	Cl.
(1)	(2)	(3)	(4)	(5)	(6)	(7)	(8)	(9)	(10)	(11)
PARUPPU KEERAI	120	67.2	716	0.19	--	--	--	--	63	73
PONNANGANNI	46	--	--	0.19	0.46	--	--	--	13	--
RADISH LEAVES	22	--	-	0.02	0.01	--	0.08	0.002	--	--
SAFFLOWER LEAVES	51	126.4	181	0.22	--	--	--	--	--	235
SPINACH	64	58.5	206	0.10	0.56	0.010	0.30	0.005	30	54
TAMARIND LEAVES, tender	26	--	--	0.02	0.12	--	0.26	0.009	63	94
ROOTS AND TUBERS										
ARROW ROOT flour	--	30.0	20	--	--	--	--	--	--	--
BEET ROOT	9	59.8	43	0.29	0.19	--	0.91	0.012	14	24
CARROT	17	35.6	108	0.10	0.16	--	0.36	0.017	27	13
COLOCASIA	28	9.0	550	0.18	0.28	--	0.31	0.005	--	--
ONION, (big)	16	4.0	127	0.18	0.18	0.030	0.41	0.009	--	--
POTATO	30	11.0	247	0.16	0.13	0.070	0.53	0.007	37	16
RADISH, pink	196	63.5	10	0.07	0.15	--	0.68	0.009	--	--
RADISH, white	--	33.0	138	0.40	--	--	--	--	--	--
SWEET POTATO	27	9.0	393	0.02	0.22	--	0.11	0.006	--	--
TAPIOCA, chips dried	66	7.5	764	0.15	--	--	--	--	58	10
YAM, ordinary	17	9.0	237	0.12	0.12	--	0.45	0.016	--	--
YAM, wild	34	11.0	450	0.16	--	--	--	--	35	29
OTHER VEGETABLES										
BITTER GOURD (white)	36	17.8	152	0.10	0.08	--	0.46	0.005	15	8

(Contd.)

Table 3: Contd.

Name of the Foodstuff	Mg.	Sod.	Pot.	Cu.	Mn.	Mo.	Zn.	Cr.	S.	Cl.
(1)	(2)	(3)	(4)	(5)	(6)	(7)	(8)	(9)	(10)	(11)
BITTER GOURD (green)	33	17.8	152	0.10	0.08	--	0.46	0.005	15	8
BOTTLE GOURD	26	1.8	87	0.03	0.06	--	0.22	0.046	10	5
BRINJAL	15	3.0	200	0.12	0.13	--	0.22	0.007	44	52
BROAD BEANS	33	43.5	39	0.17	--	--	--	--	53	43
CAULIFLOWER	18	53.0	138	0.13	0.10	--	0.40	0.003	231	34
CLUSTER BEANS	47	--	--	0.08	0.10	--	0.36	0.004	--	--
CUCUMBER	14	10.2	50	0.09	0.14	0.070	0.23	0.002	17	15
DRUM STICK	28	--	259	0.01	0.05	--	0.16	0.003	137	423
FIELD BEANS, tender	17	55.4	74	0.10	0.12	--	0.40	0.004	40	31
FRENCH BEANS	38	4.3	120	0.06	0.12	0.020	0.42	0.006	37	10
GIANT CHILLES	12	--	--	0.12	0.06	--	0.13	0.006	--	--
JACK, tender	--	35.0	328	--	--	--	--	--	--	--
JACK FRUIT, seeds	54	63.2	246	0.19	--	--	--	--	356	14
KOVAI	36	--	--	0.07	0.22	--	0.26	0.004	--	--
KNOL-KHOL	33	112.0	37	0.05	0.11	--	0.24	0.019	143	67
LADIES FINGERS	53	6.9	103	0.11	0.15	--	0.42	0.005	30	41
LOTUS STEM, dry	168	438.0	3007	1.22	--	--	--	--	258	444
MANGO, green	16	43.0	83	0.03	0.07	--	0.07	0.050	15	2
ONION STALKS	104	2.2	109	0.45	0.74	--	2.29	0.039	33	7
PAPAYA, green	--	23.0	216	--	--	--	--	--	--	--
PARWAR	9	2.6	83	1.11	--	--	--	--	17	4

(Contd.)

Table 3: Contd.

Name of the Foodstuff	Mg.	Sod.	Pot.	Cu.	Mn.	Mo.	Zn.	Cr.	S.	Cl.
(1)	(2)	(3)	(4)	(5)	(6)	(7)	(8)	(9)	(10)	(11)
PINK BEANS	--	32.2	117	0.13	--	--	--	--	182	47
PLANTAIN, flower	54	20.1	185	0.10	--	--	--	--	68	68
PLANTAIN, green	13	15.0	193	0.03	0.30	--	0.05	0.004	15	6
PUMPKIN, fruit	38	5.6	139	0.05	0.05	--	0.26	0.005	16	4
RIDGE GOURD	32	2.9	50	0.08	0.07	--	0.38	0.003	14	7
SNAKE GOURD	28	25.4	34	0.27	0.14	--	0.31	0.004	35	21
SWORD BEANS	--	29.0	1800	--	--	--	--	--	--	--
TINDA, tender	14	35.0	24	0.12	--	--	--	--	--	44
TOMATO, green	15	45.8	114	0.19	--	--	--	--	24	38
VEGETABLE MARROW	13	27.3	94	0.22	--	--	--	--	11	9
WATER CHEST NUT, fresh	72	--	--	1.31	0.85	--	1.56	0.011	-	--
NUTS AND OIL SEEDS										
ALMOND	373	--	--	0.97	1.88	--	3.57	0.161	--	--
ARECANUT (raw)	66	--	--	0.92	1.46	--	0.81	0.473	--	--
ARECANUT (processed)	83	--	--	2.54	2.83	--	1.30	0.386	--	--
CASHEW NUT	349	--	--	1.66	1.42	--	5.99	0.163	--	--
COCONUT, dry	--	--	--	1.00	6.24	0.021	5.00	--	--	--
COCONUT, meal deoiled	355	72.5	2003	--	--	--	--	--	431	374
GARDEN CRESS SEEDS	430	--	--	--	--	--	--	--	1	41
GINGELLY SEEDS	--	--	--	2.29	1.32	0.204	12.20	0.087	--	--
GROUNDNUT	--	--	--	0.90	1.10	0.166	3.90	0.048	--	--

(Contd.)

Table 3: Conta.

Name of the Foodstuff	Mg.	Sod.	Pot.	Cu.	Mn.	Mo.	Zn.	Cr.	S.	Cl.
(1)	(2)	(3)	(4)	(5)	(6)	(7)	(8)	(9)	(10)	(11)
MUSTARD SEEDS	--	--	--	0.83	2.56	0.089	4.80	0.063	--	--
PIYAL SEEDS	373	10.2	436	0.86	--	--	--	--	186	25
SAFFLOWER SEEDS	--	--	--	1.58	1.10	0.054	5.20	0.045	--	--
WALNUT	302	--	--	1.67	2.62	--	2.32	0.101	--	--
CONDIMENTS AND SPICES										
ASAFOETIDA	80	--	--	0.43	1.12	--	0.83	0.079	--	--
CARDAMOM	173	--	--	0.47	8.92	--	2.81	0.031	--	--
CHILLIES, dry	--	14.0	530	--	--	--	--	--	--	--
CHILLIES, green	272	--	--	1.40	1.38	0.070	1.78	0.040	--	--
CLOVES, dry	130	--	--	1.01	4.75	--	1.47	0.056	--	--
CORIANDER SEEDS	239	32.0	990	1.01	1.67	--	3.26	0.050	--	--
CUMIN SEEDS	475	126.0	980	0.71	1.02	--	2.66	--	--	--
FENUGREEK SEEDS	124	19.0	530	0.71	1.03	--	3.08	0.064	--	--
GARLIC, dry	71	--	--	0.63	0.86	--	1.93	0.020	--	--
GINGER, fresh	405	--	--	0.74	5.56	--	1.93	0.057	--	--
GINGER, dry (sonti)	187	--	--	0.33	12.91	--	0.82	0.144	--	--
MACE	213	--	--	1.56	1.54	--	1.26	0.039	--	--
NUT MEG, fruit	229	--	--	0.71	1.78	--	1.22	0.234	--	--
OMUM	141	--	--	0.96	3.40	--	4.52	0.057	--	--
PEPPER, dry (black)	171	--	--	1.42	4.14	--	1.31	0.074	--	--
POPPY SEEDS (khas khas)	257	--	--	0.63	4.31	--	4.34	0.108	--	--

(Contd.)

Table 3: Contd.

Name of the Foodstuff	Mg.	Sod.	Pot.	Cu.	Mn.	Mo.	Zn.	Cr.	S.	Cl.
(1)	(2)	(3)	(4)	(5)	(6)	(7)	(8)	(9)	(10)	(11)
TAMARIND PULP	41	--	--	0.20	0.55	--	--	0.056	--	--
TURMERIC	278	--	--	0.39	8.38	--	2.72	0.069	--	--
FRUITS										
AMLA	--	5.0	225	--	--	--	--	--	--	--
APPLE	7	28.0	75	0.10	0.14	--	0.06	0.008	7	1
APRICOTS, fresh	--	--	430	0.11	--	--	--	--	--	--
BAEL FRUIT	--	--	600	0.21	--	--	--	--	--	--
BANANA, ripe	41	36.6	88	0.16	0.20	--	0.15	0.004	7	8
BILIMBI	--	--	130	0.05	--	--	--	--	--	--
CAPE GOOSBERRY	31	0.9	320	0.19	--	--	--	--	43	12
CHERRIES, red	27	--	320	0.08	0.08	--	0.33	0.005	--	--
DATES, fresh	12	--	--	0.05	0.03	--	0.03	0.004	--	--
GRAPES, pale green variety	82	--	--	0.20	0.11	--	0.10	0.007	--	--
GUAVA, country	24	5.5	91	0.14	0.14	--	0.16	0.009	14	4
JACK FRUIT, ripe	24	--	--	0.12	0.06	--	0.07	0.013	69	9
JAMBU FRUIT	39	26.2	55	0.07	0.15	--	0.16	0.005	13	8
KORUKKEPALLI	40	37	377	0.60	--	--	--	--	109	51
LEMON	19	--	270	0.06	0.07	--	0.07	0.007	--	--
LEMON SWEET	--	--	210	0.11	--	--	--	--	--	--
LICHI	10	124.9	159	0.30	--	--	--	--	19	3
LIME sweet, malta	--	--	170	0.51	--	--	--	--	--	--

(Contd.)

Table 3: Contd.

Name of the Foodstuff	Mg.	Sod.	Pot.	Cu.	Mn.	Mo.	Zn.	Cr.	S.	Cl.
(1)	(2)	(3)	(4)	(5)	(6)	(7)	(8)	(9)	(10)	(11)
LIME sweet, mosambi	--	--	490	0.17	--	--	--	--	--	--
LOQUAT	--	--	390	0.13	--	--	--	--	--	--
MANGO, ripe	270	26.0	205	0.11	0.13	--	0.27	0.006	17	3
MELON, musk	31	104.6	341	0.03	--	--	--	--	32	80
MELON, water	13	27.3	160	0.05	--	--	--	--	42	21
ORANGE	9	4.5	9.3	0.58	--	--	--	--	7	5
PAPAYA, ripe	11	6.0	69	0.20	--	--	--	--	13	11
PEACHES	21	2.0	453	0.06	--	--	--	--	26	0
PEARS	7	6.1	96	0.40	--	--	--	--	14	1
PHALSA	72	4.4	351	0.12	--	--	--	--	13	86
PINE APPLE	33	34.7	37	0.13	--	--	--	--	33	0
PLUMS	147	0.8	247	0.13	--	--	--	--	33	0
POMEGRANATE	44	0.9	133	0.34	0.77	--	0.82	0.022	12	2
ROSE APPLE	4	34.1	50	0.01	--	--	--	--	13	4
SAPOTA	25	5.9	269	0.08	0.68	--	0.16	0.008	17	26
SEETHAPHAL	84	--	--	0.43	0.64	--	0.80	0.026	--	--
TOMATO, ripe	--	12.9	146	0.19	0.26	--	0.41	0.015	11	6
TOMATILLO.	23	0.4	243	0.09	--	--	--	--	27	14
TREE TOMATO	34	1.7	539	0.17	--	--	--	--	37	10
WOOD APPLE	41	--	--	0.21	0.18	--	0.46	0.006	--	--
ZIZYPHUS	13	--	--	0.12	0.17	--	0.10	0.007	--	--

(Contd.)

Table 3: Contd.

Name of the Foodstuff	Mg.	Sod.	Pot.	Cu.	Mn.	Mo.	Zn.	Cr.	S.	Cl.
(1)	(2)	(3)	(4)	(5)	(6)	(7)	(8)	(9)	(10)	(11)
FISHES AND OTHER SEA FOODS										
AIR	--	--	--	0.06	--	--	--	--	--	--
BACHA	--	--	--	0.11	--	--	--	--	--	--
BAMI	--	--	--	0.06	--	--	--	--	--	--
BATA, small varieties	--	--	--	0.17	--	--	--	--	--	--
BHEKTI	--	66.0	173	0.11	--	--	--	--	--	--
BHOLA	--	--	--	0.05	--	--	--	--	--	--
CHELA, dried	--	--	--	0.08	--	--	--	--	--	--
CHINGRI, goda dried	--	--	--	1.40	--	--	--	--	--	--
CHITAI	--	34.0	119	0.17	--	--	--	--	--	--
HILSA	--	52.0	183	0.14	--	--	--	--	--	--
KATLA	--	50.0	151	0.12	--	--	--	--	--	--
KHORSULA	--	--	--	0.13	--	--	--	--	--	--
KOI	--	64.0	195	0.16	--	--	--	--	--	30
MAGUR	--	58.0	147	--	--	--	--	--	--	--
MAHASOLE	--	--	--	0.12	--	--	--	--	--	--
MRIGAL	--	--	--	0.12	--	--	--	--	--	--
PABDA	--	--	--	0.09	--	--	--	--	--	--
PANGAS	--	--	--	0.05	--	--	--	--	--	--
PARSEY, fresh	--	--	--	0.14	--	--	--	--	--	--
PRAWN	--	66.0	262	--	--	--	--	--	--	--

(Contd.)

Table 3: Contd.

Name of the Foodstuff	Mg.	Sod.	Pot.	Cu.	Mn.	Mo.	Zn.	Cr.	S.	Cl.
(1)	(2)	(3)	(4)	(5)	(6)	(7)	(8)	(9)	(10)	(11)
ROHU	13	101.0	288	0.13	--	--	--	--	103	3
SARPUTI	--	--	--	0.08	--	--	--	--	--	--
SINGHI	--	53.0	223	0.15	--	--	--	--	--	--
SOLE	--	--	--	0.11	--	--	--	--	--	--
TAPRA, dried	--	--	--	0.71	--	--	--	--	--	--
TAPSI, dried	--	--	--	1.20	--	--	--	--	--	--
TENGRA, dried	--	--	--	0.58	--	--	--	--	--	--
MEAT AND POULTRY										
BEEF MUSCLE	--	52.0	214	--	--	--	--	--	--	--
LIVER GOAT	--	73.0	160	--	--	--	--	--	--	--
MUTTON, muscle	--	33.0	270	--	--	--	--	--	--	--
MILK AND OTHER PRODUCTS										
MILK buffalo's	--	19.0	90	--	--	--	--	--	--	--
MILK, cow's	--	73.0	140	--	--	--	--	--	--	--
MILK, goat's	--	11.0	110	--	--	--	--	--	--	--
CURD (cow's milk)	--	32.0	130	--	--	--	--	--	--	--
BEVERAGES (ALCOHOLIC)										
PACHWAI (Assam)	51	--	110	--	--	--	--	--	25	-

Table 4 : Oxalic Acid, Phytin Phosphorus and Dietary Fibre in Foods

Name of the foodstuff	Oxalic acid mg/100 gms.	Phytin P mg/100 gms.	Phytin P as percent of total P	Total Dietary Fibre
(1)	(2)	(3)	(4)	(5)
CEREAL GRAINS AND PRODUCTS				
BAJRA	21	141	48	--
BARLETY	2	101	47	--
ITALIAN MILLET	0	198	68	24.71
JOWAR	10	172	77	12.69
MAIZE, dry	6	306	85	--
MAIZE, tender	9	66	5	--
PANIVARAGU	0	83	40	30.48
RAGI	0	209	74	19.08
RICE, parboiled, milled	1	83	58	--
RICE, raw, milled	3	83	52	--
RICE, flakes	0	151	63	--
RICE, puffed	0	47	31	--
SAMAI, (whole)	0	57	26	38.93
VARAGU, (whole)	0	135	72	37.76
WHEAT, bulgar	7	198	67	--
WHEAT, whole	8	238	80	11.40
WHEAT, flour (refined)	0	38	81	--
WHEAT, vermicelli	0	19	21	--
PULSES AND LEGUMES				
BENGAL GRAM, (whole)	2	158	51	--
BENGAL GRAM, dhal	5	133	40	--
BENGAL GRAM, roasted, dehusked	3	159	47	--
BLACK GRAM, (whole)	--	--	--	16.54
BLACK GRAM, dhal	16	169	43	--
COW PEA	9	185	45	--
FIELD BEAN, dry	--	248	57	--
GREEN GRAM, whole	3.	148	46	9.75
GREEN GRAM, dhal	1	209	52	--
HORSE GRAM,	417	114	37	--
KHESARI dhal	122	108	31	10.44
LENTIL	14	100	34	--
MOTH BEANS	0	25	11	--
PEAS	14	55	40	--
PEAS, dry	0	135	45	--

(Contd.

Table 4 : Contd..

Name of the foodstuff	Oxalic acid (mg/100 gms.)	Phytin P (mg/100 gms.)	Phytin P as percent of total P	Total Dietary Fibre
(1)	(2)	(3)	(4)	(5)
PEAS roasted	0	136	40	--
RED GRAM, dhal	9	170	56	--
RED GRAM, whole	--	--	--	10.26
RED GRAM, tender	16	--	--	--
LEAFY VEGETABLES				
AMARANTH, tender	772	2	3	--
BRUSSELS SPROUTS	4	5	6	--
CABBAGE	3	3	7	--
CELERY LEAVES	37	6	4	--
COLOCASIA LEAVES (green variety)	43	0	0	--
CORIANDER LEAVES	47	0	0	--
CURRY LEAVES	132	35	61	--
DRUMSTICK LEAVES	101	44	·63	--
FENUGREEK LEAVES	13	0	0	--
GOGU	148	--	--	--
MINT	33	4	6	--
PARSLEY	--	16	9	--
PARUPPU KEERAI	1,679	4	9	--
SAFFLOWER LEAVES	3	--	--	--
SPINACH	658	0	0	--
SPINACH STALK	1	--	--	--
TAMARIND LEAVES tender	196	0	0	--
ROOTS AND TUBERS				
BEET ROOT	40	0	0	--
CARROT	5	0	0	--
ONION, big	1	--	--	--
ONION, small	1	--	--	--
PARSNIP	20	4	10	--
POTATO	20	14	35	10.16
RADISH, pink	20	13	65	--
RADISH, white	9	0	0	--
SWEET POTATO	--	--	--	13.04
TAPIOCA	17	--	--	--

(Contd

Table 4 : Contd..

Name of the foodstuff	Oxalic acid	Phytin P	Phytin P as percent of total P	Total Dietary Fibre
	mg/100 gms.			
(1)	(2)	(3)	(4)	(5)
TAPIOCA CHIPS, dried	31	17	24	--
YAM, (elephant)	--	4	12	--
YAM, wild	15	7	9	--
OTHER VEGETABLES				
BITTER GOURD	0	4	6	--
BITTER GOURD, small variety	0	26	19	--
BRINJAL	18	3	6	--
BROAD BEANS	1	--	--	--
CAULIFLOWER	19	10	18	--
CLUSTER BEANS	--	3	6	--
CUCUMBER	15	0	0	--
DOUBLE BEANS	--	8	5	--
DRUM STICK	101	44	40	--
FIELD BEANS, tender	1	--	--	--
FRENCH BEANS	33	0	0	--
JACK FRUIT seeds	4	40	42	--
KNOL-KHOL	10	0	0	--
LADIES FINGERS	8	0	0	--
LOTUS STEM, dry	422	0	0	--
MANGO, green	6	5	26	--
ONION STALKS	14	19	38	--
PARWAR	7	8	20	--
PINK BEANS	--	38	54	--
PLANTAIN FLOWER	420	--	--	--
PLANTAIN GREEN	480	11	37	--
RIDGE GOURD	27	11	28	--
SNAKE GOURD	34	0	0	--
TINDA, tender	2	--	--	--
TOMATO, green	2	0	0	--
VEGETABLE MARROW	56	--	--	--
NUTS AND OIL SEEDS				
ALMOND	407	--	--	--
CASHEWNUT	318	--	--	--

(Contd

Table 4 : Contd..

Name of the foodstuff	Oxalic acid (mg/100 gms.)	Phytin P (mg/100 gms.)	Phytin P as percent of total P	Total Dietary Fibre
(1)	(2)	(3)	(4)	(5)
COCONUT MEAL DEOILED	--	285	44	--
GARDEN CRESS SEEDS	149	442	61	--
GINGELLY SEEDS	1,700	--	--	--
PIYAL SEEDS	2	158	30	--
SAFFLOWER CAKE (defatted)	--	--	--	24.80
CONDIMENTS AND SPICES				
ARISITHIPPILI	--	56	17	--
CHILLIES, dry	--	71	19	--
CHILLIES, green	67	7	9	--
CORIANDER	--	320	81	--
CUMIN SEEDS	--	153	30	--
FENUGREEK SEEDS	--	151	41	--
OMUM	--	296	67	--
PEPPER, dry	--	115	58	--
TURMERIC	--	97	34	--
FRUITS				
AMLA	296	--	--	--
APPLE	10	0	0	--
BANANA RIPE	--	4	10	--
CAPE GOOSEBERRY	1	18	27	--
GUAVA, country	14	15	54	--
JACK FRUIT	27	17	41	--
JAMBU FRUIT	89	2	13	--
LICHI	19	--	--	--
MANGO RIPE	26	--	--	--
MELON, musk	2	--	--	--
MELON, water	11	--	--	--
ORANGE	10	1	5	--
PAPAYA, ripe	1	4	31	--
PEACHES	1	1	2	--
PEARS	4	1	10	--
PHALSA	200	13	33	--
PINEAPPLE	5	2	22	--

(Contd.

Table 4 : Contd..

Name of the foodstuff	Oxalic acid mg/100 gms.	Phytin P	Phytin P as percent of total P	Total Dietary Fibre
(1)	(2)	(3)	(4)	(5)
PLUM	1	0	0	--
POMEGRANATE	14	11	28	--
SEETHAPHAL	30	--		--
TOMATO ripe	4	--	--	--
TOMATILLO	0	7	18	--
TREE TOMATO	·1	6	13	--
FISHES AND OTHER SEA FOODS				
ROHU	5	18	10	--
OTHER FLESH FOODS				
BEEF MEAL	--	90	28	--
BEEF MUSCLE	25	--	--	--
MUTTON	7	--	--	--
MILK AND MILK PRODUCTS				
MILK, cow's	2	--	--	--
MISCELLANEOUS FOOD STUFFS				
BANTI (whole)	--	--	--	31.06
BUCK WHEAT	--	322	91	--
RAJKEERA SEEDS	29	--	--	12.72
BAMBOO, tender shoots	2	--	--	--
JUNGLI BADAM	0	197	48	--
THAVITTUPAZHAM	42	11	73	--
VIKKIPAZHAM	272	--	--	--

Table 5 : Conversions to and from Metric Measures

If Measure Is In	*Multiply By*	*To Find*
Length		
inches	25.4	millimeters
inches	2.54	centimeters
feet	30.48	centimeters
feet	0.305	meters
centimeters	0.394	inches
meters	3.281	feet
Weight		
grains	64,799	milligrams
ounces (Av.)	28.35	grams
pounds (Av.)	454	grams
pounds	0.454	kilograms
grams	15.432	grains
grams	0.035	ounces (Av.)
grams	0.0022	pounds (Av.
kilograms	2.205	pounds
Capacity (liquid)		
teaspoons	4.7	milliliters
tablespoons	14.1	milliliters
fluid ounces	29.573	milliliters
cups (8 ounces)	238	milliliters
pints	0.473	liters
quarts	0.946	liters
milliliters	0.034	fluid ounces
liters	1.057	quarts
Energy units		
kilocalories	4.184	kilojoules
kilojoules	0.239	kilocalories
Temperature		
Fahrenheit	subtract 32; then multiplyby $^5/_9$	Celsius (Centigrade)
Celsius	multiply by $^9/_5$; then add 32	Fahrenheit

Metric equivalents

1 kilograms (kg)	=	1,000 grams
1 gram (gm)	=	1,000 milligrams
1 milligram (mg)	=	1,000 micrograms
1 microgram (mcg, mg, g)	=	1,000 nanograms
1 nanogram (ng)	=	1,000 picograms (pg)

Multiples

deca-	10
hecto-	10^2 (100)
kilo-	10^3 (1,000)
mega-	10^6 (1,000,000)

Submultiples

deci-	=	one tenth	10^{-1}	(0.1)
centi	=	one hundredth	10^{-2}	(0.01)
milli	=	one thousandth	10^{-3}	(0.001)
micro	=	one millionth	10^{-6}	(0.000,001)
nano	=	one billionth	10^{-9}	(0.000,000,001)
pico	=	one trillionth	10^{-12}	(0.000,000,000,001)

Table 6 : Synopsis of Fat-Soluble and Water-Soluble Vitamins

Name of Vitamins, Empirical and Structural Formulae	Properties	Distribution	Functions	Effects of Deficiency	Daily Requirement
Vitamin A Retinol Retinal Retinyl ester Retinoic Acid α, β and γ Carotene	Soluble in fat-solvents. Insoluble in water. It is a viscid colourless oil but by careful fractionation it has also been isolated as pale yellowish needles. Easily destroyed on exposure to air or ultra-violet rays. Heat stable	*Animal sources*—cod-liver oil, halibut-liver oil, milk, butter, eggs, fishes. *Vegetable sources*—(as carotene) carrots, spinach, vegetable oils, green leaves, yellow fruits.	Essential for growth. It is a component of rhodopsin, hence essential for night vision. Helps in the preservation of structural integrity and the normal permeability of membranes. Maintains the health and activity of epithelial tissues and glands. Prevents infection. Maintains nutrition and functions of the nervous tissue. Controls the action of the bone cells, formation and sulphation of mucopolysaccharide. Helps in normal fertility.	Night-blindness (Nyctalopia). Xerophthalmia. Keratinisation of skin and mucous membrane with increased susceptibility to infections entering by way of epithelial tissues. Retardation of growth in children Defective growth of bone and teeth.	3,000 i.u. for adults. 1,000–5,000 i.u. for growing children and during puberty, lactation and pregnancy.

Table 6 : (Contd.)

Name of Vitamins, Empirical and Structural Formulae	Properties	Distribution	Functions	Effects of Deficiency	Daily Requirement
Vitamin D (Calciferol) Vitamin D_2 (Ergocalciferol) Vitamin D_3 (Cholecolciferol) Antirachitic factor	Soluble in fat-solvents but insoluble in water. Heat-stable. There are a group of D vitamins of which D_2 (ergo-calciferol) are chief. D_2 is a white, crystalline material, soluble in fat and stable in heat, acids and alkalis, and oxidation. D_2 is made by ultra-violet irradiation of 7-dehydrocholesterol (provitamin D) and is also close isomer of cholesterol. D_3 is also a white, odourless, crystalline compound, soluble in fats and in common fat-solvents.	Richest sources are fish-liver oils, e.g., cod-liver oil, halibut-liver oil, etc. Butter, milk, eggs, liver, etc	Favours calcium and phosphorus absorption from the intestine. Helps in the bone formation by direct action on bone cells. Helps in the development of the normal teeth. Activates the alkaline phosphatase in bone, kidney and intstine.	Defective bone growth, condition known as rickets in infants and children and osteomalacia in adults. The formation of teeth becomes defective and leads to the development of dental caries. Tetany in infants.	200–300 i.u. in growing children and during pregnancy and lactation.

Table 6 : (Contd.)

Name of Vitamins, Empirical and Structural Formulae	Properties	Distribution	Functions	Effects of Deficiency	Daily Requirement
Vitamin E (tocopherols) α-Tocopherol β-Tocopherol γ-Tocopherol	Soluble in fat and fat-solvents. Heat-stable. Exists naturally as a yellow oil. In food, acts as an antioxidant. There are three varieties of tocopherols α, β and γ. The most active compound is α-tocopherol.	*Animal sources*—egg, milk, fish and muscles. *Vegetable sources*—vegetable seed oils, especially wheat, soyabean and corn. It can also be produced synthetically.	Tocopherols act as a cofactor in the electron transport system acting between cytochromes *b* and *c* and have got antioxidative effects and prevent oxidation (unwanted in the body). Prevent sterility. Essential for foetal development. Required for normal function of muscles. Maintains the physiological equilibrium in vascular and nervous system.	Vitamin E therapy is of some promise in the prevention of habitual miscarriage in women.	Average daily intake in diet is about 15 to 20 mgm, which satisfies the requirement.

Table 6 : (Contd.)

Name of Vitamins, Empirical and Structural Formulae	Properties	Distribution	Functions	Effects of Deficiency	Daily Requirement
Vitamin K K_1 (Phylloquinone) K_2 (Flavinoquinone)	Fat-soluble. Heat-stable. More than one member of K family, such as K_1, K_2, etc. which are synthesised by green plants and bacteria. The synthetic product is 2-methyl-1 : 4-naphthoquinone (K_3). K_1 is a yellow viscid oil, but K_2 is a yellow, crystalline solid.	*Vegetable sources*—cabbage, spinach, alfalfa, tomato, soyabean, etc. It can also be produced synthetically.	It catalyses the formation of prothrombin and factor VII in the blood and helps in the normal coagulation of blood. It has been suggested that this vitamin acts as a coenzyme for some enzymes responsible for normal clotting reactions. It plays an important role in oxidative phosphorylation in the mitochondria. Bile salts are necessary for the absorption of vitamin K.	Defective blood coagulation due to reduction of prothrombin and factor VII in the blood causes haemorrhages. The haemorrhagic disease in the new-born in believed to be due to lack of vitamin K.	Normal mixed diet supplies adequate amount. In the treatment of certain haemorrhagic diseases, 5 mgm is given either orally or by injection.

Table 6 : (Contd.)

Name of Vitamins, Empirical and Structural Formulae	Properties	Distribution	Functions	Effects of Deficiency	Daily Requirement
Thiamine (aneurine, vitamin B_1) Thiamine hydrochloride	White, crystalline substance. Water-soluble. Heat-labile. Unstable at high temperature and in alkaline medium. Stable in acid medium. On oxidation it gives a yellowish dye with fluorescence known as *thiochrome*.	*Vegetable sources*—cereals (in the husk and embryo), pulses, nuts, yeast, beets, carrots, turnips, lettuce, cauliflower, pears, beans, etc. Polished rice or white flour is poor in this vitamin. *Animal sources*—egg-yolk contains fair amount. It has also been produced synthetically.	Acts as a coenzyme of the carboxylase which helps in the oxidative decarboxylation of pyruvic acid (α-keto acid). In tissues thiamine exists as thiamine pyrophosphate and helps in oxidative decarboxylation of α-ketonic acid as a coenzyme. In the absence of this vitamin, pyruvic and lactic acids fail to be broken down, and accumulate in blood and tissues. Helps the enzyme system for the synthesis of fats from carbohydrates and proteins. It helps in transketolation reaction. It is also called *anti-neuritic* factor.	Beriberi—dry, wet, cardiac or mixed type. (a) Dry beriberi is associated with disorders of nervours systems, (*b*) Cardiac beriberi is associated with signs of congestive cardiac and circulatory failure, (*c*) In wet beriberi, polyneuritis is accompanied by oede-ma, (*d*) In mixed beriberi there is a combination of the above conditions. Loss of appetite, atony of the gastro-intestinal tract and hypo-chlorhydria. In addition to these signs heart becomes weak and enlarged and oedema of the legs occurs. Cardiac failure may also occur in some subjects. In rats, marked bradycardia occurs.	About 1–4 mgm. In pregnancy, lactation, heavy muscular work, high carbohydrate diet, etc. increase the requirement.

Table 6 : (Contd.)

Name of Vitamins, Empirical and Structural Formulae	Properties	Distribution	Functions	Effects of Deficiency	Daily Requirement
Lipoic Acid (Thioctic acid)	6,8-dithio-octanoic acid. Sulphur-containing fatty acid.	Widely deistributed in nautre.	Along with thiamine and some other members of vitamins B helps in the oxidative decarboxylation of pyruvic acid and α-ketoglutaric acid to acetyl CoA and succinyl CoA respectively.	Deficiency signs not known in higher animals.	Probably not required from the dietary source in higher animals.
Riboflavin (Vitamin B_2, Lactoflavin) Riboflavin phosphate or FMN FAD (FADN)	Yellow crystals, Sparingly soluble in water. Heat-stable in neutral and acid media. Destroyed by light.	*Animal sources*—milk (lactoflavin), liver, kidney, muscle, raw egg-white, etc. *Vegetable sources*—whole grains and green-leafy vegetables. It has been synthetically produced.	Essential for growth. Constituent of yellow enzyme' of Warburg, hence essential for tissue oxidation. In the tissues, riboflavin mononucleotide (FMN) and flavin adenine dinucleotide (FAD). These two coenzymes in	In man—oral fissures at the corners of the mouth—Cheilosis. Ulcers on the lips. Angular stomatitis. Glossitis. Keratitis, corneal opacities, vascularisation of cornea and photophobia. Loss of hair. Skin becomes dry and scaly.	In adults—1.2 to 2.3 mgm.

Table 6 : (Contd.)

Name of Vitamins, Empirical and Structural Formulae	Properties	Distribution	Functions	Effects of Deficiency	Daily Requirement
			combination with protein are termed flavoprotein which have a major functional role as a number of enzyme system act as hydrogen-carrier to the cytochromes which further carry the same to molecular oxygen where hyrogen finally combines with it to form H_2O.		
Nicotinic acid (Niacin) Niacin	White, crystalline substance. Moderately soluble inwater. Heat-stable.	*Vegetable sources*—dried legumes, peas, beans, tomatoes, whole wheat meal, green vegetables, etc.	Acts as a *pellagra-preventing* factor. Essential for growth. Remains as a part of at least two enzymes—NAD(DPN) and NADP (TPN). They act along with	Dermatitis, diarrhoea and dementia. Pellagra—Characteristic dermatitis specially on the exposed parts of the body. The dermatitis begins with erythema resembling sunburnt	16–26 mgm for adult males and a little less in adult females. Requirement varies with the protein content of diet, as amino acid tryptophan gives rise to niacin.

Table 6 : (Contd.)

Name of Vitamins, Empirical and Structural Formulae	Properties	Distribution	Functions	Effects of Deficiency	Daily Requirement
Nicotinic acid amide (Niacinamide, Nicotinamide) Nicotinamide		*Animal sources*—meat, fish, liver, milk, eggs, yeast, kidneys, heart, etc. It has been produced synthetically.	dehydrogenase and take part in tissue oxidation. Helps in the formation of fats from carbohydrates. Stimulates the central nervous system.	areas. Gradually these areas become reddish brown, rough, scaly and keratotic. Gastro-intestinal disorders. Polyneuritis.	
Pantothenic acid (vitamin B_3)	White, crystalline substance. Highly soluble in water. Hygroscopic. Heat-stable.	*Animal sources*—liver, kidney, egg-yolk, meat, milk, yeast, etc. *Vegetable sources*—molasses, wheat bran, peas, sweet potatoes, etc. It has also been produced synthetically.	Plays a fundamental role in the metabolism as coenzyme A (CoA). Its acetyl derivative (acetyl CoA) called active acetate, a pivot on which transfer of acetyl mechanism depends.	Various issues affected, e.g., gastro-intestinal disturbances, alopecia, cornification of the skin and hypo-function of adrenal cortex.	Not exactly known.

Table 6 : (Contd.)

Name of Vitamins, Empirical and Structural Formulae	Properties	Distribution	Functions	Effects of Deficiency	Daily Requirement
Pyridoxine (vitamin B_6)	Two allied compounds—*pyridoxal* and *pyridoxamine*, (natural) and synthetic, have the same action and the three vitamins are known as vitamin B_6. White crystal, soluble in water. Heat-stable in both acidic and alkaline solutions.	*Vegetable sources*—germs of various grains and seeds, leafy vegetables, etc. *Animal sources*—liver, egg-yolk, meat, kidney, yeast, etc. It has been produced synthetically.	Helps in the normal metabolism of tryptophan. Acts as a coenzyme for (*a*) transaminases or aminotransferases, (*b*) decarboxylases, (*c*) deaminases or dehydrases, and (*d*) desulphy-drases. Related to the metabolism of unsaturated fatty acids. Helps in the synthesis of fats from proteins and carbohydrates. It is also called antidermatitis factor.	In man its role is not exactly known. But in subjects suffering from pellagra and beriberi, synthetic B_6 can easily cure insomnia, irritability, abdominal pain, difficulty in walking, etc., which cannot be cured by other vitamins.	0.3 mgm per day in infants and in adults 2.0 mgm daily.

Table 6 : (Contd.)

Name of Vitamins, Empirical and Structural Formulae	Properties	Distribution	Functions	Effects of Deficiency	Daily Requirement
Folic acid *Pteroylglutamic acid (PGA)*	Yellow compound. Slightly soluble in water, and destroyed by light.	*Animal sources*—liver, kidney, etc. Vegetable sources—widely distributed in plants, and in green vegetables.	Essential for the synthesis of deoxyribonucleic acid (DNA) in the nuclei of the cells. Along with vitamin B_{12} it helps in the synthesis of nucleic acid.	In man—Megaloblastic anaemia, especially occurring during pregnancy. Combined system disease, i.e., pernicious anaemia and neurological symptoms, i.e., pernicious anaemia may develop as a result of deficiency of this vitamin along with vitamin B_{12} deficiency.	100 μg. Need in pregnancy and lactation is more.
Leucovorin Folinic acid (CF)			Reduced form of folic acid, i.e., tetrahydrofolic acid (FH_4) is converted into folinic acid in the body, a formyl derivative of FH4 (single carbon carrier) which acts as a coenzyme in the transfer of formyl and hydroxymethyl group in various biological systems. Related to phospholipid metabolism (choline synthesis) and amino acid metabolism.		

Table 6 : (Contd.)

Name of Vitamins, Empirical and Structural Formulae	Properties	Distribution	Functions	Effects of Deficiency	Daily Requirement
Cyanocobalamin (vitamin B_{12})	Red crystalline substance. Soluble in water. Contains metallo-porphyrin nucleus and cobalt. Three different cobalamin compounds having common prosthetic group possess vitamin B_{12} activity which are as follows: (i) Cyanocobalamin, in which cobalt attached to cyanide group. (ii) *Hydroxycobalamin*, (B_{12a}) in which cyanide group is replaced by hydroxyl group.	Absent in plants but present in almost all animal tissues. Rich sources are liver, kidney, eggs, beef extract, milk, etc. Also found in fungus—*Streptomyces griseus*. Hence vitamin B_{12} is obtained as a by-product in the manufacture of Streptomycin.	*Antipernicious anaemia* factor. Essential for the formation and maturation of red blood cells. Recent idea is that vitamin B_{12} is Castle's extrinsic factor. The intrinsic factor helps in its absorption from the intestine. Plays an essential role in the synthesis of nucleic acid. Increase the white cell count and the platelets through its action in the bone-marrow. Concerned with the maintenance of nor-	Pernicious or Macrocytic anaemia. Brings about Hyperglycaemia	The requirement is about 1 μ gm per day.

(Contd.)

Table 6 : (Contd.)

Name of Vitamins, Empirical and Structural Formulae	Properties	Distribution	Functions	Effects of Deficiency	Daily Requirement
	(iii) Nitrocobalamin in which cyanide group is replaced by nitro group. B_{12}, is must active and enzyme system requiring B_{12}.		mal health and activity of certain parts of nervous system. Cures pernicious anaemia and also neurological manifestations of pernicious anaemia. Helps in the growth of *Lactobacillus lactis*. Hyperglycaemia due to deficiency of B_{12} can be corrected after administration of vitamin B_{12} or glutathione (GSH).		
Biotin (vitamin H)	It is a valeric acid derivative. Soluble in water and alcohl.	Widely distributed in all common article of food—specially in yeast, egg-yolk, kidney, liver,	Biotin acts as coenzyme in CO_3 fixation for the urea (carbamyl phosphate) formation as	Experimental deficiency in man causes (1) peculiar dermatitis, (2) symptoms resem-	Average daily diet contains sufficient amount.

(Contd.)

Table 6 : (Contd.)

Name of Vitamins, Empirical and Structural Formulae	Properties	Distribution	Functions	Effects of Deficiency	Daily Requirement
Biotin (vitamin H) *(contd..)*	Heat-stable. Resistant to acids and alkalis. It contains sulphur.	cauliflower, peas, etc. Raw egg-white contains **avidin** (antivitamin of biotin) which antagonises and prevents its action.	well as for the biosynthesis of pyrimidines and fatty acids. Helps in deamination of threonine, serine and aspartic acid.	bling thiamine deficiency, and (3) rise of blood cholesterol. Deficiency does not occur normally but may be induced by either (1) feeding raw egg white or (2) intake of sulphur drugs which interferes with the biosynthesis of this vitamin in the intestine.	
Choline and Lipotropic factor	Water-soluble. Component of lecithin and other phospholipids, acetylcholine, etc.	Butter, nervous tissues, eggs, etc.	Lipotropic action. Synthesis of lecithin, sphingomyelin, acetylcholine, etc. Acts as a methyl donor in transmethylation.		Not essential for man, because freely synthesised in the body.

Table 6 : (Contd.)

Name of Vitamins, Empirical and Structural Formulae	Properties	Distribution	Functions	Effects of Deficiency	Daily Requirement
Para-amino-benzoic acid (PAB)	White crystalline substance. Slightly soluble in water but highly soluble in alcohol.	Widely distributed in animal tissues. Also found in wheat germ, rice bran and polishings and milk.	Prevents the bacteriostatic properties of sulpha drugs due to structural similarities.	Might produce (1) achromotrichia in man due to changes in intestinal microflora, (2) premature graying of hair, (3) Some rickettsial infection.	——
Inositol Myo-inositol or Meso-inositol	Soluble in water. Sweet taste. The natural variety is known as meso-inositol or myo-inositol (i.e., insoitol present in muscle) or muscle sugar.	Rich sources are muscles, liver, kidney, brain, etc. In cereals present as phytic acid.	Its role in human nutrition is not definitely known.	Alopecia in mice. Peculiar eye condition known as 'Spectacle eye', in rats.	Human requirement not known. Daily diet contains about 1 gm which seems enough.
Ascorbic Acid (vitamin C)	White crystals. Soluble in water. Insoluble in fat-solvents. Heat labile	*Vegetable sources*—fresh (cirus) fruits, e.g., emblic myrobalan (amlaki), orange, lemon, tomato, etc.	Regulates oxidation—reduction potential inside the cell, probably by acting as hydrogen-carrier.	*Scurvy*—Increased fragility of the capillaries causing haemorrhages—under the skin, periosteum, intestine, kidney, etc.	In adults normally 40 mgm on the average, during pregnancy, lactation and adolescence 100 mgm approximately.

Table 6 : (Contd.)

Name of Vitamins, Empirical and Structural Formulae	Properties	Distribution	Functions	Effects of Deficiency	Daily Requirement
Ascorbic acid (Vitamin C) (Contd.)	Easily oxidised at 100°C. in presence of oxygen. Cannot stand cooking and canning. Destroyed by alkali and cooper salts.	Fresh vegetables, e.g., cabbage, cauliflower, lettuce, etc. Properly sprouted pulses, germinating grams, etc. *Animal sources*—generally contains a negligible amount, e.g., adrenal.	It helps in the oxidation of ρ-hydroxyphenyl pyruvic acid to homogentisic acid which is the intermediate metabolic product of tyrosine metabolism. Related to carbohydrate metabolism. In ascorbic acid deficiency, reduced production of insulin takes place. On the other hand, dehydroascorbic acid (oxidation product of this vitamin), when injected in animals produces diabetes. Essential for the proper functioning of the formative cells of various tissues.	The gums show erosion of the mucous membrane at their margins and due to increased fragility of the capillaries there is frequent bleeding. The osteoblasts remain functionless. Many of them are reverted to fibroblasts. There is irregular deposition of bone salts. The functions of the odontoblast are impaired. New dentine is not formed and the tissue becomes spongy and porous.	

Table 7 : Synopsis of Macro and Micro Elements

Minerals	Function in the Body	Metabolism	Food Sources
Calcium	Hardness of bones, teeth Transmission of nerve impulse. Muscle contraction. Normal heart rhythm Activate enzymes Increase cell permeability Catalyze thrombin formation	*Absorption* : about 15–40 per cent, according to body need; aided by gastric acidity, vitamin D, lactose; excess phosphate, fat, phytate, oxalic acid interfere. *Storage* : trabeculae to bones; easily mobilized. *Utilization* : needs parathyroid hormone, vitamin D *Excretion* : 60–85 per cent of diet intake in feces; small urinary excretion; high protein intake increases urinary excretion. *Deficiency* : retarded bone mineralization; fragile bones; stunted growth; rickets; osteomalacia; osteoporosis	Milk, hard cheese Ice cream, cottage cheese Greens : turnip, collards, kale, mustard, broccoli Oysters, shrimp, salmon, clams
Chlorine	Chief anion of extracellular fluid Constituent of gastric juice Acid-base balance; chloride-bicarbonate shift in red cells.	*Absorption* : rapid, almost complete *Excretion* : chiefly in urine; parallels intake *Deficiency* : with prolonged vomiting, drainage from fistula, diarrhoea	Table salt
Chromium	Efficient use of insulin in glucose uptake; glucose oxidation, protein synthesis, stimulation of fat, and cholesterol synthesis Activation of enzymes	Usable form in organic compound : glucose tolerance factor	Liver, meat Cheese Whole-grain cereals

Table 7 : Contd.

Minerals	Function in the Body	Metabolism	Food Sources
Copper	Aids absorption and use of iron in synthesis of hemoglobin Electron transport Melanin formation Myelin sheath of nerves Purine metabolism.	*Transport*: chiefly as protein, ceruloplasmin *Storage* : liver, central nervous system *Excretion* : bile into intestine *Deficiency* : rare; occurs in sever malnutrition Abnormal storage in Wilson's disease	Liver, shelfish Meats Nuts, legumes Whole-grain cereals Typical diet provides 1 to 5 mg
Fluorine	Increases resistance of teeth to decay; most effective in young children Moderate levels in bone may reduce osteoporosis	*Storage*: bones and teeth *Excretion* : urine Excess leads to mottling of teeth	Fluoridated water : 1 ppm
Iodine	Constituent of diiodotyrosine, triiodothyronine, thyroxine; regulate rate of energy metabolism.	*Absorption*: controlled by blood level of protein-bound iodine *Storage*: thyroid gland; activity regulated by thyroid-stimulating hormone *Excretion*: in urine *Deficiency*: simple goiter; if sever, cretinism	Iodized salt is most reliable source Seafood Foods grown in non-goitrous coastal areas
Iron	Constituent of hemoglobin, myoglobin, and oxidative enzymes : catalase, cytochrome, xanthine oxidase	*Absorption*: about 3 to 23 per cent, depending on food source and body need; aided by gastric acidity, ascorbic acid. *Transport*: bound to protein, transferrin *Storage*: as ferritin in liver, bone marrow, spleen	Liver, organ meats Meat, poultry Egg yolk

Table 7 : Contd.

Minerals	Function in the Body	Metabolism	Food Sources
Iron (*Contd.*)		*Utilization*: chiefly in hemoglobin; daily turnover about 27 to 28 mg; iron used over and over again. *Excretion*: men, about 1 mg; women, 1 to 2 mg; in urine, perspiration, menstrual flow; fecal excretion is from unabsorbed dietary iron. *Deficiency*: anemia; frequent in infants, pre-school children, teen-age girls, pregnant women.	Enriched and whole-grain breads, cereals Dark-green vegetables Legumes Molasses, dark Peaches, apricots, prunes, raisins Diets supply about 6 mg per 1,000 kcal.
Magnesium	Constituents of bones, teeth Activates enzymes in carbohydrate metabolism Muscle and nerve irritability	*Absorption*: parallels that of calcium; competes with calcium for carriers. *Utilization*: slowly mobilized from bone *Excretion*: chiefly by kidney *Deficiency*: seen in alcoholism, severe renal disease; hypomagnesemia, tremor.	Whole-grains cereals Nuts; legumes Meat Milk Green leafy vegetables
Manganese	Activation of many enzymes; oxidation of carbohydrates, urea formation, protein hydrolysis Bone formation	*Absorption*: limited *Excretion*: chiefly by feces *Deficiency*: seen in alcoholism, severe renal disease; hypomagnesemia, tremor	Legumes, nuts Whole-grain cereals

Table 7 : Contd.

Minerals	Function in the Body	Metabolism	Food Sources
Molybdenum	Cofactor for flavorprotein enzymes; present in xanthine oxidase	Absorbed as molybdate Stored in liver, adrenal, kidney Related to metabolism of copper and sulfur	Oran meats Legumes Whole-grain cereals
Phosphorus	Structure of bones, teeth Cell permeability Metabolism of fats and carbohydrates : storage and release of ATP Phospholipids in transport of fats Buffer salts in acid-base balance	*Absorption*: about 70 per cent; aided by vitamin D *Utilization*: about 85 per cent in bones; controlled by vitamin D, parathormone *Excretion*: about one third of diet in feces; metabolic products chiefly in urine *Deficiency*: poor bone mineralisation; poor growth; rickets	Milk, cheese Eggs, meat, fish, poultry Legumes, nuts Whole-grain cereals
Potassium	Principal cation of intracellular fluid Osmotic pressure; water balance; acid-base balance Nerve irritability and muscle contraction, regular heart rhythm	*Absorption*: readily absorbed *Excretion*: chiefly in urine; increased with aldosterone secretion *Deficiency*: following starvation, correction of diabetic acidosis, adrenal tumors; some diuretics; muscle weakness, nausea, tachycardia, glycogen depletion, heart failure.	Widely distributed in foods Meat, fish, fowl Cereals Fruits, vegetables.
Selenium	Antioxidant Constituent of glutathione oxidase	Stored especially in liver, kidney Spares vitamin E	Meat and seafoods Cereal foods

Table 7 : Contd.

Minerals	Function in the Body	Metabolism	Food Sources
Sodium	Principal cation of extracellular fluid Osmotic pressure; water balance Acid-base balance Regulate nerve irritability and muscle contraction "Pump" for active transport such as for glucose.	*Absorption*: rapid and almost complete *Excretion*: chiefly in urine; some by skin and in feces; parallels intake; controlled by aldosterone *Deficiency*: rare; occurs with excessive perspiration and poor diet intake; nausea, diarrhea, abdominal cramps, muscle cramps	Table salt Processed foods Milk Meat, fish, poultry
Sulfur	Constituent of proteins, especially cartilage, hair, nails Constituent of melanin, glutathione, thiamin, biotin, coenzyme A, insulin High-energy sulfur bonds Detoxication reactions	Absorbed chiefly as sulfur-containing amino acids Excreted as inorganic sulfate in urine in proportion to nitrogen loss	Protein foods rich in sulfur-amino acids Eggs Meat, fish, poultry Milk, cheese Nuts
Zinc	Constituent of enzymes : carbonic anhydrase, carboxypeptidase, lactic dehydrogenase	*Absorption*: limited; competes with calcium for absorption sites *Storate*: liver, muscles, bones, organs *Excretion*: chiefly by intestine	Seafoods Liver and other organ meats Meats, fish Wheat germ Yeast Plant foods are generally low Usual diet supplies 10 to 15 mg

Glossary

Absorption : The transfer of nutrients across cell membranes; following digestion, nutrients are transferred from the intestinal lumen into the blood and lymph circulation.

Acetoacetic acid : A 4-carbon keto acid; one of the acetone bodies in diabetic urine.

Acetone : Dimethyl ketone produced when fats are incompletely oxidized as in diabetes mellitus; gives fruity odor to the breath.

Acetylcholine : An acetic acid ester of choline; involved in nerve transmission.

Acetyl coenzyme A : Condensation product of acetic acid and coenzyme A; form by which 2-carbon fragment eneter the tricarboxylic acid cycle.

Achlorhydria : Absence of hydrocholoric acid in gastric juice.

Acid : A substance that gives off or donates protons.

Acidosis : Condition caused by accumulation of an excess of acids in the body, or by excessive loss of base from the body.

Acrolein : An irritating volatile decomposition product of glycerol that results from overheating fat.

Active transport : The movement of substance across cell membranes by pumping against a concentration gradient; requires source of energy.

Active immunity : Immunity acquired as a result of individual's own reactions to pathogenic microorganisms or their antigens; attributable to the presence of antibody or immune lymphoid cells formed in response to an antigenic stimulus.

Acquired Immune Deficiency Syndrom (AIDS) : An infectious disease syndrome caused by HIV retrovirus, characterized by the loss of normal immune response system functions, followed by various opportunistic infections.

Acquired Immunity : The ability of an individual to produce specific antibodies in response to antigens to which the body has been previously exposed based on the development of a memory response.

Adenine : One of the purines that are constituents of nucleic acid.

Adenosine Triphosphate : A compound consisting of 1 molecule each of adenine and ribose and 3 molecules of phosphoric acid; two of the phosphate groups are held by high-energy bonds; ATP.

Aflatoxin : A carcinogenic poison produced by some strains of the fungus Aspergillus flavus.

Agar : An indigestible polysaccharide prepared from moss and seaweed; has property of holding water and is often used to relieve constipation and is used as a solidifying agent in microbiological media.

Agglutin : An antibody capable of causing the clumping or agglutination of bacteria or other cells.

Airborne transmission : Route by which pathogens are transported to a susceptible host via the air; main route of trasmission of pathogens that enter via the respiratory tract through the air.

Albumin : A protein in tissues and body fluids soluble in water and coagulated by heat; protein in blood.

Aldehyde : Any of a large group of compounds containing the grouping—CHO.

Aldohexose : A 6-carbon sugar containing a -CHO grouping; glucose, galactose.

Aldosterone : A steroid hormone produced by the adrenal cortex; increases sodium retention and potassium loss.

Alkalosis : Increased alkali reserve of the blood and other body fluids; caused by excessive ingestion of sodium bicarbonate, persistent vomiting, or hyperventilation.

Allergen : Substance capable of producing altered response of cell. resulting in manifesration of allergy.

Amino acid : An organic acid containing an amino group; the building blocks of protein molecules.

Amylase : Salivary or pancretic enzyme that hydrolyzes starch.

Amylopectin : Polysaccharide found in starch consisting of branched chains of glucose.

Amylose : Polysaccharide of starch consiting of unbranched chains of glucose.

Anabolism : Processes for building complex substances from simple substances.

Androgen : A substance such as testosterone that produces male sex characteristics.

Anemia : Deficiency in the circulating hemoglobin, red blood cells, or packed cell volume.

Anorexia : Loss of appetite.

Antibiotic : A substance that inhibits the growth of bacteria.

Antibiotics : Substances of microbial origin that in very small amounts have antimicrobial activity; current usage of the term extends to synthetic and semisynthetic substances that are closely related to naturally occuring antibiotics and that have antimicrobial activity; current usage of the term extends to synthetic and semi-synthetic substances that are closely related to naturally occuring antibiotics and that have antimicro-bial activity.

Antibody : A protein substance produced in an organism as a response to the presence of an antigen.

Antigen : Any substance such as bacteria or foreign proetin that, as a result of contact with tissues of the animal body, produces an immune response.

Antioxidant : A substance that prevents deterioration by hindering oxidation.

Anuria : Lack of urinary secretion.

Apathy : Indifference; lack of interest.

Apoenzyme : The protein part of an enzyme.

Arachidonic acid : A 20-carbon fatty acid with four double bonds; the physiologically functioning essential fatty acid.

Arginine : A diamino acid; required for growth but not required by adults.

Arteriosclerosis : Thickening and hardening of the inner walls of the arteries.

Ascites : Accumulation of fluid in the abdominal cavity.

Ascorbic acid : Water-soluble vitamin required for collagenous intercellular substance; also known as vitamin C.

Aspartic acid : A non-essential diabasic amino acid.

Ataxia : Loss of ability of muscular coordination.

Atherosclerosis : Thickening of the walls of blood vessels by desposits of fatty materials, including cholesterol.

Atrophy : A wasting away of cell, tissue or organ.

Autoclave : Apparatus in which objects or materials may be sterilized by air-free saturated steam under pressure at temperatures in excess of 100°C.

Autolysis : Self digestion : The break down of the cell and/or its contents by the action of enzymes produced within it.

Autosome : Any chromosome other than a sex chromosome.

Avidin : Protein substance in raw egg white which binds and prevents its absorption from the digestive tract.

Azotemia : Elevated levels of nitrogenous constituents in the blood.

B lymphocytes : White blood cells that are able to produce specific immunoglobulins; their surfaces carry specific immunoglobulin antigen binding receptor sites.

Bacteriophate : A virus whose hose is a bacterium; a virus that replicates within bacterial cells.

Bacterium : Unicellular microscopic organisms, containing no chlorophyll; they can multiply rapidly by simple fission in suitable conditions.

Basal metabolic rate : The rate at which energy is used to maintain body processes and body temperature when the subject is completely at rest and in a comfortably warm room.

Basal metabolism : Energy expenditure of the body at rest in the postabsorptive state.

Benign : Mild nature of an illness; with reference to a neoplasm, not malignant.

Beriberi : A deficiency disease caused by lack of thiamin and characterized by extreme weakness, polyneuritis, emaciation, edema, and cardiac failure.

Beta-hydroxybutyric acid : A 4-carbon intermediate in oxidation of fatty acids; one of the acetone bodies excreted in the urine in uncontrolled diabetes.

Biochemistry : The study of the chemical composition and chemical processess of living things.

Bioassay : Testing of activity or potency, as a of a vitamin or hormone, on an animal or micro-organism.

Biological oxygen demand (BOD) : The amount of dissolved oxygen required by aerobic and facultative micro-organisms to stabilize organic matter in sewage or water, also known as biochemical oxygen demand.

Biopsy : Examination of a piece of tissue removed from a living subject.

Bitot's spots : Gray, shiny spots on the conjunctiva resulting from vitamin A deficiency.

Blood serum : The fluid expressed from clotted blood or clotted blood plasma.

Botulism : Frequently fatal poisoning caused by toxin produced in inadequately sterilized canned food by the Clostridium botulinum.

Bran : The outer covering of wheat grain, consisting of several distinct layers and makes 12 per cent by weight of whole grain.

Bronchitis : Inflammation occuring in the mucous membranes of the bronchi, often caused by Streptococcus pneumoniae, Haemophilus influenzae, and certian viruses.

Buffer : A mixture of an acid and its conjugate base that is capable of neutralizing either an acid or a base without appreciably changing the original acidity or alkalinity, e.g., H_2CO_3/HCO_3^-.

Calcification : Hardening of tissue by a deposit of calcium and also magnesium salts.

Calcitonin : Hormone secreted by the thyroid gland; opposes action of parathormone.

Calorie : A unit of heat measurement; in nutrition, the kilocalories is the amount of heat required to raise the temperature of 1 kg. water 1 °C = 4186 Joules.

Canning : Method for the preservation of foodstuffs in which suitably prepared foods are placed in metal containers that are heated, exhausted, and hermetically sealed.

Carbohydrate : A compound containing carbon, hydrogen and oxygen in which the ratio of the numbers of hydrogen and oxygen atoms is 2:1.

Carboxylase : A thiamin-containing enzymes that catalyzes the removal of the carboxyl group of alpha keto acids, e.g., decarboxylation of pyruvic acid.

Carboxypeptidase : An intestinal enzyme which catalyzes the splitting of peptides.

Carotene : Precursor of vitamin A; occuring abundantly in dark green leafy and deep yellow vegetables.

Casein : Principal protein in milk; a phosphoprotein.

Catabolism : Process for breaking down complex substances to simpler substances; usually yields energy.

Cation : An ion that carries a positive charge and migrates to the negatively charged pole.

Cell : A mass of protoplasm within a membrane, constituting either a part or whole of an organism.

Cell-mediated immunity : Specific acquired immunity involving T cells, primarily responsible for resistance to infectious diseases caused by certian bacteria and viruses that reproduce within host cells.

Cellulose : The structural fibers of plants; an indigestible polysaccharide.

Ceruloplasmin : Copper-containing protien in blood plasma.

Cheilosis : Lesions of the lips and the angles of the mouth; characteristic of riboflavin deficiency.

Cholecystitis : Inflammation of the gall-bladder

Cholecystokinin : Hormone produced in duodenum in presence of fat; stimulates contraction of gall-bladder and release of bile.

Cholesterol : The commonest member of the sterol group; found in animal foods and made within the body.

Choline : A nitrogenous base that donates methyl groups; a component of lecithin and acetylcholine; classed as a B-complex vitamin.

Chylomicrons : Large molecules of fat occuring in lymph and plasm after a fatrich meal; consist of triglycerids attached to a small amount of protein.

Chymotrypsin : Enzyme produced in pancreas for the hydrolysis of protein.

Citric acid : An organic acid containing three carboxyl groups; one of compounds in the Krebs or citric acid cycle; a constituent of citrus fruits.

Citrulline : An amino acid formed from ornithine in the urea cycle.

Clostridium : A genus of bacteria, chiefly anaerobic, found in soils and in the intestinal tract, e.g., botulinum, perfringens.

Coagulation : Process of changing into a clot, as in heating of an egg, curdling of milk.

Cocarboxylase : Thiamin-containing coenzyme of carboxylase.

Coenzyme : The prosthetic group of an enzyme.

Collagen : Widely distributed protein that makes up the matrix of bone, cartilage, and connective tissue.

Colony : The micro-scopically visible growth of micro-organisms on a solid culture medium.

Colostrum : Milk secreted during the first few days after the birth of a baby.

Combustion : The union of oxygen with a fuel, with the production of energy in the form of heat and light.

Complementarity : The ability of one substance to supply a missing substance in another.

Congenital : Existing at or before birth with reference to certain physical or mental traits.

Cortisone : Hormone of the adrenal cortex.

Cretine : A nitrogenous constituent of muscle; phosphorylated form essential for muscle contraction.

Creatinine : A nitrogen-containing substance derived from catabolism of creatine and present in the urine.

Crude fiber : Plant fiber that remains after sample has been treated with sulfuric acid and sodium hydroxide; chiefly cellulose and lingnin.

Crytoxanthine : A yellow pigment present in some foods; precursor of vitamin A.

Cyanobacteria : Prokaryotic, photosynthetic organisms containing chlorophyll a, capable of producing oxygen by splitting water; formerly known as blue-green algae.

Cystine : Sulfur-containing non-essential amino acid.

Cytology : The anatomy, chemistry, physiology, and pathology of the cell.

Cytoplasm : Substance within the cell exclusive of the nucleus.

Deamination, deaminization : Removal of the amino group from an amino acid.

Debility : Weakness

Deficiency disease : A condition caused by the lack of sufficient amounts of a particular nutrient in diet or by the body's in ability to absorb it.

Dehydrocholesterol, 7: Cholesterol derivative in the skin that is converted to vitamin D.

Dehydrogenases : Enzymes that catalyze oxidation by transferring hydrogen to a hydrogen acceptor.

Denaturation : The alteration of the natural properties of a susbtance by physical or chemical means.

Deoxypyriodoxine : A compound similar in structure to pyriodoxine that is antagonistic to the action of pyriodixine.

Deoxyribonucleic acid : Gaint molecule in cell nucleus which determines hereditary traits; consists of four bases attached to ribose and phosphate.

Dermatitis : Inflammation of the surface of the skin.

Dextrin : Intermediate product in breakdown of starches; a polysaccharide.

Diffusion : The movement of particles from an area of higher concentration to one of lower concentration.

Digestion : The hydrolysis of foods in the diegstive tract to simpler substances so they can be used by the body.

Diglyceride : A fat containing 2 fatty acid molecules.

Disaccaridase : Enzyme which hydrolyzes disaccharides.

Disaccharide : A carbohydrate that yileds two simple sugars upon hydrolysis; sucross, maltose, lactose.

Disease : A condition of an organ, part, structure, or system of the body in which there is incorrect functioning due to the effect of heredity, infection, diet, or environment a physiologically impaired state of a plant or animal resulting from microbial infection, microbial products, or microbial activities; a physiological condition that occurs when micro-organisms overcome host defense systems.

Dissemination : The scattering of dispersion of micro-organisms or disease, e.g., the spread of disease associated with the dispersal of pathogens.

Distal : Part of structure farthest from the point of attachment.

Duodenum : First portion of the small intestine, extending from the pylorus to the jejunum.

Dysentery : An infectious disease marked by inflammation and ulceration of th lower part of the bowels, with diarrhoea that becomes mucous and hemorrhagic; disease condition characterized by diarrhoea.

Dysgeusia : Perverted sense of taste; "bad" taste.

Dysosmia : Impaired sense of smell, obnoxious odor.

Dyspepsia : Indigestion or upset stomach.

Dysphagia : Difficulty in swallowing.

Dyspnea : Difficulty or distress in breathing.

Eclampsia : Convulsions occurring during pregnancy and associated with edema, hypertension, and proteinuria.

Edema : Presence of abnormal amounts of fluid in intercellular space.

Electrolyte : Any substance which dissociates into ions when dissolved and thus conducts and electric current.

Embryo : An organism in the process of development from a fertilized ovum; in man, the term is only used for the first few weeks after fertilization.

Emulsion : A system of two immiscible liquids in which one is finely divided and held in suspension by another.

Endemic : Prevalence of a disease in a given region.

Endocrine : Pertaining to glands that secrete substances into the blood for control of metabolic processes.

Endogenous : Originating in the cells or tissues of the body.

Endosperm : Reserve food material of the plant; the starchy center of the cereal grain.

Enteritis : Inflammation of the intestine.

Enterogastrone : Hormone secreted by duodenal mucosa upon stimulation by fat, inhibits secretion of gastric juice and reduces motility.

Enterokinase : Enzyme of intestinal juice that converts trypsinogen to trypsin.

Enzyme : An organic compound of protein nature produced by living tissue to accelerate metabolic reactions; hydrolases, oxidases, transferases, dehydrogenases, peptidases etc.

Epidemiology : The science of epidemic diseases; factors that influence frequency and distribution of disease.

Epinephrine : Secrettion of the medulla of the adrenal gland that stimulates energy metabolism; adrenaline.

Epithelium : The covering layer of the skin and mucous membranes.

Ergotism : A condition of intoxication that results from the ingestion of grain contaminated by ergot alkaloids produced by the fungus claviceps purpurea.

Erythrocyte : Mature red blood cell.

Erythropoieses : Formation of red blood cells.

Essential amino acid : An amino acid that must be supplied in the diet to provide the body's need for it.

Essential fatty acid : A fatty acid that must be present in the diet and that prevents certain deficiencies of the skin and blood capillaries; linoleic acid, arachidonic acid.

Estrogen : Hormone secreted by the ovary.

Etiology : Cause of a disease.

Exogenous : Originating or produced from the outside.

Excretion : The removal of th waste products of metabolism from the body.

Extrinsic factor : Vitamin B-12; term used by Castle prior to identification of the nature of the compound.

Fatty acids : Open-chain mono-carboxylic acids containing only carbon, hydrogen, and oxygen.

Favism : Condition caused by eating certain species of beans, e.g., Vicia faba; symptoms include fever, abdominal pain, headache, anemia, coma.

Febrile : Feverish; having a fever.

Ferritin : Water-soluble storage form of iron in the body; composed of protein and colloidal ferric iron.

Fetor hepaticus : Offensive odor to the breath present in persons with severe liver disease.

Fibrosis : Formation of fibrous tissues in repair processes.

Fistula : A tubelike ulcer leading from an abscess cavity or organ to the surface, or from one abscess cavity to another.

Flatulence : Distention of stomach or intestines with gases.

Flavin adenine dinucleotide, FAD : A coenzyme consisting of riboflavin and adenosine diphosphate required for the action of various dehydrogenases.

Flavin mono-nucleotide, FMN : A riboflavin-containing coenzyme involved in the action of dehydrogenases.

Flavoprotein : A conjugated protein that contains a flavin and is involved in tissue respiration.

Foetus : The term used for the embryo of a mammal. Once its characteristic features can be recognised, in man, this is after about eight weeks of pregnancy.

Folic acid : A vitamin of the B complex necessary for the maturation of red blood cells and synthesis of nucleproteins; also known as folacin and pteroylglutamic acid.

Follicle : Small excretary sac or gland, e.g., hair follicle ovarian follicle.

Food additive : A substance or mixture of substance other than the basic foodstuff, which is intentionally present in food as a result of any aspect of production, processing, storage, or packaging.

Food intoxication : Disease resulting from the ingestion of toxins produced by micro-organisms that have grown in a food.

Food poisoning : A general term applied to all stomach or intestinal disorders due to food contaminated with certain micro-organisms, their toxins, chemicals, or poisonous plant materials; disease resulting from the ingestion of toxins produced by micro-organisms that have grown in a food.

Fortification : The addition of one of more nutrients to a food to make it richer than the unprocessed food, e.g., vitamin D milk.

Galactosemia : Accumulation of galactose in the blood owing to a hereditary lack of an enzyme to convert galactose to glucose; accompanied by severe mental retardation.

Gastrectomy : Surgical removal of part or all of the stomach.

Gastrin : Hormone secreted by pyloric mucosa that stimulates secretion of hydrochloric acid by parietal cells.

Gland : A cell or group of cells specialized for the production and secretion of a chemical substance or substances required by the organism.

Gliadin : A protein fraction of wheat gluten.

Globulin : A class of proteins insoluble in water and alcohol; serum globulin, lactoglobulin, myosin.

Glomerulus : The tuft of capillaries at the beginning of each tubule in the kidney.

Glossitis : Inflammation of the tongue.

Glucagon : Hormone produced by the alpha cells of the islets of Langerhans; raises blood sugar by increasing glycogen breakdown.

Glucocorticoid : Hormone produced by the adrenal cortex that influence glucose metabolism.

Glucogenic : Glucose forming.

Gluconeogenesis : Formation of glucose from non-carbohydrate sources, namely, certain amino acids and the glycerol fraction of fats.

Glucose : A single sugar occuring in fruits and honey; also obtained by the hydrolysis of starch, sucrose, maltose, and lactose; the sugar found in the blood; dextrose, grape sugar.

Glutamic acid : A dibasic non-essential amino acid widely distributed in proteins.

Glutathione : A tripeptide of glycine, glutamic acid, and cystine; can act as hydrogen acceptor and hydrogen donor.

Glutathione peroxidase : A selenium-containing enzyme believed to deactivate lipid peroxides.

Gluten : Protein in wheat and other cereals that gives elastic quality to a dough.

Glyceride : Organic ester of glycerol; fats are esters of fatty acids and glycerol.

Glycerol : A 3-carbon alcohol derived from the hydrolysis of fats.

Glycine : Aminoacetic acid; a non-essential amino acid.

Glycogen : Polysaccharide produced from glucose by the liver or the muscle, "animal" starch.

Glycogenesis : Formation of glycogen from glucose by the liver or muscle.

Glycogenolysis : Enzymatic breakdown of glycogen to glucose.

Glycolysis : The anaerobic conversion of glucose to pyruvic and lactic acids, an energy-yielding process.

Glycosuria : Presence of sugar in the urine.

Goiter : Enlargement of the tyroid gland.

Goitrogen : A substance that leads to goiter.

Gram stain : Differential staining procedure in which bacteria are classified as Gram-negative or Gram-positive, depending on whether they retain or lose the primary stain when subject to treatment with a decolorizing agent; the staining procedure reflects the underlying structural differences in the cell wall of Gram-negative and Gram positive bacteria.

Hematocrit : Separation of red cells from the plasma.

Hematuria : Condition in which urine contains blood.

Heme : Deep red pigment consisting of ferrous iron linked to protoporphyrin.

Heme iron : Form of iron in hemoglobin and in myoglobin which is absorbed intact.

Hemicellulose : A class of indigestible polysaccharides that form the cell wall of plants.

Hemoglobin : The iron-protein pigment in the red blood cells; carries oxygen to the tissues.

Hemolytic : Causing separation of hemoglobin from the red blood cells.

Hemopoietic : Concerned with the formation of blood.

Hemorrhage : Loss of blood from the vessels; bleeding.

Hemosiderin : Water-insoluble storage form of iron in the body.

Heparin : A mucopolysaccharide that prevents clotting of blood.

Hepatomegaly : Enalrgement of the liver.

Heterozygous : Possessing dissimilar pairs of genes for any hereditary trait.

Histidine : An essential amino acid.

Homeostasis : Tendency to maintain equilibrium in normal body states.

Homozygous : Having identical pairs of genes for any given pair of hereditary traits.

Hormone : Substance produced by an organ to produce a specific effect in another organ.

Hydrogenation : The addition of hydrogen to a compound, such as an unsaturated fatty acid to produce a solid fat.

Hydrolystate : The product of hydrolysis; e.g., protein hydrolystate is a mixture of the constituent amino acids when the protein molecule is split by acids, alkalies, or enzymes.

Hydrolysis : The splitting up of a product by the addition of water.

Hydroxyproline : A non-essential amino acid occurring abundantly in collagen.

Hypercalcemia : Abnormally high calcium level in the blood.

Hypercalciuria : Abnormal calcium excretion in the urine.

Hyperchlorhdria : Increased hydrochloric acid secretion by stomach cells.

Hyperchromic : Abnormally high colour.

Hyperchromic : Abnormally high colour.

Hyperesthesia : Increased sensitivity to touch or pain.

Hyperglycemia : An excess of sugar in the blood.

Hyperkalemia : An increased level of potassium in the blood.

Hyperlipoproteinema : Increased concentration of lipoproteins in the blood.

Hyperplasia : Abnormal multiplication of normal cells.

Hypertriglyceridemia : Increased levels of triglycerides in the blood.

Hypervitaminosis : Condition produced by excessive ingestion of vitamins, especially vitamins A and D.

Hypoalbuminemia : Low albumin level of the blood.

Hypochlorhydria : Decreased secretion of hydrochloric acid by the cells of the stomach.

Hypochromic : Below normal colour; e.g., pale red blood cells lacking hemoglobin.

Hypogeusia : Diminished sense of taste.

Hypoglycemia : A lower than normal level of glucose in the blood.

Hypokalemia : Decreased potassium level in the blood.

Hyposmia : Diminished sense of smell.

Hypothalamus : A group of nuclei at the base of the brain; includes centers of appetite control, cells that produce anti-diuretic hormone.

Idiopathic : Pertaining to a disease of unknown origin.

Idiosyncrasy : A susceptibility to action of food or drugs that is characterised or peculiar to an individual person.

Ileum Lower portion of the small intestine extending from the jejunum to the cecum.

Immunity : The relative unsusceptibility of a person or animal to active infection by pathogenic micro-organisms or the harmful effects of certain toxins; resistance to disease by a living organism.

Infarction : The formation of an area of dead tissue resulting from obstruction of blood vessels supplying the part.

Ingest : To take food into the body.

Insulin : Hormone secreted by beta cells of the islets of Lnagerhans of the pancreas; promotes utilization of glucose and lowers blood sugar.

Interstitial : Situated in spaces between tissues.

Intracellular : Within the cell.

Intravenous : Into a vein.

Intrinsic factor : Mucoprotein in gastric juice which facilitates absorption of vitamin B_{12}; deficient in patients with pernicious anemia.

Iodopsin : Pigment found in cones of the retina; visual violet.

Ionize : To separate molecules into electrically charged atoms or groups of atoms; the number of negative charges exactly equals the number of positive charges.

Ischemia : A local deficiency of blood, chiefly from narrowing of the arteries.

Isoleucine : An essential amino-acid.

Isotopes : Atoms of the same element having the same atomic numbers and chemical properties but differing in the nuclear masses.

Jaundice : Condition characterised by elevated bilirubin level of the blood and deposit of bile pigments in skin and mucous membranes.

Jejunum : Middle portion of small intestine; extends from duodenum to ileum.

Keratin : An insoluble sulfur-containing protein found in the skin, nails, hair.

Keratomalacia : Dryness and ulceration of the cornea resulting from vitamin A deficiency.

Ketogenesis : Formation of ketones from fatty acids and some amino acids.

α-ketoglutaric acid : One of the intermediate in the tricarboxylic acid cycle; also the product of oxidative deamination of glutamic acid.

Ketone : Any compound containing a ketone grouping; ketone bodies include acetone, beta-hydroxybutyric acid, and acetoacetic acid.

Ketosis : Condition resulting from incomplete oxidation of fatty acids, and the consequent accumulation of ketone bodies.

Kilocalorie : The unit of heat used in nutrition; the amount of heat required to raise 1,000 gm water 1°C.

Kwashiorkor : Deficiency disease related principally to protein lack and seen in severely malnourished children; characterized by growth failure, edema, pigment changes in the skin.

Labile : Chemically unstable.

Lactalbumin : A protein in milk.

Lactic Acid : 3-carbon acid produced in milk by bacterial fementation of lactose; also produced during muscle contraction by anaerobic glycolysis.

Lactose : A disaccharide composed of glucose and galactose; the form of carbohydrate in milk.

Lean body mass : A measure of body composition which excludes adiposetissue, extracellular fluids and the skeleton.

Lecithin : A phospholipid occuring in nervous and organ tissues, and in egg-yolk; effective emulsifer.

Leucine : An essential amino acid.

Lignin : Woody part of plants; a non-carbohydrate component of dietary fiber.

Limiting amino acid : The amino acid in a protein which is present in the least amount in proportion to what is needed, thus limiting the biological value of the protein.

Linoleic acid : An 18-carbon fatty acid with two double bonds; essential for growth and skin health.

Linolenic acid : An 18-carbon fatty acid with three double bonds, not an essential fatty acid.

Lipase : An enzyme that hydrolyzes fat.

Lipid : A term for fats including neutral fats, oils, fats, oils fatty acids, phospholipids, cholesterol.

Lipogenesis : Formation of fat.

Lipoic acid : Thictic acid; protogen; a factor that functions with thiamin pyrophosphate in removing the carboxyl group from alpha keto acids such as pyruvic acid.

Lipolysis : The splitting up of fat.

Lipoprotein : A conjugated protein that incorporates lipids to facilitate transportation of the lipids in an aqueous medium.

Lipotropic : Pertaining to substances that prevent accumulation of fat in the liver.

Low-density lipo-proteins : Complexes of triglycerides, cholesterol, and phospholipids with proteins in the blood; account for about three fourths of the cholesterol in the blood.

Lymph : The colourless fluid found in the lymph vessels, containing the water soluble components of blood and some cells; it is produced by the continual filtering of blood through the thin walls of the capillary blood vessels, and is returned to the blood stream through the lymphatic system.

Lysine : A diamino essential amino acid.

Lysosomes : Structures of cell cytoplasm that contain digestive enzymes.

Macrocyte : An abnormally large red blood cell.

Malignant : Occuring in severe form, frequently fatal, in tumors refers to uncontrollable growth as in cancer.

Malnutrition : Disturbance of form or function of an organism resulting from a deficiency or excess of one of more nutrients in its diet.

Maltose : A disaccharide resulting from starch hydrolysis; yields 2 molecules glucose on further hydrolysis.

Maramus : Extreme protein-calorie malnutrition marked by emaciation, especially severe in young children who receive insufficient amounts of food.

Mastication : The process of cheuring.

Matrix : The groundwork in which something is cast; for example, protein is the bone matrix into which mineral salts are deposited.

Metabolism : Physical and chemical changes occuring within the organism; includes synthesis of biologic materials and breakdown of substances to yield energy.

Metabolite : Any substance that results from physical and chemical changes within the organism.

Methionine : An essential sulfur containing amino acid; supplies labile methyl groups.

Micelle : A microscopic particle of lipids and bile salts.

Microvilli : Minute structures visible by electron microscope, present on surface on mucosal epithelium; the "brush border"

Micro organism : An animal or plant which is so small that it is only visible with a microscope.

Mitochondria : Rod-shaped or round structures in cell that trap energy-rich ATP.

Monoglyceride : An ester of glycerol with one fatty acid.

Monosaccharide : A single sugar not affected by hydrolysis; includes glucose, fructose, galactose.

Morbidity : The proportion of disease to health in a community.

Motility : Ability to move spontaneously.

Mucin : A substance containing muco-polysaccharides secreted by goblet cells of the intestine and other glandular cells; has a protective and lubricating action.

Mucopolysaccharide : Any of a group of polysaccharides combined with other groups such as protein.

Mucoprotein : A conjugated protein containing a carbohydrate group such as chondrotin sulfuric acid.

Mucosa : Membrane lining the gastro-intestinal, respiratory, and genito-urinary tracts.

Mumps : An acute infectious disease caused by a virus, characterized by swelling of the salivary glands.

Myocardium : The heart muscle.

Mycotoxins : Toxic substances produced by fungi, including aflatoxin, amatoxin, and ergot alkaloids.

Myoglobin : An iron-protein complex in muscle that transports oxygen; somewhat similar to hemoglobin.

Myosin : A soluble protein in muscle; combines with actin to form actomyosin, an enzyme that catalyzes the dephosphorylation of ATP during muscle contraction.

Nausea : Sickness at the stomach; inclination to vomit

Necrosis : Death of a cell or cells or of a portion of tissue.

Neonatal : Pertaining to the newborn.

Neoplasm : New or abnormal, uncontrolled growth such as a tumor.

Nephron : The functional unit of the kidney consisting of a tuft of capillaries known as the glomerulus attached to the renal tubule.

Neuritic : Pertaining to inflammation of a nerve.

Neutopathy : Disease of the nervous system.

Niacin equivalent : The total niacin available from the diet including preformed niacin plus that derived from the metabolism of tryptophan; 60mg tryptophan = 1 mg niacin.

Nicotinamide adenine dinucleotide, NAD : Coenzyme for a number of enzymes, chiefly dehydrogenases.

Necturia : Excessive urination at night.

Non-heme Iron : The form ofiron in furits, vegetables, cereals eggs, and dairy products as well as the iron in meat, poultry, and fish not associated with hemoglobin or myoglobin.

Nucleic acid : Complex organic acid containing four bases—adenine, guanine, cytosine, and thymine—attached to ribose and phosphate.

Nucleoprotein : Conjugated protein in the nuclei of cells, yields a protein fraction and nucleic acid.

Nucleotide : A hydrolytic product of nucleic acid; contains one purine or pyrimidine base and a sugar phosphate.

Nutrient : Chemical substance in foods which nourishes, e.g., amino-acid, fat, calcium.

Nutrient density : The ratio of the nutritive value of a food or diet to its caloric contribution.

Nyctalopia : Nigh blindness.

Obesity : A condition in which an excess amount of fat accumulates in the body; it may be expressed relative to a standard body weight or as the percentage of the total body weight which is made up of fat.

Oil immersion lens : A high-power objective lens of a microscope designed to work with the space between the objective and the specimen, filled with oil to enhance resolution.

Oleic acid : An 18-carbon fatty acid containing one double bond, widely distributed in foods.

Oliguria : Seanty secretion of urine.

Organelles : The various structures of the cell such as lysosomes, mitochondria.

Ornithine : An amino acid formed from arginien when urea is split off.

Osmosis : Passage of a solvent from the lesser to the greater concentration when two solutions are separated by a membrane.

Ossification : Formation of bone.

Osteomalacia : Softening of the bone, chiefly in adults.

Osteoporosis : Reduction of the quantity of bone, occurring principally in women after middle age; the remaining bone is normally mineralized.

Oxalic acid : A dicorboxylic acid present in foods such as spinach, chard, rhubarb, forms insoluble salts with calcium.

Oxaloacetic acid : A-3 carbon ketodicarboxylic acid; an intermediate in the tricarboxylic acid cycle.

Oxidation : Increase in positive charges on an atom or loss of negative charges.

Palmitic acid : A 16-carbon saturated fatty acid widespread in foods.

Pancreozymin : Hormone produced in duodenal mucosa that stimulates secretion of pancreatic enzymes.

Parathormone : Secretion of parathyroid gland that regulates calcium and phosphorus metabolism.

Parenchyma : Functional tissue of an organ or gland as distinct from its supporting framework.

Parenteral : By other means than through the gastro-intestinal tract; introduction of nutrients by vein or into subcutaneous.

Paresthesia : Abnormal sensation such as numbness, burnign, pricking.

Pasteurization : Reduction in the number of micro-organisms by exposure to elevated temperatures but not necessarily the killing of all micro-organisms in a sample; a form of heat treatment that is lethal for the casual agents of a number of milk-transferable diseases, as well as for a proportion of normal milk microbiota, which also inactivates certain bacterial enzymes that may cause deterioration in milk.

Pathology : Science dealing with disease; structural and functional changes causes by disease.

Pectin : A polysaccharide found in many fruits and having properties.

Pellagra : A deficiency disease of the skin, gastrointestinal tract, and nervous system caused by lack of niacin and associated with other nutritional deficiencies.

Peptone : An intermediate product of protein digestion.

Peristalsis : The rhythmic, wave like movement produced by muscles of the small intestine to move food forward.

pH : Measure of acidity or alkalinity; the scale goes from Oto 14, with pH=7 as the neutral point, so that pH values above 7 indicate alkalimity and those less than 7 acidity.

Phagocyte : A cell capable of ingesting bacteria or other foreign material.

Phenylalanine : An essential amino acid; consists of a pheny group attached to alanine.

Phynylketonuria : Excretion of phenylpyruvic acid and other phenyl compounds in urine because of congenital lack of an enzyme required for conversion of phenylalanine to tyrosine; characterized by mental retardation.

Phospholipid : A fat like compound that contains a phosphate and another group such as a nitrogen base in addition to glycerol and fatty acids, e.g., lecithin, cephalin.

Phosphoprotein : A conjugated protein that contains phosphorus e.g., nucleoprotein, casein.

Phosphorylate : To introduce a phosphate grouping into an organic compound, e.g., glucose mono-phosphate produced by action of enzyme phosphorylase.

Photosynthesis : The process whereby the chlorophyll in green plants utilizes the energy from the sun to synthesize carbohydrate from carbon dioxide and water.

Physiology : The study of the normal functions and chemical processes which go on within a living organism.

Phytic acid : A phosphoric acid ester of inositol found in seeds, interferes with absorption of calcium, magnesium, iron, zinc.

Pica : A hunger for substances not fit for food.

Pinocytosis : The taking up of droplets by a cell by surrounding the liquid with part of the membrane.

Plaque : Any patch or flat area; atherosclerotic plaque is a deposit of lipid material in the blood vessel.

Plasma : Fluid portion of the blood before clotting has taken place. Polyneuritis : Inflammation of a number of nerves.

Polypeptide : A compound consisting of more than three amino acids; an intermediate stage in protein digestion.

Polyphagia : Excessive eating.

Polysaccharide : A class of carbohydrates containing many single sugars; includes starch glycogen, dextrins, pectins, cellulose and others.

Polyunsaturated fatty acid : Fatty acids containing two or more double bonds, linoleic, linolenic, and arachidonic acids.

Porphyrin : A pigmented compound containing four pyrrole neclei joined in a ring structure; combines with iron in hemoglobin.

Precursor : Anything that precedes another or form which another is derived; for example, carotene is a precursor to vitamin A.

Primary Immune Response : The first immune response to a particular antigen that has a characteristically long lag period and a relatively low titer of antibody production.

Processed foods : Cheese products to which water has been added, thereby diluting their nutritional vlaue.

Progesterone : Hormone of corpus luteum which prepares endometrium for reception and development of the fertilized ovum.

Prophylaxis : Prevention of disease.

Prosthetic group: Chemical group attached to a molecule such as protein; non-protein part of an enzyme.

Protease : An enzyme that digests protein.

Proteins : Complex compounds built up from some thousands of amino-acid units; the properties of a particular protein depend on the number, type and arrangement of amino acid units within the molecule.

Protein Efficiency Ratio : A measure of the quality of a protein by calculating the weight gain of an experimental animal per gram of protein fed.

Proteinuria : Excretion of protein in the urine.

Proteolytic : Effecting the hydrolysis of protein.

Prothrombin : Factor in blood plasma for blood clotting; precursor of thrombin.

Protoplasm : Form of living matter in all cells.

Protoporphyrin : A porphyrin combined with iron and globin forming hemoglobin.

Provitamin : Precursor of a vitamin.

Proximal : Nearest to the head or point of attachment.

Purine · Organic compounds containing heterocyclic nitrogen structures that are catabolized to uric acid; supplied especially by flesh foods and synthesized in the body.

Pyridoxal Phosphate : A coenzyme that contains vitamin B_6.

Pyridoxine : One of the forms of vitamin B_6.

Pyruvic acid : A 3-carbon keto acid; an intermediate in glucose metabolism.

Rancid : Term that describes rank taste or smell that results from decomposition of fatty acids.

Reagins : A group of anti-bodies in serum that react with the allergens responsible for the specific manifestations of human hypersensitivity; heterophile antibody formed during syphilis infections.

Reflex Action : An involuntary or automatic response by an organism to a change in its environments.

Remission : A lessening of the severity or temporary abatement of symptoms.

Renal threshold : The level of concentration of a substance in the blood beyond which it is excreted in the urine.

Reinin : Enzyme produced by the kidney.

Residue : Remainder; the contents remaining in the intestinal tract after digestion of food: includes fiber and other unabsorbed products.

Resorption : A loss of substance.

Reticulocyte : A young red blood cell occuring during active blood regeneraion.

Reticuloendothelium : A system of macrophages concerned with phagocytosis; present in spleen, liver, bone marrow, connective tissues, and lymph nodes.

Retinol : Vitamin A alcohol.

Retinopathy : Degenerative disease of the retina.

Rhodopsin : Visual purple; pigment of the rods of the retina bleached by light; vitamin A required for regeneration.

Ribonucleic acid, RNA : Molecules in cytoplasm which serve for transfer of amino acid code from nucleus and the synthesis of protein.

Ribose : 5-carbon sugar; a constituent of nucleic acid.

Rickets : A deficiency disease of the skeletal system caused by a lack of vitamin D or calcium or both, and often resulting in bone deformities.

Saccharin : A sweetening agent that is 300 to 500 times as sweet as sugar; yields no calories.

Salmonella : Group of bacteria causing intestinal infection; frequently contaminates foods.

Saponification : The action of alkali on a fat to form a soap.

Satiety : Feeling of satisfaction following meals.

Saturated : A state in which a substance holds the most of another substance that it can.

Scurvy : A deficiency disease caused by lack of ascorbic acid and leading to swollen bleeding gums, hemorrhages of the skin and mucous membranes, and anemia.

Secretin : A hormone secreted by the epithelium of the duodenum upon stimulation by the acid chyme; stimulates secretion of pancreatic juice and bile.

Serine : One of the amino acids occuring in protein; non-essential.

Serosa : The membranes lining the peritoneal, pericardial, and pleural cavities and covering their contents.

Serum : The fluid portion of the blood that separates from the blood cells after clotting.

Siderophilin : An iron-trasferring protein; transferrin.

Soap : A salt of a fatty acid usually with an alkali metal; for example, sodium stearate.

Sorbitol : A 6-carbon sugar alcohol with a sweet taste; used commercially to maintain moisture and inhibit crystal formation.

Sour : Tart test due to the presence of acid in foods; can be evidence of microbial spoilage or the desired result of controlled fermentation to produce a food product; caused by accumulation of acidic products of microbial metabolism.

Sphincter : A muscle surrounding and closing an orifice.

Spore : A cell, or goup of cells, which become detached from the parent organism and which can eventually develop into a new individual; some spores are resting forms of the organism which enable it to survive unfavourable environmental conditions.

Starch : A polysaccharide which is a mixture of two dissimilar polysaccharides, any lose and any lopectin, both consisting of chains of glucose units it is the chief food reserve substance of plants.

Steapsin : A hormone in pancreatic juice that hydrolyzes fat, lipase.

Stearic acid : A saturated fatty acid containing 18 carbo atoms.

Steatorrhea : Excessive amount of fat in the feces.

Steroid : A group of compounds similar in structure to cholesterol; includes bile acids, sterols, sex hormones.

Sterol : An alcohol of high molecular weight; cholesterol, ergosterol.

Stomatitis : Inflammation of the mucous membranes of the mouth.

Substrate : Substance upon which an enzyme acts.

Succinic acid : A 3-carbon dicarboxylic acid that is an intermediate in the tricarboxylic acid cycle.

Sucrose : Cane or beet sugar, a disaccharide that yields glucose and fructose when hydrolyzed.

Symptom : A physiological disorder that results in a detectable deviation from the normal healthy state and is usually indicated by compalints from a patient.

Syndrome : A set of symptoms occuring together.

Synthesis : Process of building up a compound.

Tachycardia : Rapid beating of the heart.

Testosterone : Testicular hormone responsible for male secondary sex characteristics.

Tetanus : Lock jaw, a disease of humans and other animals in which the symptoms are due to a powerful neurotoxin formed by the casual agent, clostridum tetani, present in an anaerobic would or other lesion, characterized by sustained involuntary contraction of the muscles of the jaw and neck.

Thermogenesis : The capacity to dissipate some of the energy provided by food as heat, after it has been eaten.

Threonine : An essential amino acid.

Thrombus : A clot in a blood vessel formed by coagulation of blood.

Thymine : One of the four nitrogenous bases in nucleic acid.

Throxine : Iodine-containing hormone produced by the thyroid gland; regulates the rate of energy metabolism.

Tocopherol : Vitamin E; antioxidant alcohol occurring in vegetable germ oils; alpha-, beta-, gamma-, delta- tocopherol.

Toxicity : The quality of being toxic; the kind and quantity of a poison produced by a micro-organism or possessed by a non-biological chemical.

Toxin : A poisonous substance produced by the metabolism of a plant or animal, especially certain bacteria.

Toxemia of pregnancy : A disorder of pregnancy characterized by hypertension, edema, albuminuria.

Toxoid : A modified protein exotoxin that has lost its toxicity but has retained it specific anti-genicity.

Transamination : Transfer of an amino group to another molecule, e.g., transfer to a keto acid, thus forming another amino acid.

Transferase : An enzyme that transfers a chemical grouping from one compound to another, for example, transaminase, transphosphorylase.

Transferrin : Iron-binding protein for transport of iron in blood siderophilin.

Trauma : Wound or injury usually inflicted suddenly.

Triglyceride : An ester of glycerol and three fatty acids.

Trypsin : A protein-digesting enzyme secreted by the pancreas and released into the small intestine.

Trypsinogen : Inactive form of trypsin

Tryptophan : An essential amino acid that contains the indole ring; a precursor of niacin.

Tuber : The part of an underground stem which is swollen with food deserves; it carries buds which can give rise to new plants.

Tyrosine : Semi-essential amino acid; spares phenylanine; the amino acid in thyroxine.

Urea : Chief nitrogenous consistent of the urine; formed by the liver when amino acids are deaminized.

Uremia : Presence of urinary constituents in the blood resulting from deficient secretion of urine.

Uric acid : A nitrogenous costituent formed in the metabolism of purines; excreted in the urine; blood levels increased in gout.

Vaccine : Any antigenic preparation administered to stimulate the recipent's immune defense mechanisms with respect to given pathogens or toxic agents.

Valine : An essential amino acid.

Vegetable : A plant or part of a plant which is used as a foodstuff, the word is also used as an adjective to indicate plant orisins, as in vegetable oil, vegetable protein.

Villus : Fingerlike projection of the intestinal mucosa.

Vinegar : A condiment prepared by the microbial oxidation of ethanol to acetic acid.

Virus : A non-cellular entity that consists minimally of protein and nucleic acid and than can replicate only after entry into specific types of living cells; it has no intrinsic metabolism, and its replication is dependent on the direction of cellular metabolism by the viral genome; within the host cell, viral components are synthesized separately and are assembled intracellularly to form mature infectious viruses.

Visual purple : Photosensitive pigment found in the rods of the retina; rhodopsin.

Vitamin : Organic compound occurring in minute amounts in foods and essential for numerous metabolic reactions; fat-soluble A, D,

E, and K; water-soluble ascorbic acid and B complex.

Xanthine : An intermediate in the metabolism of purines; related to uric acid.

Xanthomatosis : Accumulation of lipids in the form of tumors in various parts of the body.

Xerophthalmia : Dry infected eye condition caused by lack of vitamin A.

Xerosis : Abnormal dryness of skin and eye.

Xylose : A 5-carbon aldehyde sugar that is not metabolized by the body.

Yeast : Single-celled fungi, many of which produce ethane and carbondioxide as the products of their metabolism of carbohydrate foods.

Zein : A protein of low biologic value present in corn.

Zymogen : The inactive form of an enzyme.

Bibliography

Abidi SA and Allen ER, "Impaired jejunal absorption rates of essential amino acids induced by either dietary caloric or protein deprivation in man", Gastroenterology 1970; 59:404–13.

Agus ZA, Wasserstein A, Gold Farb S. "Disorders of Calcium and Magnesium Homeostasis", Am. J. Med 1982; 72 : 473–88.

Allison J B and Wannamacher R N Jr. "The concept and significance of Labile and Overall Protein Reserves of the Body", Am. J. Clin. Nutr 1965; 16:445–52.

Alton I R "Nutrition Services for Pregnant Adolescents within a Public High School", J. Am. Diet. Assoc. 1979; 74 : 667–69.

Anonymous, "Advances in Biotechnology of Lysine Production", Nutr Rev. 1985; 43 : 88–90.

Anonymous. "Growth of Vegetarian Children", Nutr. Rev. 1979; 37 : 108–09.

Anonymous. "Clouds over Galactosemia", Lancet 1982; ii : 1379–80.

Anonymous. "Clay Eating", Lancet 1978; ii:614–15.

Anonymous. "Recent Advances in Research of Flouride Toxicity and Flourosis", ICMR Bull 1979; 9:1–5.

Anonymous "Hot peppers and substance P (Editorial)" Lancet 1983; i:1198.

Arvanitakis C, Chen GH, Folscroft J, Greenberger N J : "Effect of Aspirin on Intestinal Absorption of Glucose, Sodium and

Water in Man", Gut 1977; 18:187–90.

Asatoor A M, Cheng B, Edwards KDG, et al : "Intestinal Absorption of Two Dipeptides in Hartnup Disease", Gut 1970; 11:380–87.

Babu S, Srikantia S G "Availability of Folates from Some Foods", Am. J. Clin. Nutr 1976; 29:376–79.

Bapurao S, Krishna Swamy K. "Vitamin B_6 Nutritional, Status of Pellagrins and Their Leucine Tolerance", Am. J. Clin. Nutr. 1978; 31:819–24.

Boland R L : "Plants as a Source of Vitamin B_3 Metabolites", Nutr. Rev. 1986; 44:1–8.

Brook C E and Anast C S : "Oral Fluid and Electrolytes", JAMA. 1962; 179:792–97.

Burkitt D P, et al : "Dietary Fibre and Disease", JAMA 1974; 229:1068–74.

Cahill C F Jr., Herrera M G, Morgan A P, et al : "Hormone—Fuel Interrelationships during Fasting", J. Clin. Invest. 1966; 45:1751–69.

Campbell C H : "The Severe Lactic Acidosis of Thiamine Deficiency : Acute Pernicious or Fulminating Beri Beri", Lancet 1984; ii:466–49.

Chandra R : "Imminological Aspects of Human Milk", Nutr. Rev. 1978; 36:265–72.

Committee on Drugs and on Nutrition, American Academy of Pediat rics : "The Use and Abuse of Vitamin A", Nutr. Rev. 1974; 32:41–43.

Condon J R, Nassim D R, Millard F J C, Hilbe A, Slainthrope E M : "Calcium and Phosphorus Metabolism in Relation to Lactose Tolerance", Lancet 1970; i: 1027–29.

Connor W E, Lin D.: "The Intestinal Absorption of Dietary Cholesterol by Hypercholesterolaemic and Normal Humans", j. Lab. Clin. Med. 1970; 76:870.

Cook J D, Monsen E F : "Food Iron Absorption in Human Subjects III Comparison of the Effect of Animal Proteins on Non-heme Iron Absorption", Am. J. Clin. Nutr. 1976; 29: 859–67.

Cook J D, Reusser M E : "Iron Fortification and Update", Am. J. Clin. Nutr. 1983; 38:648–49.

Consolazio C F : "Comparison of Nitrogen, Calcium and Iodine Excretion in Arm and Total Body Sweat", Am. J. Clin. Nutr. 1966; 18:443–48.

Consolazio C F, et al : "Protein Metabolism During Intesive Physical Training in the Young Adult", Am. J. Clin Nutr. 1975; 29:29–35.

Crossby W H : "Pica", JAMA 1976; 235 : 2765.

Costill D L, Sherman W M, Fink W J, Maresh C, Witten M, Miller J M : "The Role of Dietary Carbohydrates in Muscle Glycogen Resynthesis after Sternous Running", Am. J. Clin. Nut 1981; 34:1831–36.

Cottrell R C : "Vitamin E", Nutr. Bull 1984; 9:143–54.

Coursin D B : "Convulsive Seizures in Infants with Pyridoxine Deficient Diet", JAMA 1954; 154:406–08.

Daniel W A Jr., et al : "Dietary Intakes and Plasma Concentrations of Folate in Healthy Adolescents", Am. J. Clin. Nutr. 1975; 28 : 363–70.

Debongnie J C, Phillips S F : "Functional Reserve Capacity of the Human Large Bowel (Abstract)", Gastroenterology 1976; 70:A18/876.

Deluca H F : "The Vitamin D System in the Regulation of Calcium and Phosphorus Metabolism", Nutr. Rev. 1979; 37:161–93.

Deosthale YG : "Home Processing : A Nutritive Value of Pulses", Nutrition News, Hyderabad, NIN, 1982; Vol. 3, No. 1.

Descouich G C, Ceredic, Gaddi A, et al : "Multicentre Study of Soybean Protein Diet for Out Patient Hypocholes Ferolaemic Patients, Lancet 1980; ii : 709–12.

Dreyfus P M : "Thiamin and Nervous System : An Over View". J. Nutr. Sci. Vitamin nol, 1976; 22: 13–16.

Dwyer J T, et al : "Pre-schoolers on Alternate Life Style Diets", J. Am. Diet. Assoc. 1978; 72: 264–70.

Felig P, Cherif A Minagawa A, Wahren J : "Hypologycemia During Prolonged Excercise in Normal Mena", N. Engl. J. Med. 1982; 306 : 895–900.

Filer L J : "Salt in Infant Foods", Nutr. Rev. 1971; 29:27–30.

Finch C A and Monsen E R: "Iron Nutrition and Fortification of Food with Iron", JAMA 1972; 219:1462–65.

Foman S J et al : "Recommendations for Feeding Normal Infants", Pediatric, 1979; 63: 52–59.

Fradkin J E, Wolff J : "Iodine Induced Thyrotoxicosis. Medicine", 1983; 62:1–20.

Fraser D R and Kodicek E : "Unique Biosynthesis by Kidney of Biochemically Active D Metabolite", Nature 1970; 228:764–66.

Gilsanz. V, Alvarez J L , Serrano S, Simon J : "Evolution of the Ailmentary Toxic Oil Syndrome Due to Ingestion of Denatured Rape Seed Oil", Ann. Intern. Med. 1984, 144:254–56.

Glueck C J : "Appraisal of Dietary Fat as Causative Factor in Atherogensis", Am. J. Clin. Nutr. 1979; 32:2637–43.

Glusman N "The Syndrome of 'Burning Fee' as a Manifestationof Nutritional Deficiency", Am. J. Med. 1947; 3:211–23.

Goldsmit H S : "Coconut Water for Intraveneous Therapy," Br. J. Surg. 1962; 4: 421–22.

Gotto A M : "Is Atherosclerosis Reversible", J. Am. Diet. Assoc. 1979; 74:551–57.

Gubler C J : "Absorption and Metabolism of Iron", Science, 1956; 123 : 87–90.

Gupta N N, Mehrotra R M L, Sircar A R : "Effect of Onion on Serum Cholesterol, Blood Coagulation Factors and Fibrinolytic Activity in Ailmentary Lipemia", Indian J. Med. Res. 1966; 54: 48–53.

Hardinge M G, et al : "Nutritional Studies of Vegetarians. V. Proteins and Essential Amino Acids", J. Am. Diet. Assoc. 1966; 48: 25–28.

Hardinge M G, et al : "Carbohydrates in Foods, J. Am. Diet. Assoc. 1965; 46 : 197–204.

Hegsted D M : "Assessment of Nitrogen Requirements, Am. J. Clin. Nutr. 1978; 31: 1669–71.

Henkin R I , et al : "Idiopathic Hypogeusia, Hyposmia and Dysosmia A New Syndrome", JAMA 1971; 217: 434–40.

Het Zel B S : "Iodine Deficiency Disorders and their Eradication",

Lancet 1983; ii: 1126–29.

Heyssel R M, et al : "Vitamin B_{12} Turnover in Man", Am. J. Clin. Nutr. 1966; 18: 176–84.

Hook E B : "Dietary Cravings and Aversions During Pregnancy", Am. J. Clin. Nutr. 1978; 31: 1355–62.

Horwitt M K et al : "Correlation of Urinary Excretion of Riboflavin with Dietary Intake and Symptoms of a Riboflavinasis", J. Nutr. 1950; 41: 247–64.

Huenemann. R L, et al : "A Congitudinal Study of Gross Body Composition and Body Conformation and Their Association with Food and Activity in a Teen Age Population. View of Teen Age subjects on body conformaiton, food and activity", Am. J. Clin. Nutr. 1966; 18: 325–38.

Hussey H H : "Taste and Smell Deviations : Importance of Zinc", JAMA 1974; 228: 1669–70.

Issacs G : "Permanent Local Anaethesia and Anhidrosis After Clover Oil Spillage", Lancet 1983; i:882.

Jackson R L "Maternal and Infant Nutrition and Health in Later Life", Nutr. Rev. 1979; 37: 33–37.

Jenkins D A J, Wolever T M, Jenkins A L, Josse R G, Wong G S : "The Glycaemic Response to Carbohydrate Foods", Lancet, 1984; ii:388–91.

Johnston F A : "Calcium Retained by Young Women before and After Adding Spinach to the Deit", J. Am. Diet. Assoc. 1952; 28: 933–38.

Jungalwala F B, Cama H R: "Carotenoids in Mango Fruit", Indian. J. Chem. 1963; i:36–40.

Kabara J J: "Lipids as Hast Resistance Factors in Human Milk", Nutr. Rev. 1980; 38: 65–73.

Karlowski T R , Chalmers T C, Frenkel L D, Kapikian A Z, Lewis T L, Lynch J M. "Ascorbic Acid for the Common Cold, A Prophy lactic and Theropentic Trail", JAMA 1975; 231: 1038–42.

Kerilin P, Wong L, Harris B, Capra S : "Rice Flour, Breath Hydrogen, and Malabsorption", Gastroenterology 1984; 87: 578–85.

Kopple J D, Swendeseid M E : "Evidence that Histidine is an Essential Amino Acid in Normal and Chronically Uremic Man", J. Clin.

Invest. 1975; 55: 881–91.

Leeds A R, Ralphs D N L, Ebied F, Metz G, Dilawari J B. "Pectin in Dumping Syndrome : Reduction of Symptoms and Plasma Volume Changes", Lancet 1981; i: 1075–8.

Levine A S, Silvis S E: "Absorption of Whole Peanuts, Peanut Oil and Peanut Butter", N. Engl. Med. 1980; 303: 917–18.

Lion O K, Jay L T, Rose C S, Prawiranegare D D, Gyorgy P : "Red Pal Oil in the Prevention ofVitamin A Deficiency—A Trial on Pre-School Children in Indonesia", Am. J. Clin. Nutr. 1967; 20:1267–74.

Macy I G : "Metabolic and Biochemical Changes in Normal Pregnancy", JAMA 1958; 168: 2265–71.

Martinez-Torres C; Romano E, Lay Risse M: "Effect of Cysteine on Iron Absorption in Man", Am. J. Clin. Nutr. 1981; 34: 322–7.

Mattson F A, Grundy S M, Crouse J E : "Optimizing the Effect of Plant Sterols on cholesterol Absorption in Man", Am. J. Clin. Nutr. 1982; 35: 697–700.

Mc Cance R A , Widdowson E M : "Old Thoughts and New Work on Breads White and Brown", Lancet 1955; ii: 205–10.

Mc Collum E V and Davis M : "The Necessity of Certain Lipids in the Diet during Growth", Jol. Biol. Chem 1913; 15: 167–75 See Nutrition Classic. Nutr. Rev. 1973; 31: 280–81.

Mc Curdy P R "B_{12} Shots", JAMA 1974; 229:703.

Mc Ganity W J, et al "Vanderbilt co-operative Study of Maternal and Infant Nutrition XII Effect of Reproductive Cycle on Nutritional Status and Requirements, JAMA 1958; 168: 2138–45.

Mc Gill H C Jr. "Appraisal of Cholesterol as a Curative Factor in Atherogenesis", Am. J. Clin. Nutr. 1979; 32: 2632–36.

Mc Millan M, Thomson J G : "An Outbreak of Suspected Solanine Poisoning in School Boys. Examination of Criteria of Solanine Poisoning" A. J. Med. 1979; 48:227–43.

Mc Millan J A, Landon S A, Oski F A: "Iron Sufficiency in Breast Fed Infants and Availability of Iron from Human Milk", Pediatrics 1976; 58: 686–91.

Minot G R and Murphy WP : "Treatment of Pernicious Anemia by a

Special Diet", JAMA 1926; 84: 470–76 Reproduced in Part in Nutr. Rev. 1978; 36: 50–52.

Monson E R, et al : "Estimation of Available Dietary Iron", Am. J. Clin. Nutr. 1978; 31: 134–41.

Morck T A, Lynch S R, Cook J D: "Reduction of Soy induced Infribition of non heme Iron Asborption", Am. J. Clin. Nutr. 1982; 36:219–28.

Morck T A, Lynch S R, Cook J D. "Reduction of Soy Induced Infribition of non-heme Iron Absorption", Am. J. Clin. Nutr. 1982; 36: 219–28.

Morck T A, Lynch S R, Cook J D: "Inhibition of Food Iron Absorption by Coffee", Am. J. Clin. Nutr. 1983; 37: 416–20.

Ngindu A, Johnson B K, Kenya P R, et al :"Outbreak of Acute Hepatiris caused by Aflatoxin Poisoning in Kenya", Lancet 1982; i : 134–48.

Nicholus Butkus and Mahan "Food Allergies : Immunological Reactions to Food", JADA 1986; 86: 601–608.

Nomenclature Policy : Generic Descriptions and Trivial Names for Vitamins and Related Compounds, J. Nutr. 1980; 110 : 8–15.

Oomen HAPC : "Vitamin A Deficiency, Xeropthalmia and Blindness", Nutr. Rev. 1974, 32: 161–70.

Osborne T B and Mendel L B: "The Relation of Growth to the Chemical Constituents of the Diet", J. Biol. Chem. 1913; 15: 311–26.

parsons H T, et al : "Inter-relationship between Dietary Egg white and Requirements for Protective Factor in Cure of Nutritional Disorder due to Egg white", Biochem. J. 1937; 31: 424–32.

Pasricha J S "Food Allergy" Indian. Journal. Pediatrics 1981; 48: 47–50.

Pelletier O and Keith MO : "Bio Availability of Synthetic and Natural Ascorbic Acid}, J. Am. Diet. Assoc. 1974; 64: 271–75.

Pelletier O: "Vitamin C and cigerette Smokers", Ann. N. Y. Acad. Sci. 1975; 258: 156–62.

Pereira S M, Begum A : "Studies in the Prevention of Vitamin A Deficiency, Indian. J. Med. Res. 1968; 56: 362–69.

Porikas K P, Vanitalie T B: "Diet Induced Changes in Serum Transaminose and Triglyceride Levels in Healthy Adult Men. Role of Sucrose and Excess Calories", Am. J. Med. 1983; 75: 624–30.

Ravich W J, Bayless T M, Thomas M: "Fructose in Complete Intestinal Absorption in Human", Gastroenterology 1983; 84:26–9.

Reeds P J, James WPT : "Proteinutur", Lancet 1983; i: 571–4.

Report of the Working Group on Fortification of salt with iron use of common salt fortified with iron in the control and prevention of anemia—a collaborative Study. Am. J. Clin. Nutr. 1982; 35:1442–51.

Ritchine J H, et al "Edema and Hemolytic Anemia in Pre-mature infants: A Vitamin E Deficiency Syndrome", N. Engl. J. Med. 1968; 279: 1185–90.

Rivlin R S: "Hormones Drugs and Riboflavin", Nutr. Rev. 1979; 37: 241–46.

Rivers J M: "Oral Contraceptives and Ascorbic Acid", Am. J. Clin. Nuts 1975; 28: 550–54.

Roberts H J : "Vitamin E and Thrombophlebitis", Lancet 1978; i: 49.

Rose W C, et al : "Further Experiments on the Role of Amino Acids in Human Nutrition", J. Biol. Chem 1943; 148: 457–58.

Rose W C, Wixom R L, Lockhart HB, Lambert G R : "The Amino Acid Requirements of Man. XV. The Valine Requirement; Summary and Final Observations", J. Biol. Che. 1955; 217: 987–1004.

Rungruangro K, Tosukh Wong P, Panijpan B, Vimokesant S L. "Chemical Interactions Between Thiamine and Tannic Acid. I. Kinetics, Oxygen Dependence and Inhibition by Ascorbic Acid", Am. J. Clin. Nutr. 1977; 30: 1680–85.

Schaumburg H S, Kaplan J, Winde Bank A, et al : "Sensory Neuropethy from Pyridoxine Abuse. A new Mega Vitamin Syndrome", N. Engl. J. Med. 1983; 309: 445–48.

Stearns A : "Nutritional State of the Mother Prior to Conception", JAMA 1958; 168: 1655–59.

Shank R E "A Chink in Our Armous", Nutr. Today 1970; 5: 3–11

Smith I, Lobascher M E, Stevenson J E, et al : "Effect of Stopping Low Phenyl Alanine Diet on Intellectual Progress of Children with Phenyl Ketonuric", Br. med. J. 1978; 2: 723–6.

Snyderman S E et al : "Pyridoxine Deficiency in Human Infant", Am. J. Clin. Nutr. 1954; 1 : 200-07.

Solomons N W Russell R M : "The Interaction of Vitamin A and Zinc : Implications for Human Nutrition", Am. J. Clin. Nutr. 1980; 33: 2031–40.

Stoff J S : "Phosphate Homeostasis and Hypophosphatemia", Am. J. Med. 1982; 72: 489–95.

Stokes P L. et al : "Folate Metabolism in Scurvy", Am. J. Clin. Nutr. 1975; 28: 126-29.

Sur. A M, Bhati. A : "Indian Childhood Cirrhosis : An Inherited Disorder of Tryptophan Metabolism ?", Br. Med. J. 1978; 2:529-31.

Tanaka K, Kean E A, Johnson B. "Jamaican Vomiting Sickness--Biochemical Investigation of Two Cases", N. Engl. J. Med. 1976; 295: 461-67.

Taylor L "Food Allergies and Sensitivities" JADA 1986, May; 86: 599–600.

Teotia S P S, Teotia M, Singh R K, Taves D R, Heels S : "Endocrine Aspects of Endemic Skeletal Fluorosis", J. Assoc. Physicians, India 1978; 26: 996–1000.

Trowell K "Ischemic Heart Disease and Dietary Fibre", Am. J. Clin. Nutr. 1972; 25: 926–32.

Tsai A C et al "Study on the Effect of Megavitamin E Supplementation in Man", Am. J. Clin. Nutr. 1978; 31: 831-37.

Tsai A C, Kelley J J, Peng B, Cook N. "Study on the Effect of Mega Vitamin Supplementation in Man", Am. J. Clin. Nutr. 1978; 31 : 831–37.

Vickery H B : "The Origin of the Word Protein", Yale. J. Biol. Med. 1950; 22: 387–93.

Vijayaraghavan K, Sarma K V R, Rao N P, Reddy V: "Impact of Massive Doses of Vitamin A on incidence of nutritional blindness", Lancet 1984; ii: 149–51.

Whang R, Oei TO, Aikawa J K, A, Vannatta J, Frayer A; "Predictors of Hypomagnesemia, Hypokalemia, Hypophosphatemia, Hyponatremia and Hypocalcemia", Arch. Intern. Med. 1984; 144: 1794-96.

Wheat Foods : Nutritional Implications in Health and Disease" Proceedings of a sumpasium held in Washington, DC, May, 21–22, 1984, Am. J. Clin. Nutr. 1985; 41 (Suppl.).

Williams C D : "The Story of Kwashiorkor", Nutr. Rev. 1973; 31: 334-40.

Wood B et al: "A Study of Partial Thiamin Restriction in Human Volunteers", Am. J. Clin. Nutr. 1980; 33: 848–61.

Wurtman R J : "Behavioural Effects of Nutrients", Lancet 1983; i: 1145–7.

York DA : "The Theimic Effects of Diet", Nutr. Bull 1981; 6: 22–9

Index

Adipose tissue, 37
Adulteration of food stuffs, 240–44
  Food adulterants, 242–44
  Injurious to health, 240
  Intentional additives, 242
Agmark, 240
Albuminoios, 36
Albumins, 36
Alcoholic beverages, 214–16
  Ale, 215
  Arrack, 216
  Beer, 215
  Brandy, 215
  Cider, 215
  Gin, 216
  Porter, 215
  Rum, 216
  Stout, 215
  Toddy, 215
  Vodka, 216
Ale, 215
Allergy from food, 265–73
  Antibodies molecules, 267, 270
  Assessment of, 271–73
    Diet diaries, 271–72
    Elimination diet, 271–72
    History of, 271
    Immunological list, 272
    Leukopenic index, 272
    Provocative diet, 272
    Treatment, 272–73
  Asthma, 271
  Athopic eczema, 271
  Blood involved in, 267
  Classification of, 266
  Classification of allergens, 270
  Definition of, 265–66
  Delayed, 266
  Hay fever, 270
  Immediate, 266–67
  Immunoglobulin
  Nettlerash and Odema, 271
  Perennial rhinitis, 270–71
Amino acid, 31, 32, 35, 53
Aminopeptidase, 40
Amonoia,
  Disposal of, 53–54
Amylopectin, 10
Anemia, 57, 140
Anjus, 59, 70
Ansbacher, 111
Antidiuretic hormone, 153
Army Service Corps, 240
Aromatic amino acid, 32
Arrak, 216
Asafoetide, 270

Ascorbic acid, 113, 163
Asthma, 271
Athopic eczema, 271

Bajra, 172
Barley, 173
Baumenn, 137
Bengal gram, 175
Bendur, 41
Benjamin, H., 247
Berger, Gold, 88, 93
Beri Beri, 82
Dry, 87
In fantile, 87
Wet, 87
Best, 111
Beverages, 208–16
Alcoholic, 214–16
Cocoa, 212–13
Coffee, 208–11
Non-alcoholic, 213–14
Tea, 211–12
Bioflavanoids, 113
Biolin, 102–04
Chemistry, 103
Daily requirements, 104
Deficiency, 104
History, 102–03
Hypervitaminosis, 104
Metabolism and functions, 103
Sources, 103
Vitamin H, Anti egg white injury factor, 102–03
Bishop, 77
Bitot spot's, 69
Black gram, 175
Blood glucose, 14
Blood sugar level, control, 14
Boas, 102
Bone, 67
Brain, 15
Brandy, 215
Butler, 92

Cadmium, 148–49
Calcitonin, 118–19
Calcium, 118–22
Absorption, 121
Factors enhancing, 121
Factors interfering, 121
Daily allowance, 119, 161–62
Dietary sources of, 119–21
Effect of deficiency, 122
Effect of excess of, 122
Factors regulating, 118–19
Calcitonin, 118–99
Hypercalcium, 119
Parathyroid, 118
Functions of, 118
In blood, 118
Loss of, 121
Carbohydrates, 4–15
Absorption, 12
Classification and distribution, 5
Composition of, 4–5
Digestion, 11–15
Disaccharides, 7–8
Functions of, 15
Monosaccharides, 5–7
Polysaccharides, 9–11
Cardamom, 217–18
Carotene, 64
Cartier, Jacques, 59
Cashewnut, 178
Castle, 108
Cellulose, 10
Central Advisory Board of Health and Food Adulteration Committee, 240
Central Committee for Food Standards, 240
Cereals, 166–74
Bajra, 172

Barley, 173
Maize, 172
Oats, 172–73
Ragi, 172
Rice, 167–70
Structure of, 166–67
Wheat, 170–72
CFTRI, 221, 240, 241
Chalim, 137
Chest, 75
Chevallier–Appert, 247
Chillies, 218
Cholesterol, 24, 28
Choline, 111
Christian, 88
Chromium, 147
Chromo proteins, 37
Chymotrysinogen, 40
Cider, 215
Cinnamon, 218
Cloves, 218
Coagulated proteins, 38
Cobalt, 148
Cocoa, 212–13
Curing, 212
Fermentation, 212
Grinding and defatting, 213
Powdering, 213
Processing, 212
Roasting, 212
Coconut, 178–79
Coconut mulk, 214
Coconut water, 214
Cod liver oil, 70
Coffee, 208–11
Alkaloid coffeine, 208–09
Processing of, 209–11
Nature or cherry, 209–10
Plantation, 209
Roasting, 210–11
Coindet, 137
Colormetric method, 86
Conjunctional xerosis, 68
Conklin, 77
Copper, 140–43
Absorption, 141
Corebal type, 142
Daily allowances, 141
Deficiency, 141
Dietary sources of, 141
Excess of, 141–42
Functions of 141
Hepatic type, 143
Coriander, 219
Corneal Xerosis, 68–69
Courtois, 137
Cowgill, 93
Cretinism, 140
Cumin seeds, 219

Dam, 80
Davis, 61
Dehydration, 153
Dextrins, 10
Diaminomono carboxylic acids, 32
Dietary allowances, 160–65
Calories, 161
Disadvantage of recommended tables, 161
Dietary fat, 30
Digestibility coefficient, 41
Digestion, 11–15
Absorption, 12
Absorption of fats and, 24–25
Absorption protein and, 39–40
Blood glucose, 14
Blood sugar level, control, 14–15
Liver and carbohydrate metabolism, 13
Mouth, 11
Small intenstine, 12
Stomach, 11

Disacchar. . s, 7–8
Lactose 7–8
Maltose, 7–8
Sucrose, 7–8
Doell, 41
Donath, 82
Dumas, 59

Edema, 57, 87
Eggs, 20107
Changes during storage, 205
Chemical, 205
Physical, 205
Colour of, 204
Shall, 204
White, 204
Yolk, 204
Egg shall, 204
Egg white, 203
Egg yolk, 20203
Processing, 206–07
Cold storage, 206
Drying, 206–07
Freezing, 206
Thermostablization, 207
Quality of, 204–05
Storage, 205–06
Structure of, 201–02
Eijleman, 59, 82
Electrolyte balance, 153–55
Constant level, 154
Decrease in, 154–55
Increase in, 154
Elevenjem, 93, 140
Emulsification, 23
Energy, 15, 23
Epithelial, tissue, 67
Ernengen, van, 248
Evans, 77, 78

Fair Average Quality Standards, 240
FAO, 96
Fats characteristics, 22–23
Dietary allowances, 161
Emulsification, 23
Hardness, 22
Hydrogenation, 22
Iodine number, 23
Rancidity, 23
Saponification, 23
Fats soluble vitamins, 59–81
Vitamin A, 61–70
Vitamin D, 70–77
Vitamin E, 77–80
Vitamin K, 80–81
Fats synthesis, 27–28
Fatty acids, 20, 24–25
Cholesteral, 24
Digestion and absorption acids, 24
Oxidation, 28
Phospholipids, 24
Fellenberg, 137, 138
Fernoholtz, 78
Ferry, 40
Fibrous proteins, 36
Fish, 198
Fluorine, 145–47
Absorption, 147
Deficiency, 146
Folic acid, 104–08
Assay methods, 107
Chemistry, 105
Daily requirements, 107, 163
Deficiency, 108
History, 104–05
Hypervitaminosis, 108
Metabolism and functions, 105–07
Sources of, 105
Vitamin B, 104
Folcors, 98
Follicular hyperkeratosis, 69

Food Adulteration Committee, 240
Food borne bacteria, 250–53, 257
  Aceto bacter, 250
  Acromonas, 250
  Alcatigenes, 250
  Alteromonas, 250
  Bacillus, 251, 258
  Brochothrix, 251
  Combylobacter, 251
  Citrobacter, 251
  Clostridium, 251, 257–58
  Corynebacitersum, 251
  Enterobacter, 251
  Erwinia, 252
  Escherichia, 252
  Flavobacterium, 252
  Lactobacillus, 252
  Leuconos toc, 252
  Micrococius, 252
  Moraxella, 252
  Pediococcus, 252
  Protins, 252, 253
  Pseudomonas, 253
  Salmonella, 252, 257
  Serratia, 253
  Shigella, 253
  Staphylococcus, 253, 257
  Streptococcus, 253
  Vibrio, 253
  Yerginia, 253
Food borne molds, 253–56
  Aspergillus, 255
  Botrytis, 255
  Cladosporium, 255
  Fisarium, 255
  Helminthosporium, 255
  Mucor, 255
  Penicillium, 255–56
  Rhizopus, 256
  Rhizopus, 256
  Sporotrichum, 256
Food borne yeasts, 254–55
  Brettanomyces, 254
  Candida, 254
  Debaryomyces, 254
  Hansanula, 254
  Mycoderma, 254
  Rhodotogula, 254
  Saccharomyces, 254
  Schizosa ccharomyces, 254–55
  Torula, 255
Food exchange list for India, 233–39
  Advantages of, 233
  Definition of, 234
  Indian diet, 233
  Nutritive value, 233
Food poisioning, 245–49, 259
  Bacteria in, 246–249
  Characteristics of, 245–46
  Contaminator by germs, 246
  Food hygiene, 245
  Food microbiology, 247
    Food poisoning, 248–49
    Food preservation, 247–48
    Food spoilage, 249
  Measures to control, 258–59
Foutsetal, 93
Fruit juices, 191, 214
Fruits, 184–91
  Changes occurs in, 184
    Colour, 184
    Flavour, 184
    Taste, 184
    Texture, 184
  Chemical composition of, 185–57
    Ascorbic acid, 185
    Enzymes, 187
    Other acid, 185
    Pigments, 186
    Polyphenols, 186
    Sugar, 185
  Classification of, 185

Colours, 187–89
Flavour of, 187
Prevention of enzymatic browning, 189–91
Candies, glaced, and crystallised, 191
Canning, 190–91
Cold storage, 190
Drying, 191
Flakes, 191
Freezing, 190
Preservation and processing, 189–90
Waxing, 190
Fructose, 6
Funk, 59

Galactose, 7
Galic, 219
Gastrointestinal tract, 57, 80, 86, 87
Gaut. Bussin, 137
Gin, 216
Gin jelly seeds, 179
Ginger, 218
Glisson, 74
Globulins, 36
Glucose, 6
Glutamic rezidues, 80
Glutelins, 36
Glycogen, 10
Glyco proteins, 37
Goitre, 137, 139
Green gram, 175
Grijns, 60
Groundnut, 176, 179
Gyorgy, 98, 103

Harrington, Charles, 137
Harris, 98
Hart, 140
Hay fever, 270
Head, 74–75
Heart, 15
Hemicellulose, 11
Hemoglobin, 132
Hess, 59, 70
Hetero cyclic amino acids, 32
Hexuronic acid, 113
Histones, 37
Hock, van Leuwan, 246
Holmes, 61
Hopkins, 60
Huldschinsky, 59
Huntsman, 111
Hydrochlonic acid, 40
Hydrogenation, 22
Hypercalcium, 119
Hyperkalimia, 132
Hypernatremia, 129
Hyperparathyroidism, 118
Hyper Thyroidism, 140
Hypogevsia, 144
Hypokalimia, 130–32
Hyponatremia, 127–29

Indian Council of Medical Research, 96, 160
Indian food preparations, 221–32
Cereal recipes, 222
Egg, fish and meat recipes, 222
Milk recipes, 222
Pulse recipes, 222
Ready to serve preparation, 222
Indian standard institute, 240
ISI Agricultural Marketing Association, 240
Infantile Beri Beri, 87
Cardiovascular, type, 87
Neuritic type, 87
Insotol, 112
Insulation and packing, 23–24
Iodine, 137–40

Absorption, 139
Cretinism, 140
Daily allowance, 138
Deficiency, 139–40
Dietary sources of, 138
Hyperthyroidism, 140
Myxodema, 140
Iodine number, 23
Iron, 132–36
Absorption, 135
Daily allowance, 134, 162
Deficiency, 135
Dietary sources of, 135
Excess of, 135
Functions of, 133–34
Ishizaka, kimishige, 267
Ishizaka, Teruka, 267
Isotonic contraction, 155
Itiba, 98

Jams, Jellies and marmaledes, 191
Janson, 82, 86

Karrer, 61
Kendell, 137
Keratomalacta, 69
Kerseztesy, 98
Keto acids, 53
Ketogenesis, 28
Khesari Dal, 176
Kimball, 137
King, 113
Kogl, 103
Krabs–Henseleitt urea cycle, 54
Kuhn, 61, 98
Kustner, Heinz, 267
Kwashiar kar, 56, 57, 58

Lactose, 7
Lancaster, James, 59
Lecithin, 23
Lepkosky, 98
Leproproteins, 25–27
High density, 25
Low density, 25
Lind, James, 113
Linoleic acid, 17
Lipids, 16–30
Adipose tissue, 27
Cholesterol, 28
Classification of, 20–22
Compound, 22
Derived, 22
Simple, 22
Composition of, 16–18
Fatty acids, 29
Linoleic acid, 17
Linolenic acid, 18
Oleic acid, 17
Dietary fats, 30
Fats characteristics, 22–23
Fats synthesis, 27–28
Fatty acids, 20, 24–25
Functions, 23–24
Energy, 23
Insullation and padding, 23–24
Palatability, 23
Satiety value, 23
Vitamins, 24
Ketogenesis, 28
Liproproteins, 25–27
Liver, 27
Metabolism, 25
Organic substances, 16
Oxidation of fatty acids, 28
Lipoic acid, 112–13
Liver, 15, 27, 57
Liver and carbohydrate metabolism, 13
Lunin, 59

Macro elements, 117–36
Calcium, 118–22
Chloride, 129
Iron, 132–36
Magnesium, 124–26
Minerals, 117
Phosphorus, 122–24
Potassium, 129–32
Sodium, 126–29
Magnesium, 124–26
Absorption, 124–25
Daily allowances, 124
Deficiency, 125–26
Dietary sources, 124
Functions, 124
Maize, 172
Maltose, 7
Manganese, 147
Marina, 137
Mc collum, 59, 61, 70
Mcollum, 59
Mc collum, 61
Mc collun, 70
Meat, 196–200
Composition of, 198
Cuts, 196–97
Fish, 198
Poultry, 198
Softness, 200
Structures of, 196
Mellamby, 59, 70
Mendel, 40, 61
Mental face, 57
Metabolism, 25, 52
Metallo proteins, 37
Meta proteins, 38
Micro elements, 137–49
Chromium, 147
Cobalt, 148
Copper, 140–43
Fluorine, 145–47
Iodine, 137–40
Manganese, 147
Molybdenum, 148
Seleninn, 145
Silicon, 148
Zinc, 143–45
Milk and milk products, 192–95
Evaporization, 195
Fermentation, 195
Fortification, 195
Freezing, 195
Homogenization, 194–95
Lactose, 192–93
Milk serum, 192
Pasteurization, 194
Protein, 194
Milk recipes, 222
Minot, 108
Miti, 98
Molybdenum, 148
Mono amino dicarboxylic acids, 32
Mono amino mono carboxylic acids, 32
Monosaccharides, 5–7
Disaccharides, 7
Fructose, 6
Galactose, 7
Glucose, 6
Moon face, 57
Moore, 61
Morris, 61
Mouth, 11
Mucus membrances, 69
Mulder, 31
Murphy, 108
Muscle, 15, 76
Muscle wasting, 57
Mustard seeds, 219
Myxodema, 140

Neera, 214

Net Protein Ratio, 41
Net Protein Utilization, 42
Nettla rash, 271
Neurology, 142
Niacin, 92–97
  Assay methods, 96–97
  Chemistry, 93–94
  Daily requirements, 96, 162
  Deficiency, 97
  History of, 92–93
  Hypervitaminosis, 97
  Metabolism and functions, 95
  Sources, 93
Nicotinamide, 92
Nicotinic acid, 92
Night blindness, 68
Non-alcoholic beverages, 213–14
  Coconut milk, 214
  Coconut water, 214
  Fruit beverages, 213
  Fruit juice, 214
  Neera, 214
  Sherbat, 214
  Sugar cane juice, 214
Nucleoproteins, 37
Nutmeg and mace, 218–19
Nutrients and inter-relationship, 156–59
  Carbohydrate, proteins and fats effects on vitamin A and fats, 157
    Choline and methionine, 157
    Nicotinic acid and tryptophan, 157
    Pyridoxine and fat, 157
    Thiamine and carbohydrate, 157
  Mineral–mineral relationship, 159
  Protein energy inter-relationship, 156–57
  Vitamin-vitamin inter-relationship, 158–59
    Riboflavin and Iron, 158
    Vitamin C and Iron, 158
    Vitamin C, leed, Iron and mercury, 158–59
    Vitamin D, Calcium and phosphorus, 158
Nutrition and hearth, 1–3
  Avoids deficiency, 2–3
  Decision makers for, 3
  For good health, 1
  Influence on health of, 2
  Science of food, 1, 2
Nutrition of children and adolescents, 282–83
  Adolescents influenced by peer group, 282–83
  Balanced diet for, 283–84
    Child choice, 282
    Growth pattern of, 282
    Nutrition education to, 283
    Nutrition in foods and leave nutrition foods, 283
Nutrition of normal infants, 274–78
  At birth, 274–75
  Characteristics of, 274
  Growth and development of, 274–75
  Requirements of, 275–77
    Carbohydrate, 276
    Energy, 276
    Fats, 276
    Minerals, 276
    Protein, 275–76
    Vitamins, 277
  Requirements of infants, 277–78
    Human milk, 277
    Immunoglobulins, 277–78
    Lactobacillus Bifidus factor, 278
    Lactoferrin, 278
    Lymphoid cells, 278
Nutrition of old age, 285–87

Cardiovascular system, 286
Cellular changes, 285
Daily allowances, 286
Decline in water content in, 285
Functions of gastroinstestinal tract, 285
Nervous system, 286
Principles of, 286
Renal system, 286
Skeletal changes, 286
Nutrition of pregnant and lactating woman, 288–92
Changes during pregnancy, 289–91
Basal metabolism increases, 290
Blood volume increases, 290
Progesteron, 289–90
Stages, 289
Dietary allowance for, 291
Diet for adult women, 292
Needs of, 288
Neonatal mortality, 288–89
Nutrition of pre-school children, 279–81
Growth and development of, 279
Requirements of, 279–81
Nuts and oil seeds, 178–80
Nyctalopia, 68

Oats, 172–73
Ocular lesions, 92
Odema, 271
Oleic acid, 17
Onion, 219
Oral and facial lesions, 92
Osborne, 40, 61
Osteomalacia, 76
Osteoporosis, 76
Ovary wall, 166

Palability, 23
Pantothenic acid, 101–02
Assay methods, 102
Chemistry, 101
Daily requirements, 102
Deficiency, 102
History, 101
Hypervitaminosis, 102
Metabolism and functions, 102
Para Amino Benzoic Acid, 111–12
Parathyroid, 118
Parker, 108
Pasteur, Louis, 246
Peas, 175
Pectins, 11
Pepper, 218
Peptides, 38
Perennial rhinitis, 270
Phospholipids, 24
Phospho proteins, 37
Phosphorus, 122–24
Absorption, 124
Daily allowance, 123, 162
Dietary sources of, 123–24
Functions, 122
In blood, 122
Plasma vitamin A, 65
Polyneuritis in bigenons, 86
Polysaccharides, 9–11
Cellulose, 10
Dextrins, 10
Glycogen, 10
Hemicellulose, 11
Pectins, 11
Starch, 9–10
Porter, 215
Potassium, 129–32
Absorption, 130
Contents in gastro intestinal secretions, 129
Daily allowances, 130
Dietary sources, 130

Functions of, 130
Hyperkalimia, 132
Retention of, 130
Poultry, 198
Prausnitz, carl, 267
Prevention of Food Adultration Act, 240, 241
Prolamines, 36
Protamines, 37
Protein Efficiency Ratio, 40–41
Proteins, 31–58
Biological value, 42
Chemical sore, 42
Classification of, 36–38
Conjugated, 37
Derived, 37–38
Simple, 36–37
Composition of, 31
Daily allowances, 56, 161
Deemination, 53
Digestation and absorption, 39–40
Digestibility coefficient, 41
Disposal of ammonia, 53–54
Functions of, 39
Metabolism, 52
Net Protein Ratio, 41
Net Protein utilization, 42
Nutritional properties, 38–39
Nutritional value of, 40
Protein calorie malnutrition, 56–58
Protein Efficiency ratio, 40–41
Structure of, 31–36
Transamination, 53
Urea synthesis, 54–55
Protein Sparing Action, 15
Proteoses, 38
Prout, 137
Pro Vitamin A, 61
Pulses, 175–77
Pyridoxin, 98–101
Assay methods, 99–100
Chemistry, 98
Daily requirements, 99, 163
Deficiency, 100
History of, 98
Hypervitaminosis, 100–01
Metabolism and functions, 98–99
Sources, 98
Vitamin B_6, 98

Ragi, 172
Rancidity, 23
Redgram, 175
Reed, 112
Reerick, 70
Retina, 66
Retinaldehyde, 64
Retinoic acid, 64
Retinol, 63–64
Riboflavin, 88–92
Assay methods, 90–92
Biological, 91
Mocrobiological, 92
Physio-chemical, 91
Chemistry, 88–90
Deficiency, 92
Ocular lesions, 92
Oral and facial lesions, 92
Scrotal and vulval lesions, 92
History of, 88
Hypervitaminosis, 92
Metabolism and functions, 90
Sources, 88
Vitamin B_2, lactoflavin, 88
Rice, 167–70
Processing, 167–70
Hand bouding, 168
Macine milling, 169
Parboiling, 169–70
Products, 170
Flakes, 170
Puffed, 170

Stable food, 167
Structure of, 167
Aleurone layer, 167
Brain, 167
Embryo, 167
Endoperm, 167
Husk, 167
Rickets, 59, 74, 122
Ricks, 108
Rose, William C, 38
Rousseus, 39
Rum, 216

Saporification, 23
Satiety value, 23
Sclero Proteins, 36
Scrotal and Vulval lesions, 92
Sebrell, 92
Selanium, 145
Serum Albumin, 57
Sherbat, 214
Silicon, 148
Skin and Hair changes, 57
Small intestine, 12
Smith, 93, 108
Sodium, 126–29
Absorption, 127
Daily allowance, 126–27
Dietary Sources, 127
Functions, 126
Hypernatremia, 129
Hyponatremia, 127–29
Soyabean, 175–76
Spices and Condiments, 217–20
Squash, 214
Starch, 9–10
Steenback, 59, 61
Steencock, 70
Stevens, 98
Stomach, 11
Stout, 215
Sucrose, 7
Sugar cane juice, 214
Sulpher, 32, 132
Szent-Gyorgy, 113

Takaki, 82
Tamarid, 219–20
Tea, 211–12
Cultivation, 211
Processing of, 211–12
Black, 211
Green, 211–12
Oolong, 212
Thiamin, 82–88
Assay methods, 85–86
Biological, 86
Microbiological, 86
Physio–chemical, 86
Chemistry, 83–84
Daily requirements, 84–85, 162
Deficiency, 86–88
History, 82
Hypervitaminosis, 88
Metabolism and functions, 84
Sources, 82–83
Thiochrome method, 86
Thyroid, 137
Toddy, 215
Tonnis, 103
Toxicants, in foods, 260–64
Ackee fruit poisoning, 260
American water hemlock, 262
Atriplicism, 262
Bacterial toxins, 264
Bush tea, 262
Camas, 262
Claviceps furpurea, 264
Djenkol Beans, 262
Fats and oils, 263
Favism, 260
Fungal Toxins, 263–64

Goitrogens, 262
Hemagglutinins, 261
In spices, 261–62
Lathyrogens, 261
Leu Caena glauca, 262–63
Lima beans and Cassava, 263
Minerals, 263
Mushroom poisoning, 262
Pencillium species, 264
Sea foods, 263
Solamine, 263
Toxicity, 88
Trypsinogen, 40
Turmeric, 219

Urea synthesis, 54–55

Vanadium, 149
Van Wijk, 70
Vegetables, 181–83
Flavones and flavanols, 182
Green colour of, 181–82
Green leafy, 181
Others, 181
Roots and tubers, 181
Storage of, 183
Sulphur in, 182–83
Yellow Colour of, 182
Vitamin A, 61–70
assay method, 68
Chemistry, 61–64
Carotene, 64
Retinaldehyde, 64
Ratinoic acid, 64
Retional, 63–64
Daily allowances, 67, 162
Deficiency, 68–69
Bitat spot's, 69
Follincular hyperkaratosis, 69
Keratomalacta, 69
Night blindness, 68
Xerosis of conjuctival, 68
Xerosis of cornea, 68–69
Functions, 66–67
Bone, 67
Epithelial tissues, 67
Retina, 66
History of, 61
Hypervitaminosis, 70
Measurement of, 64–65
Metabolism and functions, 65
Mucus membrances, 69
Plasma, 65
Sources, 61
Storage of, 65–66
Treatment, 69–70
Vitamin B, complex group, 82–113
Biotin, 102–04
Choline, 111
Folic acid, 104–08
Inositol, 112
Lipoic acid, 112–13
Niacin 92–97
Pantothenic acid, 101–02
Para Amino Benzoic acid, 111–12
Pyridoxin, 98–101
Riboflavin, 88–92
Thiamin, 82–88
Vitamin B_{12}, 108–11
Vitamin B_{12}, 108–11
Assay methods, 110
Chemistry, 109
Daily requirements, 110
Deficiency, 110–11
History of, 109
Hypervitaminosis, 111
Metabolism and functions, 109–10
Sources, 108–09
Vitamin C, 113–16
Assay method, 116
Dinitropheny l hydrazine, 116
Dye, 116

Chemistry, 114–15
Daily requirements, 115, 163
Deficiency, 116
History, 113–14
Hypervitaminosis, 116
Metabolism and functions, 115
Scurvy, 116
Sources, 114
Vitamin D., 70–77
Assay methods, 73
Biological method, 73–74
Boneash, 73–74
Growth, 73
Line test, 73–74
Chemical method, 73
Daily allowances, 73, 163
Deficiency of, 74–77
Chest, 75
Head, 74–75
Hypervitaminosis, 77
Long bone, 75–76
Muscles, 76
Osteomalacia, 76
Osteoporosis, 76–77
Rickets, 74
Wrist, knee and ankle joints, 75
History of, 70
Metabolism and functions, 72–73
Sources of, 70
Vitamin E, 77–80
Assay methods, 79
Chemistry, 78
Daily requirements, 79
Deficiency, 79–80
History of, 77–78
Hypervitaminosis, 79–80
Metabolism and functions, 78–79
Sources of, 78
Vitamin C, 80–81
Assay methods, 81
Chemistry, 80
Daily requirements, 81
Deficiency, 81
History, 80
Hypervitaminosis, 81
Metabolism and functions, 80–81
Sources, 80
Vitamin K, 24, 59–116
Fats soluble, 60, 61–81
Water soluble, 60–61, 82–116
History of, 59–61
Vodka, 216
Von Dirquet, Boran Clemens, 265

Warburg, 88
Water balance, 150–54
Constituent of body, 150
Dehydration, 153
Effect of excess sodium chloride, 152–53
Effect of sodium chloride depletion, 153
Fuctions of, 150–51
Regulation of, 152
Renal loss, 152
Respiration, 152
Sources to body, 151
Sweat, 152
Water intoxication, 154
Water soluble vitamins, 82–116
Vitamin B Complex, 82–113
Vitamin C, 113–16
Waught, 113
Wendt, 98
Wet Beri Beri, 87
Wheat, 170–72
Structure of, 170–72
Aleurone layer, 171
Embryo, 171
Endosperm, 171
Scutellum, 171–72
Whisky, 215